Essentials of Robotic Surgery

Essentials of Robotic Surgery

Manak Sood, MD
and
Stefan W. Leichtle, MD
Editors

SpryPublishing
ideas to life

Published by Spry Publishing LLC
2500 South State Street
Ann Arbor, MI 48104 USA

Printed and bound in the United States of America.

10 9 8 7 6 5 4 3 2 1

Hardcover ISBN: 978-1-938170-12-6
E-book ISBN: 978-1-938170-14-0

Library of Congress Control Number: 2013932494

Prepared in collaboration with the staff of SAINT JOSEPH MERCY HEALTH SYSTEM
A Member of Trinity Health

To my late parents, Sheila and Sagar Sood

Special Acknowledgments

When Richard (Dick) and Norma Sarns first became acquainted with a circle of St. Joe's doctors in the 1950s, they found themselves among pioneers exploring the boundaries of surgical care.

Dick, an engineer by trade, held just the right blend of talent, ingenuity, and passion needed to translate the doctors' ideas into hardware—new surgical tools that could surpass the limitations of the time. Norma shared their drive for transforming health care and took on the role of a volunteer and ambassador for St. Joe's. The Sarnses' desire to contribute led to the development of their successful biotechnology company, creating medical instruments and equipment that could turn groundbreaking discoveries into "standard operating procedure."

St. Joe's is grateful to the Sarnses for their relentless quest to do things better, their commitment to patients in our community and beyond, and their ongoing generosity and partnership. They have remained in St. Joe's circle of friends for more than half a century. In 2005, the Sarnses made a noteworthy gift to help purchase the hospital's first da Vinci robot and launch the robotic surgery program. Their vision and generosity continue to blaze the trail for the future of surgical care.

Another noted innovator was Dr. Joe D. Morris, a renowned leader in the field of thoracic surgery who joined St. Joseph Mercy Hospital's medical staff in 1954. Dr. Morris joined Dick Sarns on a path to improvements in biotechnology that led to the design and building of the gold standard of heart-lung machines. Dr. Morris is credited as being among St. Joe's surgical pioneers.

Contents

Editors & Contributors

Editors

Stefan W. Leichtle, MD
Resident, General Surgery, St. Joseph Mercy Ann Arbor
A History of Robotic Surgical Systems, Coronary Revascularization, General and Pediatric Surgery, The Colon and Rectum

Manak S. Sood, MD
Director, Center for Robotic Surgery, St. Joseph Mercy Ann Arbor
Section Head, Cardiothoracic Surgery
Coronary Revascularization, Mitral Valve

Contributors

Jan A. Akervall, MD
Director, Head and Neck Oncology, St. Joseph Mercy Ann Arbor
Head and Neck Cancer

Susanne L. Archer, MD
Attending Surgeon, Obstetrics and Gynecology, St. Joseph Mercy Ann Arbor
Uterine Surgery

Robert F. Casalou
President and CEO, St. Joseph Mercy Ann Arbor and Livingston
Robotic Surgery: A CEO's Perspective

Robert K. Cleary, MD
Director, Fellowship in Colorectal Surgery, St. Joseph Mercy Ann Arbor
Section Head, General Surgery
The Colon and Rectum

Rajiv J. Deenadayalu, MD
Attending Surgeon, Obstetrics and Gynecology, St. Joseph Mercy Ann Arbor
Fibroid Surgery, Uterine Surgery

James S. DeMeester, MD
Director, Cardiac Anesthesia, St. Joseph Mercy Ann Arbor
Anesthetic Considerations

Ajay Gupta, MD
Attending Surgeon, Thoracic Surgery, St. Joseph Mercy Ann Arbor
The Mediastinum, Lung Cancer, Esophageal Myotomy

M. LaWaun Hance PA-C
Cardiothoracic Surgery, St. Joseph Mercy Ann Arbor
Mitral Valve

Christina L. Harsant, MD
Resident, General Surgery, St. Joseph Mercy Ann Arbor
Lung Cancer, Esophageal Myotomy

Paul T. Hoff, MD
Section Head, Otolaryngology, St. Joseph Mercy Ann Arbor
Surgery for Sleep Apnea

Seema Kapur, MD
Attending Surgeon, General Surgery, St. Joseph Mercy Ann Arbor
General and Pediatric Surgery

Christodoulos G. Kaoutzanis, MD
Resident, General Surgery, St. Joseph Mercy Ann Arbor
Robotic Partial Nephrectomy, Robotic Prostatectomy

Crystal M. Kavanagh, MD
Resident, General Surgery, St. Joseph Mercy Ann Arbor
Robotic Partial Nephrectomy, Robotic Prostatectomy

Eduardo Kleer, MD
Section Head, Urology, St. Joseph Mercy Ann Arbor
Robotic Partial Nephrectomy, Robotic Prostatectomy

Bobby K. Kong, MD
Attending Surgeon, Cardiothoracic Surgery, St. Joseph Mercy Ann Arbor
Mitral Valve

Vita V. McCabe, MD
Director, Thoracic Surgery Program, St. Joseph Mercy Ann Arbor
The Mediastinum, Lung Cancer, Esophageal Myotomy

Brandy N. Michaels, MD
Resident, Obstetrics and Gynecology, St. Joseph Mercy Ann Arbor
Fibroid Surgery, Uterine Surgery

Lisa H. Morris, MD
Attending Surgeon, Obstetrics and Gynecology, St. Joseph Mercy Ann Arbor
Uterine Surgery

Nicolas J. Mouawad, MD, MPH, MBA
Resident, General Surgery, St. Joseph Mercy Ann Arbor
Mitral Valve

Gail S. Moyer, MD
Attending Surgeon, Obstetrics and Gynecology, St. Joseph Mercy Ann Arbor
Uterine Surgery

Daniel S. Rhee, MD
Resident, General Surgery, St. Joseph Mercy Ann Arbor
General and Pediatric Surgery

JoLyn M. Seitz, MD
Resident, Obstetrics and Gynecology, St. Joseph Mercy Ann Arbor
Fibroid Surgery, Uterine Surgery

Matthew E. Spector, MD
Fellow, Otolaryngology and Head and Neck Cancer
University of Michigan Hospital
Surgery for Sleep Apnea

Thomas A. Stark, MD
Resident, General Surgery, St. Joseph Mercy Ann Arbor
The Mediastinum

Martha M. Walsh, MD
Attending Surgeon, Obstetrics and Gynecology, St. Joseph Mercy Ann Arbor
Uterine Surgery

Walter M. Whitehouse Jr., MD
Chairman, Department of Surgery, St. Joseph Mercy Health System
Medical Doctor, Surgical Services, St. Joseph Mercy Health System
Introduction: An Evolution of Surgical Technique

Amanda Y. Yang, MD
Resident, General Surgery, St. Joseph Mercy Ann Arbor
The Colon and Rectum

Foreword

On Robotic Surgery—A CEO's Perspective

Minimally invasive surgery is quickly becoming the standard of care in multiple surgical subspecialties, which has opened up the possibilities of a quicker return to normal function for the patient, lower costs for the hospital, and a decreased burden on the health-care system overall. Open surgery and other traditional methods are becoming less common as minimally invasive options become available. Many technological innovations are revolutionizing the way we treat cardiothoracic, head and neck, gynecologic, urologic, and general surgeries through robotic procedures. This new approach greatly reduces postoperative pain and facilitates a speedier recovery for the patient. It is expected robotic surgery will surpass open surgery and become the preferred option in the near future.

All hospitals and medical centers strive to be recognized as "Centers of Excellence," facilities that provide superior health-care services with the most expert, advanced, and cost-effective procedures, thus ensuring the best possible outcomes for their patients. As an industry leader in robotic procedures, Saint Joseph Mercy Health System (SJMHS) has distinguished itself within a highly competitive marketplace by implementing futuristic performance improvements that surpass patient expectations and exceed standard levels of professional quality. The physicians at SJMHS, including the authors of this book, have succeeded at utilizing the potential offered by today's technological advancements to not only improve the quality of our care, but also to maximize our organization's economic return.

We present this book to both health-care professionals working to establish their own organizations as "Centers of Excellence" and primary care specialists who want the best surgical options for their patients. Careful analysis, justification, and implementation of a robotic surgery strategy have helped SJMHS to exceed national performance benchmarks and to give us a competitive edge within our industry. We discuss the latest developments "from the trenches" of the rapidly evolving world of minimally invasive surgery, the means by which these technologies have been adopted into the culture of SJMHS, and some of our experiences with improving patient outcomes through the use of robotic surgery. We hope that the robotics revolution you find within these pages will continue for years to come.

Robert F. Casalou
President and CEO,
St. Joseph Mercy Ann Arbor and Livingston

Chapter One

An Evolution of Surgical Technique: From Open to Robotics

Walter M. Whitehouse Jr., MD, FACS

The performance of surgical procedures has changed dramatically over the last two decades as technology has evolved. Since 1987 when laparoscopic cholecystectomy was introduced, minimally invasive surgical techniques have come to the forefront. While there was appropriate skepticism surrounding laparoscopic cholecystectomy, it was embraced and rapidly became the standard for cholecystectomy. The subsequent technological advances and refinement of laparoscopic equipment enabled broadened indications for these techniques. The introduction of robotic technology in 2001 has contributed to the ongoing evolution of minimally invasive surgical care. The adoption of surgical robotic applications has been somewhat slower than was experienced with laparoscopic procedures in the early 1990s. There is no doubt, however, that robotics will play an important role in the ongoing evolution of surgical care.

The initial application of surgical robotic techniques was in urology. Preliminary results of robotic prostatectomy suggested superior clinical outcomes. As experience increased, data became less compelling. Nonetheless, marketing of the availability of robotic procedures led to a change of traditional referral patterns and intense competition between hospitals within a market, forcing the adoption of the new technology by those who were without robots. Our institution was somewhat slow in adopting robotic prostatectomy—caution prompted by both expense and the quality of the data supporting its utilization. When our first robot was purchased, it was rapidly embraced by the urologists at our institution.

Importantly, the rapid success of this application was based on a surgeon champion leading these efforts. As more experience was gained, the data regarding outcomes were not as compelling as first perceived. Length of stay was certainly significantly reduced, but the other issues related to oncologic control and potency were not definitive. The technology was then adopted by gynecology for hysterectomy. Before further expansion of the program, we chose to establish an oversight committee with a representative from each appropriate surgical specialty.

The committee was charged with oversight of privileging, developing appropriateness criteria for inclusion of additional procedures and specialties, maximizing operating room efficiency and robot utilization, and minimizing costs. For a specialty to expand robotic technology, supporting scientific data had to be presented to the committee, and only after thorough and critical review were additional privileges granted. Under this structure, our program has expanded in what we consider to be a thoughtful and rigorous manner. The program now includes six specialties—urology, gynecology, thoracic surgery, cardiac surgery, colorectal surgery, and otolaryngology.

Dr. Manak Sood has chaired the robotics committee since its inception. It is appropriate that he is the editor of this text, as the success of our program expansion is a reflection of his enthusiastic and thoughtful leadership. The contributing authors are experienced robotic surgeons, and they present data regarding appropriate use of robotics in their specific specialties. Our institution is grateful for their contributions.

As the landscape of medical care continues to change rapidly, appropriate application of robotic technology will become more important and more challenging as population management evolves. Programmatic rigor will be essential and will require ongoing detailed outcome analysis as new procedures are considered and justified.

Chapter Two

A History of Robotic Surgical Systems

Stefan W. Leichtle, MD

On April 11, 1985, the "PUMA 200" premiered as the first surgical robot to operate on an actual human patient. Unimation, Inc.'s "Programmable Universal Machine for Assembly" (Figure 1) was an industrial robot and resembled a human worker with a sturdy "trunk" and "shoulder," "elbow joints," and "wrists." It was originally developed for assembly and materials handling, allowing for repetitive yet precise movements. The first ever robotic surgical procedure, performed by Kwoh et al. at Memorial Medical Center, Long Beach, California, was a stereotactic brain biopsy.[1] With this first "robotic surgery," science fiction had reached clinical medicine.

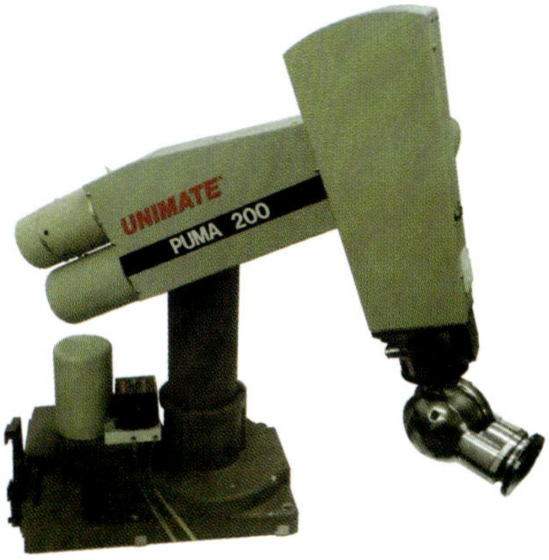

Figure 1. PUMA 200, the first robot used for a surgical procedure. Courtesy of Practical Robotic Services, Bethel, CT.

Etymology

The word *robot* was made popular by Karel Capek in his play *Rossom's Universal Robots* in 1921,[2] which described anthropomorphic machines that were mass-produced to perform industrial and agricultural work. Originally coined by his brother Josef, robot is derived from the Czech *robota*, meaning (forced) labor. Robots have long fascinated the human mind. In literature and pop culture, they have assumed roles from primitive machinery to sophisticated, super-human beings, from helpful servants to threats to humanity. In real life, their roles have been less dramatic, but no less spectacular.

From the Assembly Line to the Operating Room

The first industrial robot, "Unimate" (Figure 2), an electronically controlled hydraulic heavy-lifting arm, was used in a General Motors Corporation die-casting factory in Trenton, New Jersey, in 1961.[3] In 1978, Unimation, Inc. introduced the PUMA robotic system.

In medicine, robotic systems had a rather late career start. Surgical specialties including neurosurgery, orthopedic surgery, and urology were the first to use surgical robots, primarily for tasks that required high accuracy, but involved only a clearly defined, nonchanging operative field. After its premiere in neurosurgery in 1985,[1] the PUMA robotic system was successfully used again for prostatectomies in 1991.[4] Soon thereafter, a robot specifically designed for prostate surgery, the Probot, was developed. This robot was able to perform precise prostate resections semi-automatically, based on preoperatively constructed, three-dimensional models of the prostate.[5]

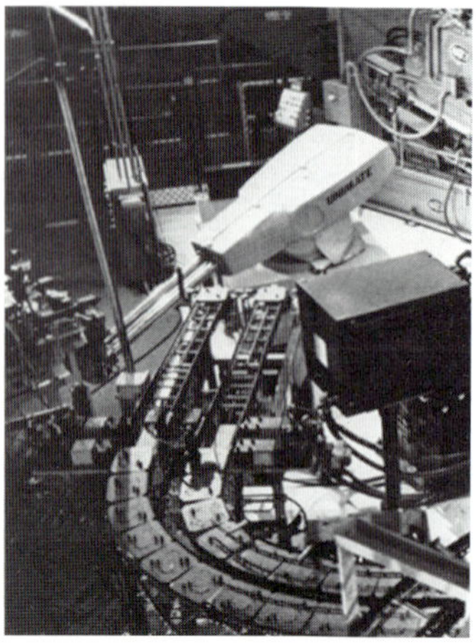

Figure 2. Unimate, the first industrial robot (1961).

In orthopedic surgery, the ROBODOC (Curexo Technology Corp.) was introduced in 1992 to improve the fit of total hip replacements.[6] As an autonomous robotic system, ROBODOC was developed for highly accurate milling of the femoral canal, following a preoperatively devised and programmed plan. However, after initial enthusiasm, concerns about technical complications and safety prevented the widespread use of the ROBODOC system,[7] and passive, merely assistive devices have come to dominate the field of robotics in orthopedics and surgery so far.[8]

The Origins of Modern Robotic Systems

With AESOP (Figure 3), Computer Motion, Inc., introduced the first ever U.S. Food and Drug Administration (FDA) approved robotic system in 1993.[9] Starting as a passive laparoscope holder, AESOP evolved into a sophisticated speech-controlled camera positioning system, and the advanced AESOP-HERMES robotic system offered additional voice-control of table position and lighting in the operating room.[10]

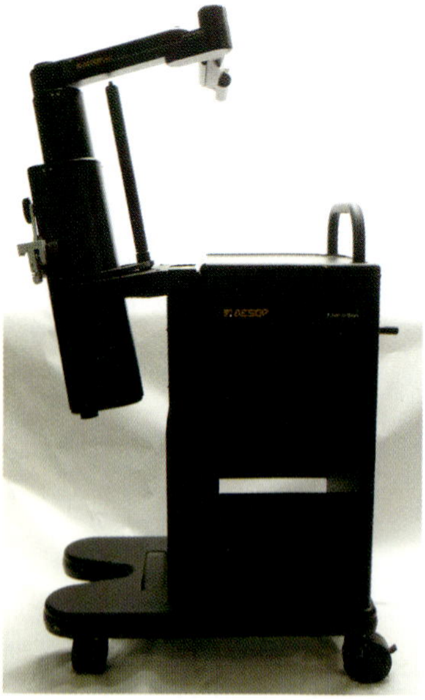

Figure 3. The Automated Endoscopic System for Optimal Positioning (AESOP). Credit: Courtesy of Rocketstar Robotics.

Based on AESOP, Computer Motion, Inc., then developed the ZEUS robotic system (Figure 4a), introduced to the commercial market in 1998 and used for the first successful coronary artery bypass operation in 1999.[11] ZEUS consisted of a surgeon's console and three table-mounted robotic arms, one of them a voice-activated camera arm based on the AESOP technology.

Surgeons operating with the ZEUS would take a comfortable seat in front of a flat, two-dimensional monitor (three-dimensional viewing was an added feature using special glasses). The instrument controls were placed at its side ergonomically, thus

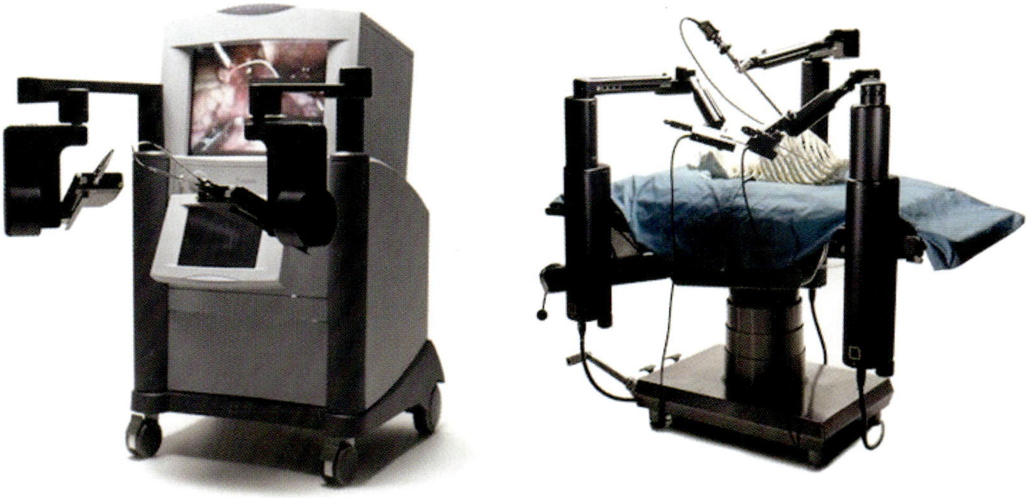

Figure 4a. The ZEUS robotic system.

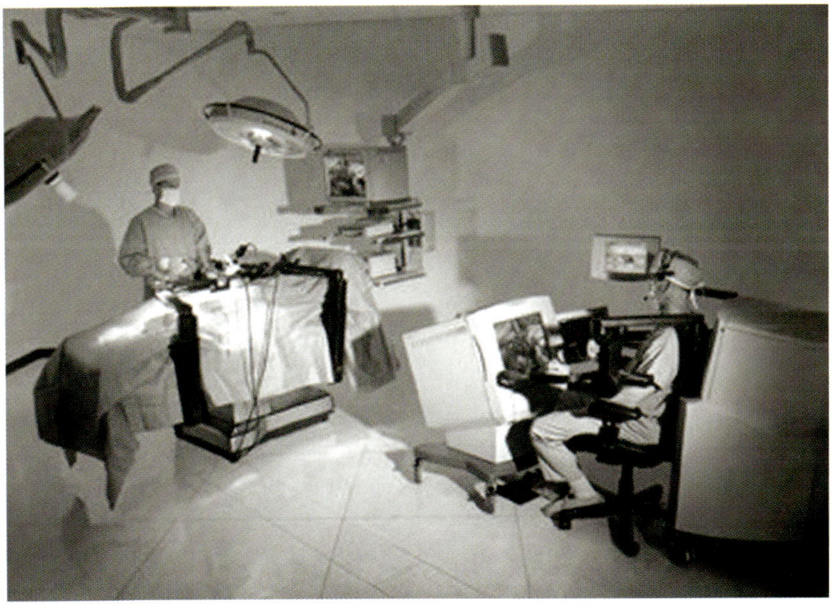

Figure 4b. ZEUS in the operating room.

providing a good view of the entire operating room (Figure 4b).[12,13] The table-mounted robotic arms of ZEUS were based on standard laparoscopic instruments and allowed for five degrees of freedom, i.e., the number of possible motions. The initial five degrees of freedom included insertion, pitch, yaw, roll, and grip, but the introduction of a "microwrist" later added a sixth degree of freedom.

Transatlantic Cholecystectomy and the Age of Telesurgery

On July 7, 2001, a 68-year-old woman underwent an uncomplicated cholecystectomy for symptomatic cholelithiasis in the Hôpital Civil in Strasbourg, France. Her surgeons, Drs. Jacques Marescaux and Michel Gagner, were 3,900 miles away in New York City.

The first "transatlantic cholecystectomy" was made possible with the ZEUS robotic system and high-speed fiber optic cables[14–16] and introduced the concept of telesurgery to the public. In telesurgery, and telemanipulation systems in general, a computer-controlled system is used to bridge the physical distance between the operator and the manipulated object. The physical distance can range from a few feet (e.g., a robotic system in an operating room) to thousands of miles, as seen in the transatlantic cholecystectomy. The operator can manipulate the distant object via a console that translates hand motions into electronic information, and eventually into movement at the side of the end-device. This "kinesthetic coupling" between input manipulator (operator) and executing manipulator (end-device) is complemented by visual and, in some systems, haptic feedback, allowing for precise manipulation of the remote object.

Further developments of the ZEUS robotic system, however, ended shortly thereafter, when Computer Motion, Inc., merged with Intuitive Surgical, Inc., in 2003, and discontinued the development of the ZEUS. A decade after the first transatlantic operation with ZEUS, telesurgery has not yet reached the relevance once anticipated. Robotic surgery, however, has advanced with the da Vinci Robotic System created by Intuitive Surgical, Inc., currently the only commercially available and FDA approved system for general surgical procedures.

The da Vinci Robotic System

The history of the da Vinci robot begins with the redesign of the Stanford Research Institute (SRI) "Green Telepresence Surgery System" by Integrated Surgical Systems (now Intuitive Surgical, Inc.) in 1997.[9,10] The system was originally designed for the military, to improve care for wounded soldiers on the battlefield and to decrease wartime mortality. The vision was that a critically injured soldier would be loaded into a battlefield ambulance, where a surgeon, potentially hundreds of miles away, would perform damage-control surgery through "telepresence," assisted by a medic on site.[9,13] Despite successful field tests, telepresence surgery has not yet reached the battlefield.[9]

In 1997, a precursor of the da Vinci system, the Mona (Intuitive Surgical, Inc.), was used to perform the first general surgical operation, a cholecystectomy, in Belgium.[17] In 2000, the da Vinci became the first robotic system approved by the FDA for general laparoscopic surgery and was successfully introduced for the treatment of gastroesophageal reflux disease,[18] diverticulitis,[19] and coronary artery disease.[20]

Rather than a true, autonomous robot, the da Vinci is a "master-slave system," in which a surgeon, sitting at a console (master), directly controls the remote

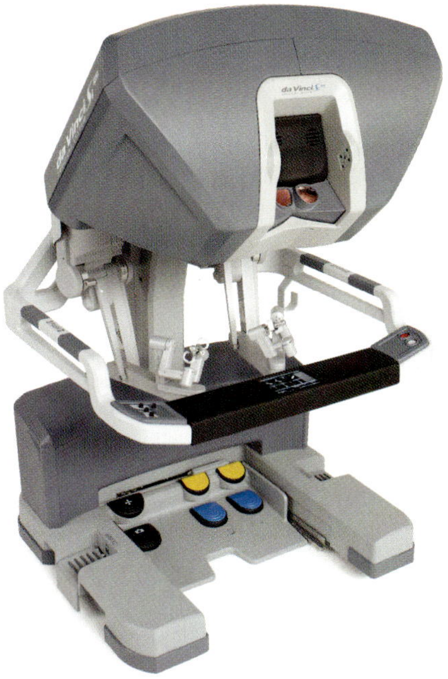

Figure 5. The da Vinci surgeon console. Credit: © 2013 Intuitive Surgical, Inc.

robotic arms (slave). The da Vinci Robotic System consists of the mobile console (Figure 5), the vision cart with a dual light source and dual 3-chip cameras, and the robot cart with three (Figure 6a) to four (Figure 6b) cable-driven robotic arms. One arm acts as a camera holder; the others are working arms and contain "endowrists," providing improved dexterity and maneuverability to a total of seven degrees of freedom (Figure 7).

The console's immersive binocular vision system allows for a magnified, three-dimensional visualization of the operative field, thus creating a feeling of "being right at the patient's side" (Figure 8). Automatic compensation of physiologic tremor and motion scaling guarantee precise control. Recent additions to the da Vinci's repertoire include the introduction of a dual console for training purposes and the development of instruments for single-site robotic surgery (VeSPA system).[19,21]

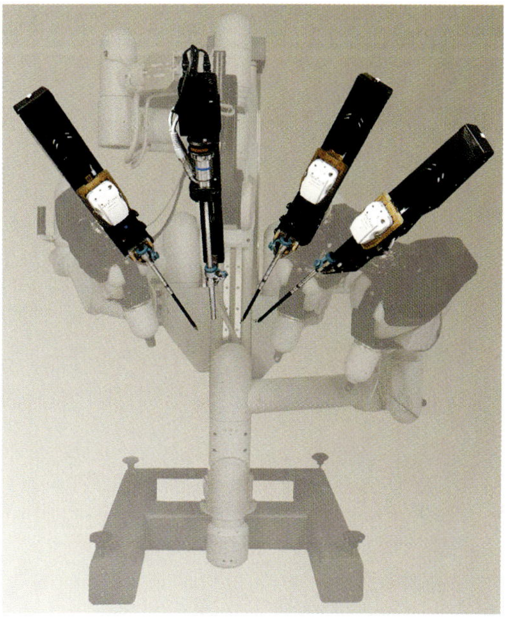

Figure 6a. The original da Vinci Robotic System. Credit: © 2013 Intuitive Surgical, Inc.

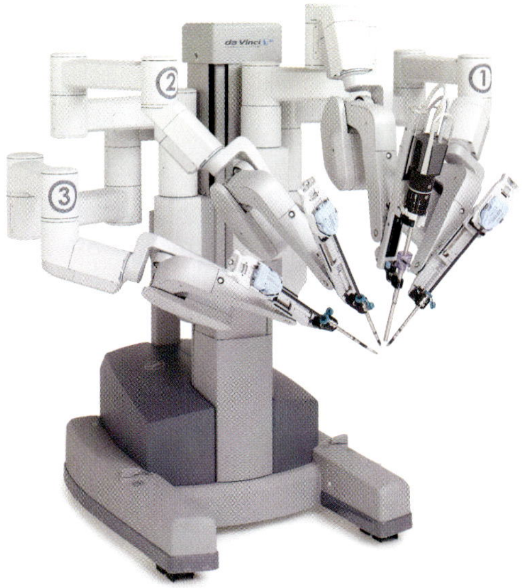

Figure 6b. The da Vinci Si Robotic System. Credit: © 2013 Intuitive Surgical, Inc.

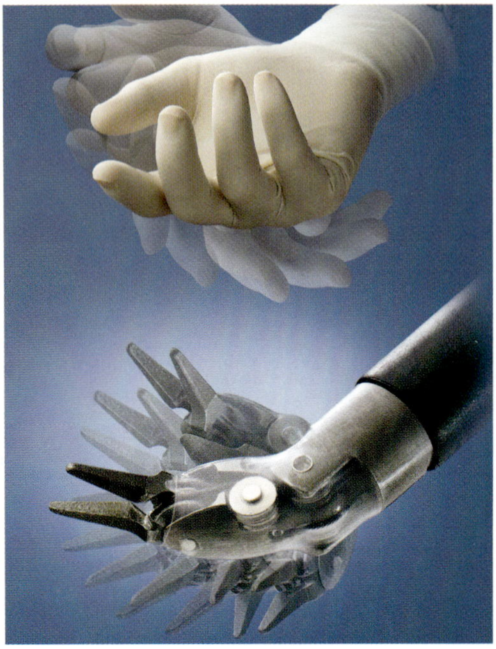

Figure 7. The EndoWrist.
Credit: © 2013 Intuitive Surgical, Inc.

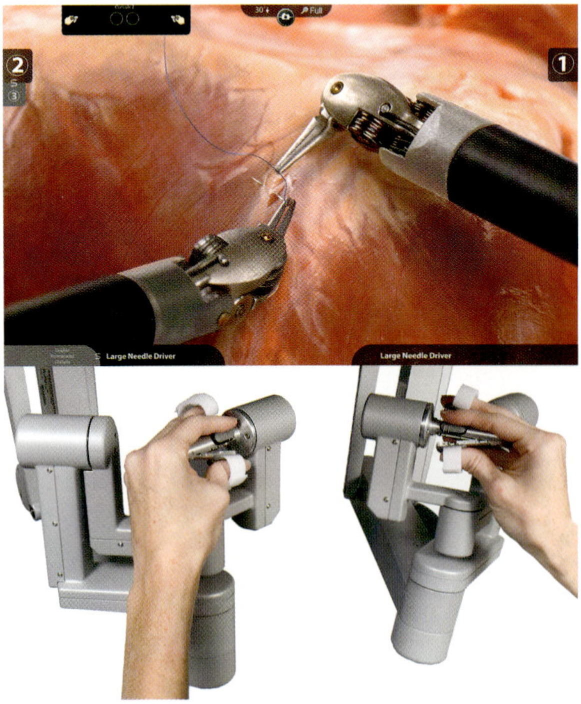

Figure 8. Operative view and controls.
Credit: © 2013 Intuitive Surgical, Inc.

From Laparoscopic to Robotic Surgery

The number of da Vinci systems and robotic-assisted procedures has grown dramatically in the last decade. The success of robotic surgery, driven by both technological advances in robotic systems as well as by consumer demands,[22] can be traced back to the introduction of minimally invasive techniques to the field of surgery in the 1980s. Since the first minimally invasive cholecystectomy in 1985,[23] the popularity of laparoscopic procedures has risen dramatically, and the scope of the procedures that can be performed using minimally invasive techniques has been growing continuously. For many elective operations, minimally invasive techniques have all but replaced open surgery.

For patients, the advantages of a minimally invasive approach, whenever feasible, are obvious. Laparoscopic surgery allows for smaller incisions and scars, decreased blood loss and risk of infection, as well as shorter hospital stays and reduced recovery time. With conventional laparoscopic surgery, however, these advantages come at a price. A two-dimensional monitor and counter-intuitive instrument movements have replaced the three-dimensional direct view, as well as the feel of the operative field experienced in traditional open surgery. Additionally, the long, inflexible instruments used in conventional laparoscopy are restricted to four degrees of motion and amplify the surgeon's physiologic tremor.

The use of surgical robots can overcome many of these limitations. The da Vinci Robotic System offers a three-dimensional view of the operative field, real depth perception, and a stable camera that is directly controlled by the operating surgeon rather than an assistant. Three cable-driven working arms are available for exposure and traction and offer seven degrees of freedom, comparable to the dexterity of the human hand. The surgeon's console enables precise control with tremor filtration and a comfortable, ergonomic position throughout the operation. Thus, the introduction of robotic systems may be viewed as an inevitable evolution of laparoscopic techniques, with surgical robots representing an advanced form of laparoscopic surgery.

Current Challenges and Future Perspectives

Despite their obvious advantages, robotic surgical systems currently face several challenges. Robotic operations have a steep learning curve and require extensive practice and training.[24,25] Operative times are usually longer and may require multiple time-consuming docking maneuvers. Perhaps the greatest challenge to overcome is the significant cost associated with robotic surgery, considering the current economic climate and health-care environment.

The fixed costs of the da Vinci Robotic System can reach one to more than $2 million per unit, with additional costs arising from maintenance contracts and expenses for robotic instruments with limited amounts of use.[22,26] These increased costs may be partially compensated for by shorter postoperative hospital stays following minimally invasive robotic surgery, and the fixed costs for surgical robots may decrease in the future with fewer expenses for disposable equipment[27] and with increasing competition, which will develop from the emergence of new robotic systems and manufacturers.

What does the future hold for robotic surgery? In addition to further advancing the field of minimally invasive surgery with robotic single-incision surgery, robotic surgery will likely expand in multiple directions. For example, improving current da Vinci systems with ceiling-mounted robotic arms[28] and employing them in Integrated Robotic Operating Rooms could pave the way toward a robotic-assisted approach to open operations. Ongoing advances and innovations in the fields of biomechanics and nanotechnology could lead to the production of injected or ingested miniature robots that could perform operations inside the patient. This concept may evoke memories of a science fiction movie plot but has recently been successfully introduced in experimental models with the "Assembling Reconfigurable Endoluminal Surgical system" (ARES), a self-assembling robot that can be used in the upper intestinal tract.[29]

Conclusion

Since their introduction to medicine in the 1980s, surgical robots have evolved from little more than modified industrial machines into sophisticated robotic systems capable of performing a wide array of complicated surgical procedures. Whether robotic surgery will eventually replace conventional laparoscopic surgery will greatly depend on the future price developments associated with robotic surgery, as well as financial constraints of our health-care system. Nevertheless, robotic surgical systems represent a tremendous advancement in surgical technology and are likely to significantly change the practice of surgery in the future.

References

1. Kwoh YS, Hou J, Jonckheere EA, Hayati S. A robot with improved absolute positioning accuracy for CT guided stereotactic brain surgery. *IEEE Trans Biomed Eng.* 1988;35:153–60.

2. Capek K. R.U.R. *Rossum's Universal Robots;* 1921.

3. Encyclopaedia Britannica. In: *Encyclopaedia Britannica.*

4. Davies BL, Hibberd RD, Ng WS, Timoney AG, Wickham JE. The development of a surgeon robot for prostatectomies. *Proc Inst Mech Eng H.* 1991;205:35–8.

5. Harris SJ, Arambula-Cosio F, Mei Q, et al. The Probot—an active robot for prostate resection. *Proc Inst Mech Eng H.* 1997;211:317–25.

6. Paul HA, Bargar WL, Mittlestadt B, et al. Development of a surgical robot for cementless total hip arthroplasty. *Clin Orthop Relat Res.* 1992:57–66.

7. Schulz AP, Seide K, Queitsch C, et al. Results of total hip replacement using the Robodoc surgical assistant system: clinical outcome and evaluation of complications for 97 procedures. *Int J Med Robot.* 2007;3:301–6.

8. Lang JE, Mannava S, Floyd AJ, et al. Robotic systems in orthopaedic surgery. *J Bone Joint Surg Br.* 2011;93:1296–9.

9. Satava RM. Surgical robotics: the early chronicles: a personal historical perspective. *Surg Laparosc Endosc Percutan Tech.* 2002;12:6–16.

10. Pugin F, Bucher P, Morel P. History of robotic surgery: from AESOP(R) and ZEUS(R) to da Vinci(R). *J Visc Surg.* 2011;148:e3–8.

11. Reichenspurner H, Damiano RJ, Mack M, et al. Use of the voice-controlled and computer-assisted surgical system ZEUS for endoscopic coronary artery bypass grafting. *J Thorac Cardiovasc Surg.* 1999;118:11–6.

12. Kim HL, Schulam P. The PAKY, HERMES, AESOP, ZEUS, and da Vinci robotic systems. *Urol Clin North Am.* 2004;31:659–69.

13. Lanfranco AR, Castellanos AE, Desai JP, Meyers WC. Robotic surgery: a current perspective. *Ann Surg.* 2004;239:14–21.

14. Marescaux J, Leroy J, Gagner M, et al. Transatlantic robot-assisted telesurgery. *Nature.* 2001;413:379–80.

15. Osborne L. Telesurgery. *The New York Times.* December 9, 2001.

16. Marescaux J, Leroy J, Rubino F, et al. Transcontinental robot-assisted remote telesurgery: feasibility and potential applications. *Ann Surg.* 2002;235:487–92.

17. Himpens J, Leman G, Cadiere GB. Telesurgical laparoscopic cholecystectomy. *Surg Endosc.* 1998;12:1091.

18. Cadiere GB, Himpens J, Vertruyen M, et al. Evaluation of telesurgical (robotic) NISSEN fundoplication. *Surg Endosc.* 2001;15:918–23.

19. Weber PA, Merola S, Wasielewski A, Ballantyne GH. Telerobotic-assisted laparoscopic right and sigmoid colectomies for benign disease. *Dis Colon Rectum.* 2002;45:1689–94; discussion 95–6.

20. Kappert U, Cichon R, Gulielmos V, et al. Robotic-enhanced Dresden technique for minimally invasive bilateral internal mammary artery grafting. *Heart Surg Forum.* 2000;3:319–21.

21. Morel P, Hagen ME, Bucher P, Buchs NC, Pugin F. Robotic single-port cholecystectomy using a new platform: initial clinical experience. *J Gastrointest Surg.* 2011;15:2182–6.

22. Barbash GI, Glied SA. New technology and health care costs—the case of robot-assisted surgery. *New Engl J Med.* 2010;363:701–4.

23. Muhe E. Long-term follow-up after laparoscopic cholecystectomy. *Endoscopy.* 1992;24:754–8.

24. Chitwood WR Jr, Nifong LW, Chapman WH, et al. Robotic surgical training in an academic institution. *Ann Surg.* 2001;234:475–84; discussion 84–6.

25. Sharma NL, Papadopoulos A, Lee D, et al. First 500 cases of robotic-assisted laparoscopic radical prostatectomy from a single UK centre: learning curves of two surgeons. *BJU Int.* 2011;108:739–47.

26. Breitenstein S, Nocito A, Puhan M, Held U, Weber M, Clavien PA. Robotic-assisted versus laparoscopic cholecystectomy: outcome and cost analyses of a case-matched control study. *Ann Surg.* 2008;247:987–93.

27. Barnett JC, Judd JP, Wu JM, Scales CD Jr, Myers ER, Havrilesky LJ. Cost comparison among robotic, laparoscopic, and open hysterectomy for endometrial cancer. *Obstet Gynecol.* 2010;116:685–93.

28. Blumenkranz S, inventor, Intuitive Surgical, Inc., assignee. *Ceiling and Floor Mounted Surgical Robot Set-up Arms.* United States. December 20, 2001.

29. Nagy Z, Flückiger M, Oung R, Kaliakatsos IK, Hawkes EW, Nelson BJ. Assembling reconfigurable endoluminal surgical systems: opportunities and challenges. *Int J Biomechatronics Biomed Robotics.* 2009;1:3–16.

Chapter Three

Coronary Revascularization

Stefan W. Leichtle, MD; Manak S. Sood, MD

History and Techniques of Coronary Artery Bypass Surgery

Though coronary artery disease (CAD) is commonly considered a problem of the twentieth century that is often associated with modern Western lifestyle, descriptions of angina pectoris (AP) date back to the eighteenth century, when "coronary-artery ossification" was suspected to be the likely cause of chest pain and sudden cardiac death.[1] Contemporary consequences of CAD are staggering, with more than one million cases of myocardial infarction (MI) in the United States annually, and one in six deaths attributable to CAD. Heart disease not only exerts a considerable toll on patients' lives, but also contributes to the ever rising costs of health care, and is responsible for $190 billion in health expenditures every year.[2]

The causality between CAD, myocardial ischemia, AP, and MI was established at the beginning of the twentieth century, but it was not until the middle of the century that medical and surgical therapies offered effective and successful treatment options. A pivotal role in the treatment of acute and chronic CAD fell to the surgical revascularization of ischemic myocardial tissue via coronary artery bypass (CAB) surgery. In 2009, an estimated 416,000 CAB procedures were performed to relieve symptoms and prolong life in patients with CAD.[2] Nevertheless, CAB surgery has to be considered a palliative procedure, as the underlying disease continues to progress and the occluded areas are not removed.

After several decades of work with experimental models and in animals, the first CAB operations were performed starting in 1960 with Goetz' successful right internal mammary artery (IMA) to right coronary artery bypass procedure.[3] Subsequently, the largest successful series of CAB operations at the time, using saphenous vein grafts (SVGs), was described by Favaloro at the Cleveland Clinic.[4] Many of the diverse techniques employed by the pioneers of CAB surgery, including the use of different autologous conduits (IMA or SVG), anastomotic techniques, and operations on the beating or arrested heart, are still in use today.[5]

Though some of the early CAB operations were performed on the beating heart (today described as "off-pump" CAB, OPCAB), the success and rapid adoption of CAB surgery in the early years would not have been possible without the invention of the heart-lung machine, allowing for extracorporeal support and operations on the arrested heart ("on-pump"). Attempts to perfuse isolated organs outside the human body can be traced back to the late nineteenth century, and, in 1935, an experiment by Nobel laureate Alexis Carrel and aviator Charles Lindbergh received nationwide attention as they used a perfusion apparatus (Figure 1) to keep a feline thyroid gland alive for 18 days. The development of more sophisticated heart-lung machines followed, but initial attempts to use cardiopulmonary bypass to repair congenital heart lesions had only very limited success. In 1953, however, John Gibbon succeeded in repairing an atrial septal defect on an arrested heart in an 18-year-old-woman.[6]

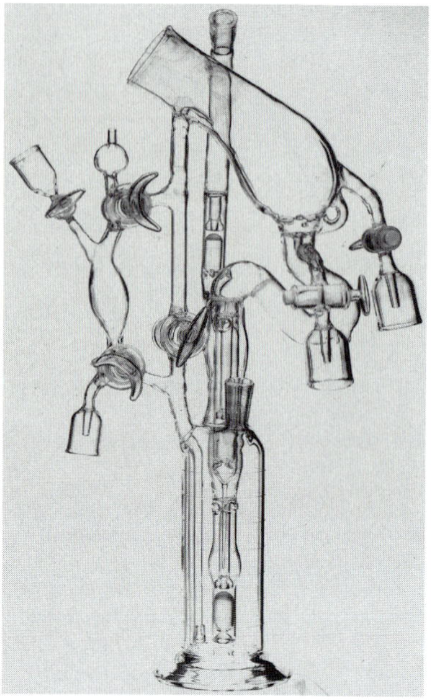

Figure 1. Perfusion apparatus developed during early attempts at extracorporeal circulation. Credit: Courtesy of the Rockefeller Archive Center.

The use of OPCAB regained increasing popularity in recent years, as the use of cardiopulmonary bypass seemed to be associated with several adverse effects including hemodynamic instability, systemic inflammation and release of cytokines, activation of the clotting cascade, microembolization, and cognitive dysfunction. The clear superiority of either method, however, has not yet been established despite multiple studies. Puskas et al. compared the outcomes of OPCAB and on-pump CAB in a large propensity matched cohort of patients, and demonstrated a significant reduction of operative mortality, stroke, and incidence of adverse cardiac events in OPCAB surgery.[7] However, in a randomized controlled trial (RCT), Shroyer et al. did not detect any significant difference between on- and off-pump CAB surgery with regard to cognitive outcomes and instead demonstrated a higher rate of complications and poorer graft patency in patients after OPCAB.[8]

Minimally Invasive Coronary Bypass Surgery

A recent major trend in CAB surgery has been the progress from "maximally invasive" operative approaches via median sternotomy to minimally invasive techniques, such as minimally invasive direct coronary artery bypass (MIDCAB),[9] totally endoscopic CAB (TECAB), and robot-assisted CAB.[10]

MIDCAB, an off-pump procedure, was pioneered in the mid 1990s. Initially, the main interest in this technique stemmed from the avoidance of cardiopulmonary bypass with its inherent complications, and MIDCAB was found to be particularly useful for the treatment of proximal left anterior descending (LAD) coronary artery disease. The advantages of MIDCAB include decreased overall morbidity and improved cosmetic results by substituting a limited, anterolateral thoracotomy for the anterior sternotomy of the traditional CAB operation (Figure 2).

In experienced hands, MIDCAB has been proven to be a very safe operation with regard to mortality, need for revascularization, and conversion to classic CAB. However, this technique requires practice, and significant improvements are not seen until after approximately 50 operations, and even more so after at least

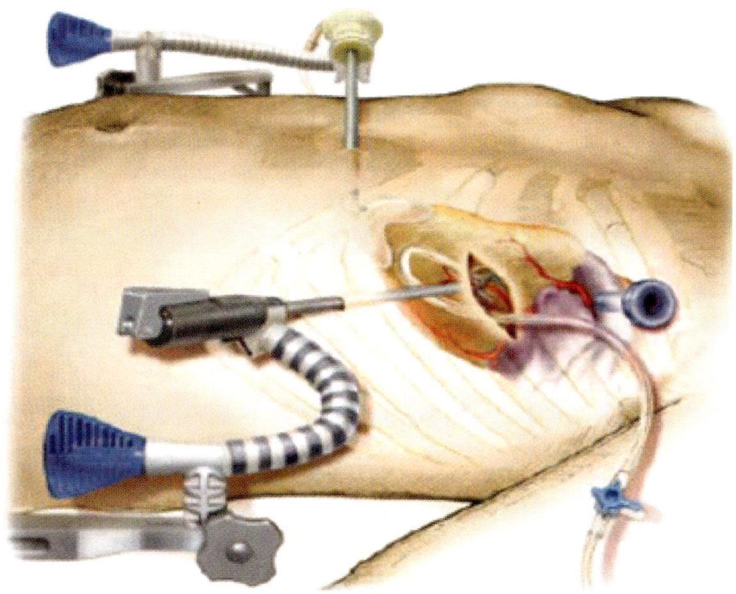

Figure 2. Operative setup for MIDCAB. The coronary stabilization device can be brought in through either an intercostal or subxiphoid location. Credit: © 2013 Intuitive Surgical, Inc.

100 cases.[11] In experienced hands, MIDCAB offers advantages even compared to contemporary percutaneous revascularization strategies employing drug-eluting stents (DES). Comparing percutaneous coronary intervention (PCI) with DES to MIDCAB in a retrospective series, Ben-Gal et al. demonstrated increased recurrence of angina (35% vs. 8.4%, $P < .001$) and a higher rate of re-interventions (16.8% vs. 3.6%, $P = .005$) in the percutaneous group, with similarly low mortality rates in both treatment arms.[12]

True minimally invasive CAB surgery arrived with the introduction of TECAB. This technique can be performed via classic endoscopy with video-assisted thoracic surgery (VATS) or with the help of a surgical robot. TECAB avoids even the limited thoracotomy of MIDCAB, but requires cardiopulmonary bypass.

Graft Options and Patency

The choice of grafts used for revascularization depends on the affected coronary artery, and their short- and long-term patency have substantial influence on outcomes and success of the CAB operation. The gold standard for grafting to the LAD is the left internal (thoracic [LITA]) mammary artery (LIMA). Patency rates for a LIMA to LAD bypass (Figure 3) remain 90%–95% even after 10 years, while the patency of the SVG decreases to 70%–80% for a similar time frame.[13,14] Interestingly, post-CAB stenoses are located mainly in the remote areas of the native coronary artery when an arterial conduit is used, while the stenosis of nonarterial grafts primarily occurs in the vein itself. The superior results of the LIMA to LAD graft are likely multifactorial and include the optimal runoff of the LAD due to its in situ location and branch septal perforators, as well as an artery-to-artery revascularization.

Radial artery (RA) grafts do not reach the patency rates of IMA grafts, but represent a viable and superior alternative to SVG.[15,16] Complications and limitations associated with RA grafts include a higher risk of vasospasm, the potential for atherosclerotic disease of the conduit at the time of harvest, and an intact ulnar artery of the ipsilateral arm as a prerequisite for harvest of the graft.

The SVG was among the first to be described for CAB surgery[4] and remains a commonly used graft due to its advantages with regard to harvest, availability, and resistance to vasospasm. Endoscopic harvesting techniques are available and confer the benefits of improved patient satisfaction due to less pain and earlier mobility, and reduced incidence of wound complications.

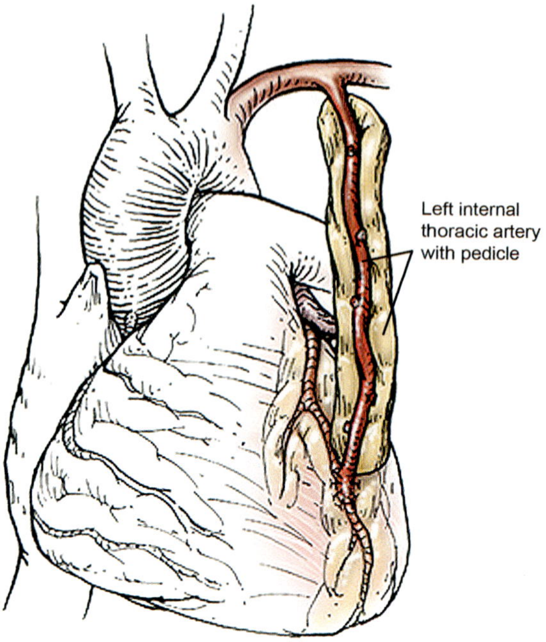

Figure 3. Diagram showing an in situ left internal thoracic artery to left anterior descending artery bypass. The LITA is a branch of the left subclavian artery.

The patency rates for common conduits are shown in Figure 4 (arterial = all arterial grafts; IMA = left and right internal mammary artery; RA = radial artery; SVG = saphenous vein graft).

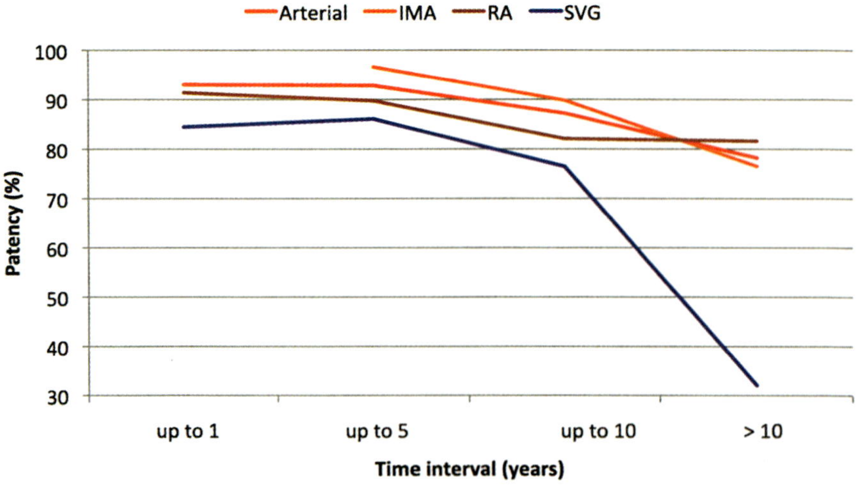

Figure 4. Graph showing patency trends for various conduits used in coronary artery bypass (CAB) grafting. Data based on references 13–18.

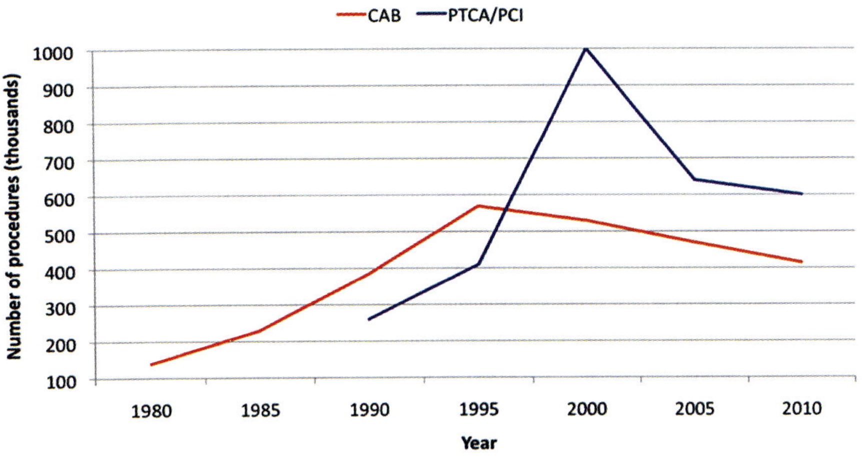

Figure 5. Graph showing trends in various approaches to coronary artery revascularization. A shift can be seen toward approaches favoring percutaneous interventions after 1995.

Percutaneous Coronary Intervention and Stenting

Advances in cardiac angiography, initially performed only for diagnostic purposes, led to the development of catheter-based interventions for the treatment of CAD. In 1977, Grüntzig introduced PCI for the treatment of coronary artery stenosis,[19] and, by 2009, more than half a million patients in the United States were undergoing this procedure annually (Figure 5, based on Roger et al.[2]).

Several large studies in the 1980s established the superiority of open surgical treatment versus PCI in the treatment for CAD,[5] but the ongoing refinement of PCI continues to challenge the superiority of surgical revascularization.

PCI with bare-metal stents (BMS) managed to achieve respectable results, but was found to be clearly inferior to CAB surgery, particularly in multivessel disease. The most prominent advantages of CAB were significantly lower rates of revascularization[20] and improved angina relief, but some studies also demonstrated a survival advantage with bypass surgery.[21,22] The rather low long-term patency rates of PCI with BMS dramatically improved with the introduction of DES,[23,24] and by 2006, 76% of stents employed were DES.[2]

Multiple studies have compared CAB surgery and PCI, but results remain variable and controversial. Nevertheless, these studies were able to delineate areas of particular strengths and weaknesses of the respective techniques.

The multicenter, randomized Synergy between PCI with Taxus and Cardiac Surgery (SYNTAX) trial attempted to establish non-inferiority of paclitaxel-eluting stents versus CAB surgery for LAD and three-vessel disease.[25] However, after one year follow-up, CAB was found to be superior with regard to major adverse cardiac and cerebrovascular events, which were defined as stroke, MI, death, or revascularization. The CAB group had significantly fewer revascularizations, albeit at the cost of a higher stroke rate with open heart surgery.

The SYNTAX trial had substantial influence on the current American College of Cardiology guidelines.[26] For left main coronary artery revascularization, they include a clear recommendation in favor of CAB to improve survival with stenosis >50%, but they also cite PCI as a reasonable alternative for patients with high surgical risk and if PCI could be performed more rapidly and safely than CAB in cases of acute MI.

For symptom relief, CAB and PCI are recommended in cases of >70% stenosis of one or more coronary arteries, if medical therapy does not resolve unacceptable angina or is not possible. For symptomatic three-vessel disease or involvement of the LAD, CAB is considered to be a reasonable choice over PCI to improve symptoms in good surgical candidates.

In summary, surgical revascularization is superior to PCI for (1) three-vessel disease with decreased left ventricular function, (2) left main coronary artery disease, and (3) in diabetics with two-vessel disease or proximal LAD disease.

Studies about short- and long-term outcomes of CAB surgery and PCI are ongoing, and several recent results continue to fuel the discussion about risks and benefits.

A comparison of quality of life after CAB and PCI demonstrated significant improvement in both groups, but PCI was superior with regard to quality of life after one month. Angina relief, however, was slightly superior in the CAB group, and long-term outcomes were equivalent.[27] Additionally, sirolimus-eluting stents were recently found to be non-inferior to CAB with regard to death, MI, and stroke, but the results also reaffirmed the need for more frequent revascularization procedures after PCI.[28] In an analysis of a large statewide database, CAB was found to be superior to PCI with DES with regard to mortality and incidence of MI in patients with two- and three-vessel disease.[29] Similar findings were reported recently in The American College of Cardiology Foundation–The Society of Thoracic Surgeons Collaboration on the Comparative Effectiveness of Revascularization Strategies (ASCERT) trial. Based on the very large Society of Thoracic Surgeons (STS) national database, CAB demonstrated a strong survival advantage versus PCI, particularly when assessing longer-term outcomes.[30,31]

Treatment of Proximal LAD Disease

Disease of the proximal LAD represents a particular challenge, and both CAB and PCI have been employed in its treatment. With PCI, there is concern for the occlusion of side branches and injury to the LAD, while CAB may seem a very invasive technique to treat single-vessel disease. A systematic analysis of comparisons between surgical and percutaneous approaches to proximal LAD disease demonstrated no differences with regard to short-term, one-year, and five-year survival, stroke, and MI rates. However, significantly fewer patients required revascularization procedures after CAB surgery (7.3% at one and five years) than after PCI (19.5% at one year, and 33.5% at five years). Furthermore, angina relief was significantly greater and longer lasting after CAB than after PCI.[32] These results were obtained mainly in trials of PCI with BMS, but a comparison between MIDCAB

(LIMA to LAD) and sirolimus-eluting stents also demonstrated the superiority of surgical revascularization.[12]

Introduction to Robotic Cardiac Surgery

With its progression toward less invasive techniques, cardiac surgery has been at the forefront of robotic technology. Starting in the late 1990s, cardiac surgeons have been experimenting with the use of robotic assistance, and step-by-step its application was expanded from camera assistance to graft harvest and anastomosis formation.[10,33] Initial studies not only confirmed the feasibility of robot assistance for individual parts of CAB operations, but also suggested several advantages.[34] Compared to conventional VATS, robotic instruments provide better range of motion and increased flexibility, while the advanced three-dimensional optic system is not limited by the fulcrum effect. Robot-assisted harvest of the IMA is generally much easier than conventional endoscopic takedown and has a shorter learning curve than the latter. Due to improved visualization, the graft is usually longer, and there is a reduced risk for chest wall fractures and costal cartilage damage as extensive sternal manipulation can be avoided.

The robot-assisted LIMA takedown quickly became a precursor for robotic MIDCAB. Through three 10-mm ports in the left second, fifth, and seventh intercostal spaces, the robot enters the thoracic cavity and is used to mobilize the entire length of the LIMA. Through a longitudinal pericardiotomy, the LAD can be identified, and a limited anterior thoracotomy provides exposure for a direct anastomosis between LIMA and LAD, using an off-pump stabilization system. Postoperatively, patients undergoing robotic MIDCAB experience a dramatic reduction in length of hospital stay (LOS) and recovery time compared to conventional open heart surgery. Surgical robots can also be utilized in the context of hybrid coronary revascularization (HR), in which robotic LIMA to LAD bypass is combined with PCI for non-LAD territories.[35]

Hybrid Procedures

The rationale for HR, i.e., the combination of surgical (CAB) and percutaneous (PCI) techniques, stems from several basic observations and concepts.[36]

- Overall survival has been shown to be similar between CAB and PCI.[20,25,28,32]
- CAB is superior to PCI with regard to angina relief and need for revascularization.[25,32]
- LIMA grafts have the highest patency rates,[18] and the LIMA to LAD bypass is the essential component responsible for the superiority of CAB surgery.
- The proximal LAD has a high rate of restenosis with PCI.
- PCI and CAB with SVG are equivalent for the revascularization of non-LAD territory.

Therefore, HR combines the efficacy and durability of surgical revascularization with the advantages of minimally invasive PCI. Ideal candidates for HR have isolated proximal LAD or multi-vessel disease, with non-LAD lesions that are amenable to PCI. As HR avoids additional SVG or RA bypass procedures, it is also well suited for the treatment of high-risk patients who might not be candidates for conventional CAB and those with a lack of adequate conduits.

HR can be performed as a one-staged or two-staged procedure. The former describes concomitant MIDCAB and PCI during the same operative session. Though the most efficient and advantageous approach, it requires a highly trained team and an advanced hybrid operating room, which currently limits its widespread use. In a two-staged HR, percutaneous procedure and surgical revascularization are performed during the same hospital stay, but not in the same procedural setting. It allows for performance of each intervention in their traditional environment, but goes along with several advantages and disadvantages depending on the order of interventions. Performing PCI first, followed by CAB, allows for multi-vessel stenting and "backup" CAB for lesions that are not amenable to percutaneous treatment. However, this technique leaves the anterior wall unprotected during PCI and necessitates a CAB operation, along with the administration of antiplatelet medication after stenting. Furthermore, there is concern for stent thrombosis upon administration of heparin reversal after CAB, and postsurgical angiographic evaluation of the LIMA to LAD bypass is not possible.

With CAB being the first intervention, followed by PCI, the LIMA to LAD bypass can be evaluated by angiography during the percutaneous procedure. Additionally, this order allows the CAB operation to be performed before administration of antiplatelet medication. However, in case of a failed percutaneous intervention, an emergency high-risk surgical procedure would have to be performed, albeit through a first-time sternotomy.

Despite its introduction more than a decade ago, data about the outcomes of HR compared to more conventional revascularization strategies are still limited and derived mostly from large single-institution experiences. The outcomes of HR have improved substantially with the evolution of percutaneous interventions, from balloon angioplasty without stenting to the use of BMS and DES, creating a considerable variability of results. Early studies employing PCI without stenting, or with BMS, reported mortality rates between 0% and 2%, and revascularization rates of up to 30%, while more recent studies utilizing PCI with DES demonstrated much lower revascularization rates up to 10%.[36–38]

Patient Selection for Robotic MIDCAB

For the most part, patient selection is predicated upon coronary anatomy, comorbidities, pulmonary reserve, and body habitus. MIDCAB patient candidates must have critical lesions in the proximal- to mid-LAD territories. A lesion of 70% or greater, confirmed by angiography, meets criteria for intervention, and more moderate lesions may be clinically relevant if flow wire testing is performed. A fractional flow reserve (FFR) of less than 0.8 is considered to be of hemodynamic significance. Intracoronary ultrasound may be performed, if degree of obstruction is in question, and can also rule out significant left main coronary artery disease, which would likely commit the patient to standard revascularization strategies via sternotomy in lieu of MIDCAB.

A da Vinci MIDCAB can be performed as an isolated procedure for single-vessel disease involving the LAD, or alternatively as part of a multi-vessel revascularization strategy in individuals with lesions in the circumflex and right coronary arteries. If a hybrid approach is being considered, it is paramount that lesions in non-LAD territories are readily amenable to PCI with DES, i.e., that they are stentable, focal lesions in larger caliber vessels. If diffuse disease is present, or if percutaneous targets are less than optimal, a standard surgical procedure is indicated. Branch-vessel disease and complex stenoses are also relative contraindications to a hybrid approach. Patient comorbidities, particularly pulmonary reserve, have to be taken into consideration, as the patient has to tolerate single-lung ventilation for an anterior thoracotomy approach.

Body habitus is another important criteria when considering robotic MIDCAB. Although there are no absolute prohibitive size criteria, individuals with a body mass index (BMI) greater than 40 kg/m^2 represent a particular challenge during surgery due to chest wall thickness and limitations of the rib-spreader. However, even though patients with a high BMI tend to have substantial abdominal girth, they may have relatively shallow chest walls, making them potential candidates for a minimally invasive approach. Therefore, a close and thorough inspection with the patient in a supine position is required before determining an individual's candidacy for robotic MIDCAB.

Target vessel size and overall preoperative left ventricular ejection fraction should also influence the decision about robotic MIDCAB. Catheterization measurements, comparing the size of the diagnostic coronary catheter (usually 1.6–2.0 mm) to the LAD on multiple views, provide a rough estimate of target vessel diameter. In our experience, target vessels less than 1.5 mm in size often prove challenging, particularly in larger patients. Patients with a low ejection fraction may be unable to tolerate the rise in intrathoracic pressure during robot-assisted LIMA harvest secondary to CO_2 insufflation. Raising the central venous pressure (CVP) above the set insufflation settings may overcome the decrease in venous return; however, patients with preoperative ejection fractions less than 30% may not tolerate these manipulations associated with OPCAB. Of note, only the anterior wall is compressed during MIDCAB, and we have successfully performed robot-assisted MIDCABs in patients with ejection fractions as low as 10%.

Absolute contraindications to a da Vinci CAB include hemodynamic instability, acute anterior wall MI, diffusely calcified or diminutive LAD by angiogram, subclavian artery stenosis, extensive pleural adhesions upon chest entry, and a deep intramyocardial vessel upon direct inspection.

Previous open heart surgery is not an absolute contradiction to robotic MIDCAB if valvular pathology prompted prior intervention, or if the LIMA was spared during previous revascularization. It is essential to obtain the previous operative records to determine if the left chest was violated during the initial operation, which could result in adhesion formation, thus precluding port placement and limited thoracotomy at reoperation. If feasible, robot-assisted LAD revascularization will allow for safer re-entry, obviating the need for repeat sternotomy. In some cases, adhesions from a previous operation may actually stabilize the anterior wall, thus facilitating exposure for a beating heart anastomosis.

Relative contraindications include severe obesity, history of pericarditis, previous radiation therapy, and significant cardiomegaly, which can potentially limit the intrathoracic excursions of the robot arms.

Determining patients' "frailty index" can provide a more individualized assessment of their ability to tolerate a standard versus robotic CAB. The STS is currently developing exact criteria determining this value as part of the preoperative risk-stratification process. However, any experienced surgeon is able to consider the overall state of a patient being evaluated for revascularization and can determine if the patient has sufficient reserve to tolerate an invasive approach via sternotomy, or would benefit from a less invasive MIDCAB. Factors contributing to the frailty index include comorbidities, functional and ambulatory status, as well as duration and nature of preoperative hospitalization. Individuals expected to have a protracted recovery from conventional surgery may benefit from minimally invasive robotic MIDCAB.

A subset of cardiac patients who may benefit from a staged interventional strategy are those with acute non-ST elevation MI (NSTEMI) without LAD involvement. The literature is replete with articles touting the benefits of delayed surgery after an acute cardiac event; ideally, CAB surgery should be delayed several days to one month after acute MI, depending on the extent of injury, overall enzyme leak, and residual ventricular function after infarction. In this setting, and assuming coronary anatomy is favorable, addressing the culprit vessel at the time of infarction using PCI may help to abort the acute event and allow for a strategy of delayed hybrid revascularization. If the residual stenosis is somewhat precarious, a BMS should be placed in the offending artery. This will allow for discontinuation of antiplatelet therapy after 30 days in anticipation of completion revascularization. Patients with less critical residual anatomy in initially non-revascularized territories may benefit from placement of a DES during initial intervention. Surgical revascularization may then be performed after 3 to 6 months of antiplatelet therapy, based on the type of DES placed.

It has been interesting to watch the evolution of robot-assisted CAB surgery at our institution over the last four years. Initially, only the healthiest candidates were selected for this procedure, ensuring excellent results. With increasing experience, we have expanded our indications, and it is now not uncommon to offer this procedure to patients who have been declined a traditional CAB operation for "prohibitive" risk factors. We feel strongly that we have been able to offer an arterial bypass to the LAD in many individuals who would otherwise have been relegated to suboptimal medical therapy or high-risk stenting.

Preoperative Testing

In addition to routine laboratory studies and chest x-ray, we include the following tests and procedures in our preoperative workup for da Vinci CAB operations.

- **Coronary Angiogram.** A critical lesion in the LAD territory must be demonstrated, and concomitant lesions must be noted. If possible, the subclavian artery and LIMA should be injected during catheterization to rule out flow-limiting stenosis and to demonstrate the course of the latter vessel.
- **Carotid Ultrasound.** Most patients presenting for surgery in our practice have generalized vascular disease. Preoperative quantification of the degree of carotid artery stenosis will aid in intraoperative hemodynamic management.
- **Pulmonary Function Testing.** Single-lung ventilation is an absolute prerequisite for MIDCAB, and, subsequently, adequate pulmonary reserve is paramount in patients selected for this procedure. In our experience, a forced expiratory volume in one second (FEV_1) of more than 700 mL and a diffusing capacity (DL_{CO}) greater than 50% predicted are sufficient to tolerate lung isolation for the duration of the operation. Continuous positive airway pressure (CPAP) of the ventilated lung may augment oxygenation if needed. Marginal candidates may benefit from optimization under the care of a pulmonologist and may be reevaluated before a final decision is made. Naturally, the overall status of the patient with regard to mobility and ambulation must be taken into account. If the patient has an oxygen saturation greater than 92% and is able to walk 15 minutes and climb stairs without difficulty, single-lung ventilation will likely be tolerated during the operation.
- **Vein Mapping.** We routinely perform an ultrasound of the greater saphenous veins in both lower extremities preoperatively. Determining which side has a higher quality vein is helpful in case conversion and standard revascularization become necessary, or if the LIMA is an inadequate conduit for the bypass.
- **Computed Tomography (CT) of the Chest.** For reoperations, particularly if the initial operation was performed at an outside institution, we obtain a non-contrast CT scan to obtain details regarding the proximity of the sternum to the right ventricle, location of the innominate vein and aorta, and to aid in port placement depending on heart size and anatomy in general.

Surgical Technique

At our institution, anesthesiologists are responsible for establishing preoperative access. A radial arterial line and internal jugular central venous catheter are standard. A Swan-Ganz catheter is placed for patients with low ejection fraction or other concerning comorbidities.

After induction of general anesthesia, the patient is positioned with the left shoulder and arm draped off the table to minimize the conflict between the right robotic arm and the protuberance of the left shoulder. The right arm is tucked close to the body, and the left arm is draped slightly off the table using side drapes, supported by an arm sling and forearm support at the elbow and wrist (Figure 6).

A double-lumen endotracheal tube is placed using a bronchoscope for guidance. Alternatively, a bronchial blocker within the left main stem bronchus can facilitate isolation in patients with small airways. Placement of an inflatable pressure cuff, or placement of a roll transversely across the midchest, may facilitate exposure by lifting the thorax and dropping the shoulder.

External defibrillator pads are placed parallel to the sternum on the right and below the left scapula, to ensure transcardiac delivery of the impulse. The area overlying the sternum is left exposed should conversion to an open procedure become necessary.

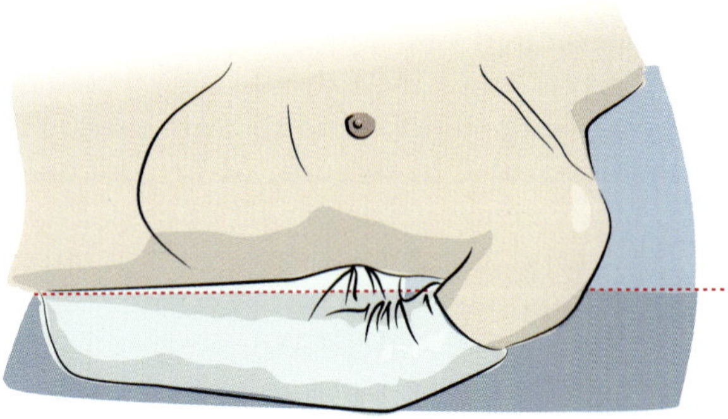

Figure 6. Patient positing for robotic-assisted MIDCAB. The left arm is draped off the operative table and the patient is rotated 15 degrees to the right. A transthoracic roll may facilitate exposure. Credit: © 2013 Intuitive Surgical, Inc.

Careful attention is directed toward addressing external landmarks prior to skin incision. Sternal notch and xiphoid process are marked for subsequent insertion of a coronary stabilization device. In women with large breasts, the course of the sternum is marked before final positioning. The femoral arteries and landmarks for endoscopic vein harvest are identified in case conversion should become necessary.

The inframammary crease serves as a landmark for anterior thoracotomy and is typically 2 cm below the nipple-areolar complex in male patients. Draping proceeds in the usual fashion, and traction on the iodinated adhesive drape toward the right shoulder helps to displace the left breast toward the midline and cephalad in those with pendulous breasts.

A transesophageal probe is placed, serving as an invaluable intraoperative tool to evaluate left ventricular function in the setting of hypotension. Confirmation of wall motion and contractility via transesophageal echocardiogram (TEE) can be helpful to guide hemodynamic management, and an anesthesiologist certified in echocardiography is integral during these minimally invasive procedures. A 5 to 10 mcg per minute nitroglycerin drip is maintained throughout the procedure to minimize spasm of the LIMA and native coronary arteries. Final positioning includes a 15-degree tilting of the table to the right. Constant communication between the surgeon at the console and the bedside assistants is critical; therefore, all participants use headsets during the robotic portion of the operation.

The initial incision is typically made in the left second or third intercostal space, in line with the lateral third of the clavicle (2 to 3 cm medial to the anterior axillary line). In patients with small thoracic cavities, a second intercostal space incision may be preferable to avoid external collisions with the camera arm.

A 15-blade is used to make a 5-mm incision and, after lung isolation, a curved tip clamp is used to penetrate the parietal pleura over the rib edge. At this point, a standard 5-mm laparoscopic port is introduced and connected to a heated CO_2 insufflator at pressures set at 8–10 mmHg, with flow rates of 2–3 L per minute. A 5-mm camera is inserted to visualize the subsequent port placements. We have found that insufflation from a superior port displaces the apex of the heart medially, making it safer to insert the lower and the larger camera ports (Figure 7).

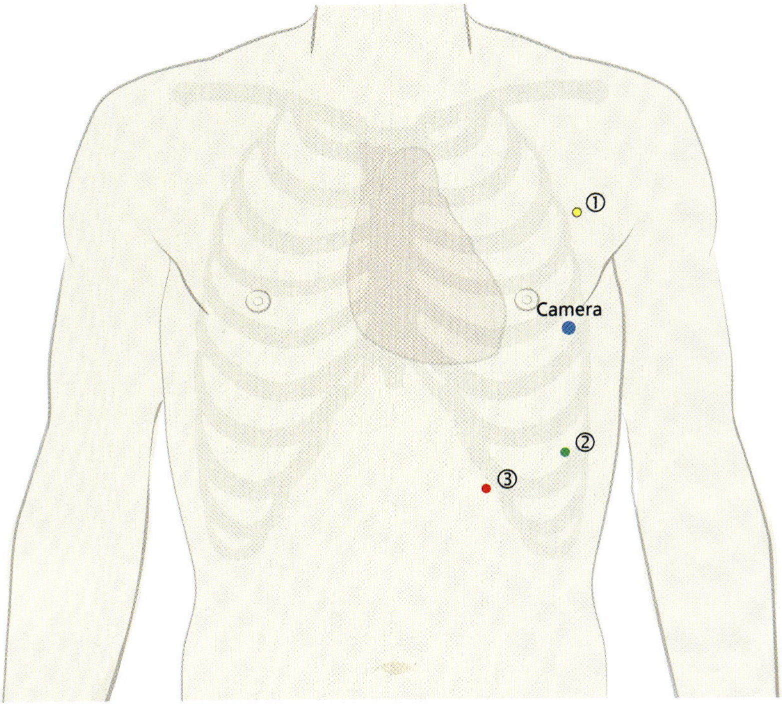

Figure 7. Port placement for robotic-assisted MIDCAB. The right arm (1) is typically in the second intercostal space, the camera arm is inserted in the fifth interspace, and the left arm is in the seventh interspace (2). The coronary stabilization device can be brought in under the rib cage or from a subxiphoid location (3). Credit: © 2013 Intuitive Surgical, Inc.

An 8-mm robotic port is introduced in the seventh intercostal space; although an alternative interspace may be chosen based on thoracic cage anatomy. A 12-mm camera port is introduced in the fourth or fifth (depending on body habitus) intercostal space, such that the balloon at its tip barely enters the chest wall (Figure 8). Balloon inflation with 5 mL of air affixes this port to the chest wall.

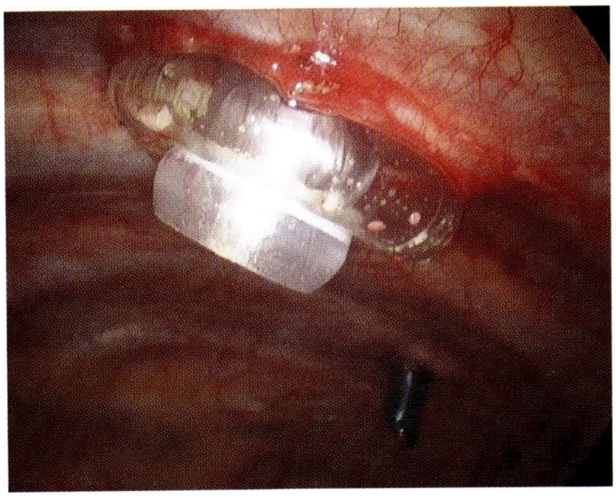

Figure 8. Intrapleural view of camera port after insufflation of balloon.

The most superior laparoscopic port is then replaced with a standard 8-mm da Vinci counterpart. We favor long left and right robotic ports for all cases, regardless of body habitus, in an effort to move the remote center of rotation further from the chest wall, thereby allowing for a greater range of motion (Figure 9). The CO_2 tubing is moved to the camera port at this time. Ideally, the three ports are placed in a gentle "V" (upright or inverted) arrangement to minimize internal collisions, and should be separated by a distance of 4 to 5 finger-breadths (approximately 10 cm).

The robotic base is then centered at the camera arm, being mindful to maintain the "sweet spot" for camera excursion (blue bar on central arm). Docking proceeds as left and right ports are locked in place, using the butterfly wings on the respective arms. The dual optic camera (30-degree up scope) is then inserted through the central port and controlled manually for the initial introduction of instruments. A unipolar spatula is inserted through the right port and a bipolar DeBakey forceps through the left. Electrocautery is set at 20 joules.

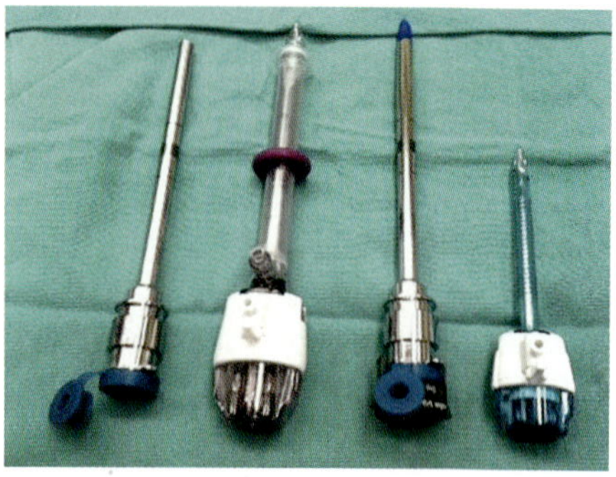

Figure 9. Ports used for robotic-assisted MIDCAB. The camera port (second from the left) has a balloon occluder at its tip. A 5-mm port (right) is used during entry and after revascularization to ensure hemostasis.

Once the surgeon is seated at the console, a brief excursion is performed along the anticipated length of the mammary bed, attempting to identify any limitations of motion at the onset of dissection. Performing a simple lift maneuver, thereby centralizing the ports within the intercostal space and altering the center of rotation, can overcome "ratcheting" of the instruments over rib surfaces. Anatomic landmarks should be identified once range of excursion has been addressed, and the left phrenic nerve and subclavian artery will help determine the proximal extent of dissection.

Mediastinal attachments between the pericardium and chest wall are taken down, and the LIMA can typically be seen in its upper third. We begin by scoring the endothoracic fascia both medially and laterally for the entire length of the artery, before initiating dissection between the conduit and the chest wall (Figure 10). It is useful to unroof the vessel by splitting the fascia overlying the distal third of the mammary artery to define its course. Often the bifurcation will become obvious at this point, and dissection typically proceeds in a lateral to medial fashion.

At this point, a decision must be made whether to take the LIMA down in a skeletonized manner or as a pedicle including both mammary veins in the dissection. Some authors favor a skeletonized LIMA harvest allowing for some extra length for subsequent anastomosis. We favor a pedicle graft, maintaining the adjacent veins to minimize the potential for thermal injury during harvest. Additionally, the presence of an intact pedicle serves as a handle for countertraction during eventual preparation of the LIMA.

Typically, we begin the dissection within an intercostal space in an area not overlying a rib (although the vessel may be more obvious over a bony protuberance). A plane is developed between the mammary artery and anterior chest wall, and special care must be taken when approaching branch intercostal vessels. Once identified, a clear space is carefully developed, 1 cm in length on either side of the branches, allowing for draping and providing maximal exposure of the branch itself.

Smaller branches can be addressed using unipolar or microbipolar electrocautery (Figure 11), whereas larger ones should be controlled with micro-titanium

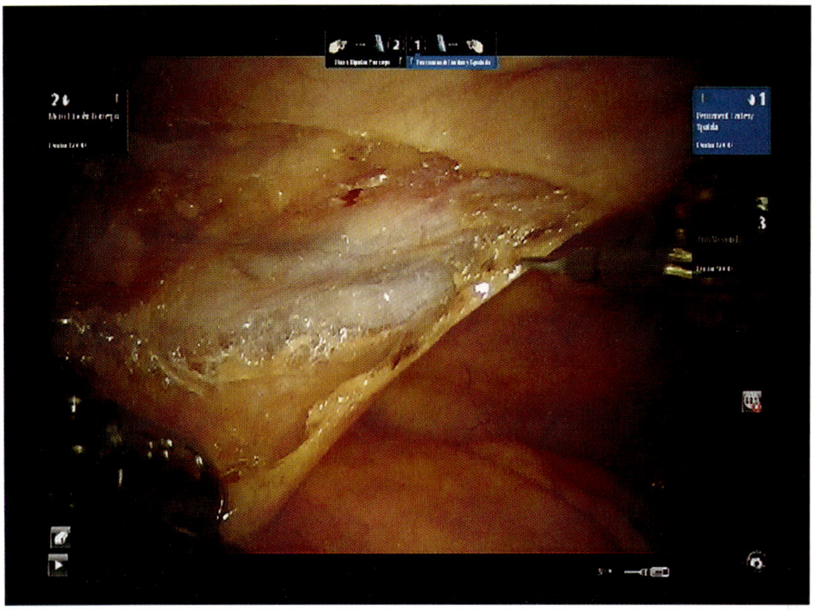

Figure 10. Dissection of thoracic pleura overlying the LIMA. The mammary artery can be seen prior to mobilization. Credit: Manak Sood, MD.

clips. In all cases, care must be taken to work as far away from the body of the LIMA as possible to prevent injury or possible kinking from the coagulation of adjacent tissues.

The LIMA bifurcation usually occurs in the sixth or seventh intercostal space, and we will typically follow the larger medial branch for another 1–2 cm to serve as a handle for subsequent manipulation. The patient is given systemic heparin commensurate with body weight (2 mg/kg) to achieve an activated clotting time (ACT) between 225 and 250 seconds. This value should be checked at 15-minute intervals during revascularization, and additional heparin administered as needed.

An anterior pericardiotomy is performed as the heparin circulates, beginning at the apex of the heart and extending toward the main pulmonary artery. A pericardial lipectomy will facilitate visualization of the pericardium at the site of entry. This can typically be performed from medial to lateral, taking care to continually visualize the phrenic nerve as it courses along the lateral edge of the pericardium. External defibrillator pads should be connected, as the delivery of an electric current upon opening the pericardium may elicit an arrhythmia, and ventilation is held upon entry.

Identification of the pulmonary artery is invaluable as a landmark, suggesting the location of the interventricular septum in those patients with multiple diagonal branches, an intramyocardial LAD, or if excessive epicardial fat is present. Palpation of the interventricular septum through the thoracotomy site may help locate the LAD if external landmarks are not obvious. Some surgeons prefer switching to a 30-degree down scope for this portion of the procedure, although this is not necessary for an anterior pericardiotomy (Figure 12).

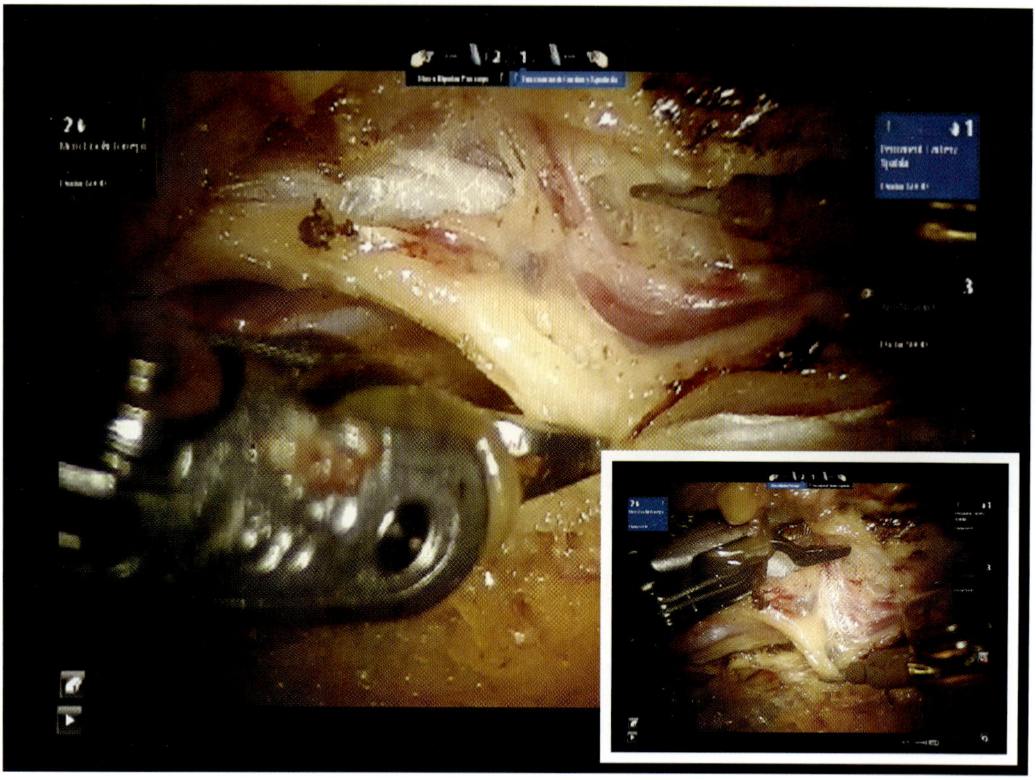

Figure 11. Dissection of the LIMA. A branch vessel can be seen as the mammary artery is mobilized. Inset: Bipolar cautery is used to coagulate larger LIMA branches.

After an adequate ACT is achieved, the distal end of the mammary vessel is divided using robotic Potts Endo-Wrist scissors (Figure 13); terminal mammary branches are clipped twice. The pedicle is then temporarily clipped to the edge of the pericardium for later identification via thoracotomy.

In those instances where multiple bypasses are being performed, the right internal mammary artery (RIMA) can be harvested via the same approach. Again, cautery takedown of mediastinal attachments to the sternum and an increase in insufflation pressures may facilitate transthoracic dissection if tolerated hemodynamically. The right endothoracic fascia is opened, and the RIMA is harvested along its entire length. Division of the right internal mammary vein proximally may help to identify the origin of the RIMA and provide extra length. The artery is then divided at both ends for later use as a composite graft.

The left arm is undocked, and the camera is directed to the most inferior region of the dissection in the area of the xiphoid process. A one-inch incision is made in a subxiphoid location, the fascia is spread, and a curved clamp is introduced into the left pleural space for subsequent placement of the stabilizer arm (Figure 14). Introducing the clamp at this juncture with camera visualization decreases the likelihood of right ventricular injury and minimizes the risk of displacement of microclips from the distal mammary bed, as CO_2 insufflation creates a greater tunnel for entry.

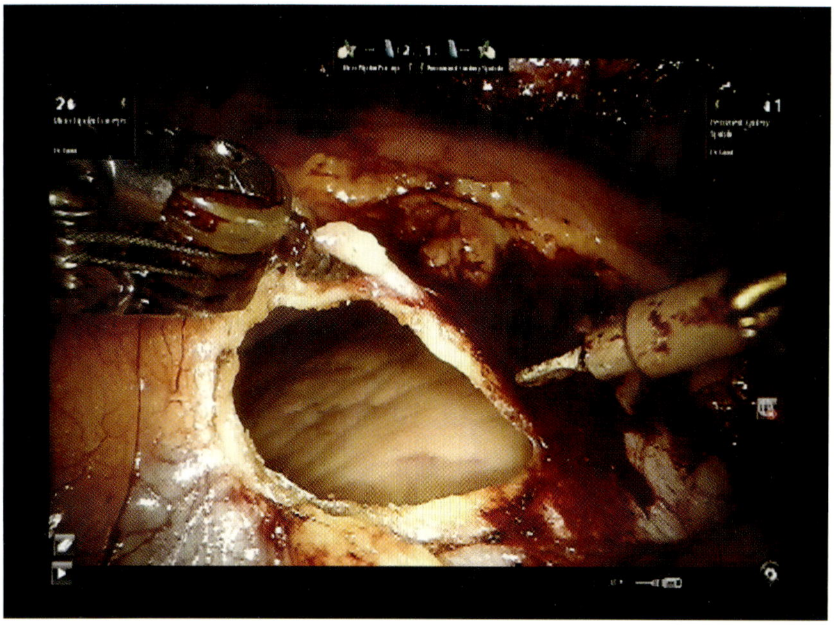

Figure 12. The pericardium is opened longitudinally beginning at the apex and extending toward the main pulmonary artery.

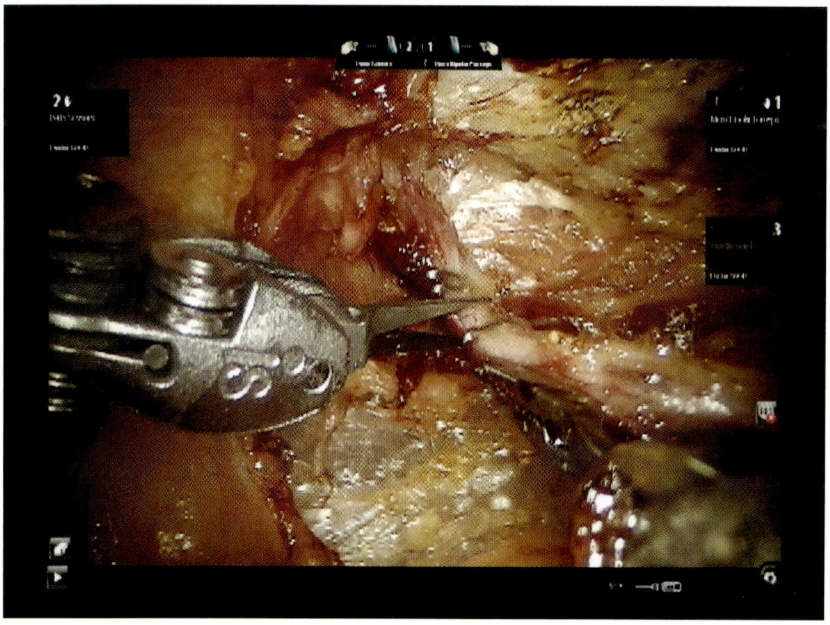

Figure 13. After systemic heparinization, the LIMA is clipped and divided using robotic Potts scissors. The free end will be temporarily clipped to the pericardium and retrieved after thoracotomy.

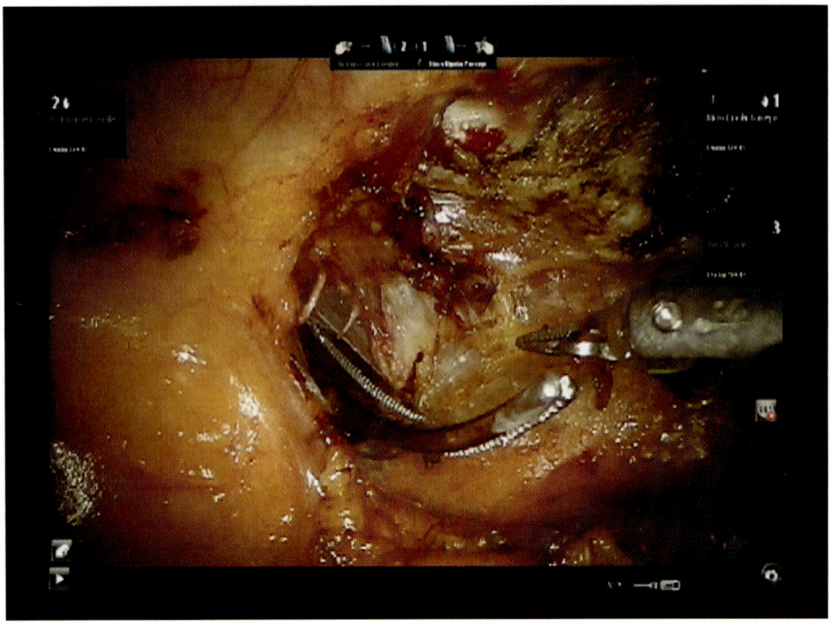

Figure 14. A curved clamp is inserted through a subxiphoid incision. Direct visualization will prevent inadvertent disruption of clips on the distal mammary stump. This clamp is secured to the skin externally using a towel clamp and will eventually be used to introduce the coronary stabilization device.

The clamp is positioned with the curve facing the chest wall and secured externally with a towel clamp.

The patient is then completely undocked from the robot, and all ports are removed. The most superior port is replaced with a simple 5-mm endoscopic port, temporarily tying it in place. This allows for subsequent revisualization of the left hemithorax after thoracotomy closure, identification of potential bleeding sites, and tracking of the course of the LIMA bypass. The middle port incision is then extended medially for a distance of 2–3 cm. The subcutaneous tissue is divided in the same line as the pectoralis muscle (muscle-sparing approach), decreasing the likelihood of lung herniation, a complication that has been described with this approach.

The fifth intercostal space is then entered, although choosing one level above or below is possible through the same incision if necessary. The pleura is undermined in both directions to allow for further rib spreading. A medium soft tissue retractor is placed to prevent skin and fat layers from obstructing the field of vision. A low-profile rib spreader is inserted to displace the ribs just enough to visualize the target vessel, and to later allow for instrument manipulation for creation of the anastomosis. Once the LAD is visualized, stabilization is optimized. Stay sutures in the medial or lateral pericardium will position the designated bypass site in the middle of the wound.

On the patient's right side, a holding bar for the endostabilizer is placed on the guardrail at the level of the iliac crest. A robotic stabilization arm is introduced through the subxiphoid location, and the vacuum stabilizer is attached through the thoracotomy incision. A blower-mister is used to achieve a bloodless field. A beaver blade is then used to dissect the overlying epicardium for a length of 2 cm, once the site for LAD anastomosis has been chosen. The epicardium on either side of the target vessel is scored 2 cm above this location, and a silastic Endoloop on a blunt curved needle is passed.

The mammary artery is injected with papaverine, and a small occlusive vascular clamp is temporarily applied several centimeters from its terminal end. The most distal portion of the LIMA is splayed in preparation for anastomosis. A coronary arteriotomy is made with an eye blade, and the vessel loop is tightened subsequently, leaving the vessel full upon initial entry to prevent back wall injury. The LAD arteriotomy is extended in both directions, and an appropriately sized shunt is placed intraluminally. The apical region on TEE beyond the arteriotomy should remain contractile, and there should be no ischemic changes on electrocardiogram (EKG) if the shunt is properly positioned and functional. Vessel loop occlusion is discontinued, and an end-to-side anastomosis is performed over the shunt between the LIMA and LAD using 7-0 nonabsorbable, monofilament suture. After the last stitch has been thrown, the shunt is removed (Figure 15).

Doppler interrogation of the bypass graft is performed to demonstrate adequate flow in diastole. The left lung is briefly inflated to ensure that there is no kinking of the graft after chest closure, and the pedicle is tacked to prevent rotation and distortion. A single straight 24-Fr chest tube is inserted through the most inferior portal incision and secured to the skin. Two heavy, absorbable pericostal sutures

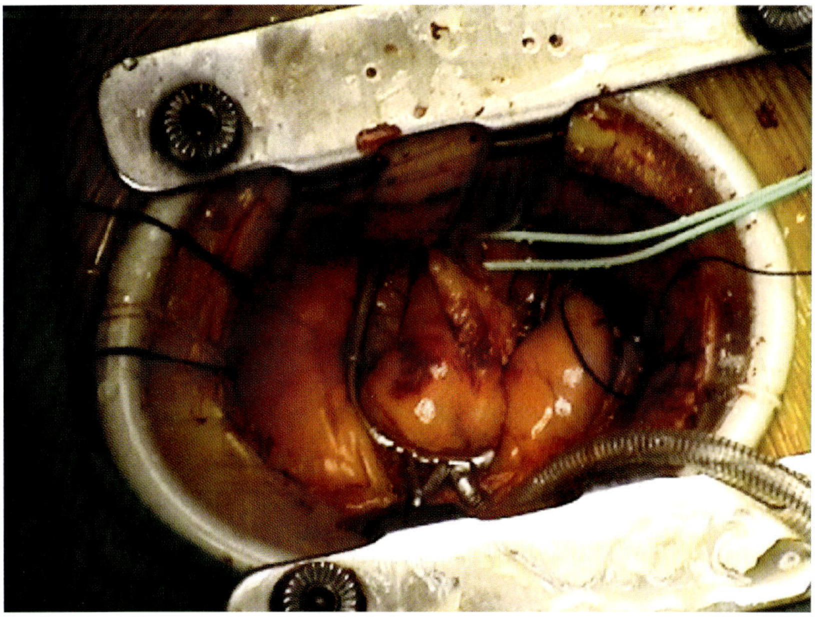

Figure 15. Completed LIMA to LAD anastomosis. The coronary artery can be seen between the skis of the stabilization device. A vessel loop occluder is placed temporarily to facilitate insertion of the intracoronary shunt.

are used for re-approximation of the ribs, and thoracotomy closure proceeds in several layers. Prior to final closure, a 5-mm laparoscopic camera is reinserted via the uppermost port site, CO_2 insufflation is reinstituted, and a general inspection of the left hemithorax is performed with emphasis on hemostasis and ensuring that the LIMA graft is not angulated or torsed. Finally, we leave it to the discretion of the anesthesiologist if extubation should be performed within the operating room. If this is not possible, a standard endotracheal tube is inserted before transfer to the ICU.

Postoperative Management

Usually, postoperative care is straightforward. In case of hemodynamic instability, we utilize radial arterial pressure waveform analysis to infer cardiac function and volume status information. Intravenous nitroglycerin is maintained until oral conversion is possible, and an antiplatelet regimen is instituted on postoperative day 1.

It has become our practice to institute patient-controlled analgesia (PCA) upon admission to the ICU, initially with delivery of a continuous dose until extubation. On postoperative day 1, chest tubes are removed and the PCA converted to oral analgesics.

Ideally, patients can be discharged on postoperative day 3 or 4, with antiplatelet therapy and oral nitrates continued for 3 months after operation. The patient is allowed to drive after 7 days, and lifting restrictions are minimal. Return to work is usually possible after 10 to 14 days.

To assess graft patency prior to discharge, CT angiography or cardiac catheterization may be performed. Numerous studies have reported excellent results using this approach. Angiographic confirmation of patency has been demonstrated to be in the range of 94% to 98% in both immediate and long-term follow-up, making robotic MIDCAB comparable to standard surgical revascularization techniques. Our data in patients tested postoperatively demonstrate a graft compromise rate of 2.8%.

Outcomes and Postoperative Complications

Despite advances in percutaneous and medical therapies, surgical revascularization will remain a mainstay in the management of coronary artery disease. Most revascularization to date is being performed on the arrested heart with cardiopulmonary bypass. Although conventional strategies are performed with very acceptable morbidity and mortality rates, an inherent complication rate associated with sternotomy, extracorporeal support, aortic manipulation, and cross-clamping remains. OPCAB avoids the potentially deleterious effects of the heart-lung machine, and MIDCAB obviates the need for sternotomy. Randomized controlled trials have shown a significant decrease in transfusion requirements, perioperative myocardial enzyme leak, and length of hospital stay (LOS) in the off-pump cohort.

Table 1. Characteristics of Conventional CAB and MIDCAB Patients at SJMHS

Patient Characteristics	Conventional CAB	da Vinci
Female gender	22.8%	23.4%
Elective operation	32.9%	67.3%
Reoperation	3.6%	4.7%
MI (1–7 days prior to operation)	21.7%	7.5%
MI (8–21 days prior to operation)	22.8%	6.5%
Preoperative IABP	4.2%	0.9%

Abbreviations: SJMHS, Saint Joseph Mercy Health System; MI, myocardial infarction; IABP, intra-aortic balloon pump.

Table 2. Thirty-Day Mortality after da Vinci MIDCAB

Parameter	STS 2011	SJMHS	O/E Ratio
Mortality	1.5%	0.9%	0.6

Abbreviations: STS, Society of Thoracic Surgeons; SJMHS, Saint Joseph Mercy Health System; O/E, observed/expected.

Additionally, several retrospective trials have shown an overall decrease in morbidity and mortality in the OPCAB group.[39] In-hospital mortality for MIDCAB has been reported to be less than 1%, compared to 1.4% for single-vessel OPCAB[40] and 2.4% from the STS.[41] Patient demographics for our conventional CAB and MIDCAB patients are shown in Table 1.

Mortality. Our all-cause 30-day robotic mortality between 2007 and 2011 was 0.93%. This compares favorably to the STS risk-stratified predicted rate of 1.52%, with an observed/expected (O/E) ratio of 0.6 (Table 2). Interestingly, our sole mortality occurred on postoperative day 4 in a patient who was turned down by two centers for conventional surgery, and postmortem analysis demonstrated a non-cardiac cause of death. Table 3 shows general postoperative complications after robotic MIDCAB at our institutions, compared to STS data.

Cerebrovascular Accident (CVA). Cardiopulmonary bypass is associated with adverse neurologic events.[42,43] There is growing evidence that neurocognitive outcome is superior in OPCAB patients, particularly in the MIDCAB subset, in which there is no manipulation of the aorta. However, within the OPCAB group, partial clamping of the aorta remains an independent predictor of CVA, and some advocate a no-touch technique.[44] The cost of CVA is high, both in terms of hospital costs, in-hospital morbidity, and longer LOS; Roach et al. noted a 21% mortality rate for patients suffering a stroke following conventional CAB and a 25-day average LOS.[43]

Risk factors for cerebrovascular injury during conventional CAB include previous CVA, smoking, diabetes, arteriosclerosis of ascending aorta, hypertension,

Table 3. Complications after Robotic MIDCAB

Complication	STS 2011	SJMHS	O/E Ratio
Reoperation for bleeding	1.8%	0.9%	0.5
Renal failure	3.8%	4.7%	1.2
Postoperative stroke	1.2%	0.0%	0.0
Atrial fibrillation	23.1%	24.0%	1.0
Wound infection	0.2%	0.0%	0.0
Prolonged ventilation	10.4%	1.9%	0.2

Abbreviations: STS, Society of Thoracic Surgeons; SJMHS, Saint Joseph Mercy Health System; O/E, observed/expected.

prolonged CPB time and low-output state, postoperative atrial fibrillation, and left main disease.

Documented preoperative carotid artery stenosis was found to be a risk factor by some authors and discounted by others. The vast majority of strokes with conventional bypass are embolic in nature; plaque rupture, local intimal damage, and thrombosis related to changes in the coagulation cascade during surgery all contribute to neurologic injury with cardiopulmonary bypass and aortic manipulation. Other sources of emboli are the carotid arteries, particles from cardiotomy suction, and left atrial thrombi. Additionally, a generalized neuropsychological decline with provocative testing has been documented in some patients after cardiopulmonary bypass, with air emboli from the bypass circuit being a suggested etiology.

MIDCAB is performed on the beating heart and requires no manipulation of the aorta. Its minimally invasive nature with minimal insult to the circulation intuitively should result in fewer neurocognitive injuries. In fact, in our series, we have yet to document a CVA in patients undergoing MIDCAB (Table 3).

Renal Complications. The etiology of renal injury during standard surgical revascularization is multifactorial and includes microembolic loads to the renal vasculature, inadequate or nonpulsatile renal perfusion, increased venous pressures with resultant tissue edema, and a generalized inflammatory response.

Risk factors for postoperative renal dysfunction include increasing age, previous renal injury, low cardiac output, inotropic/vasoconstrictor support, complexity of the operation, and bleeding and blood transfusions.

Hemodilution can attenuate some of the adverse physiologic events associated with extracorporeal support, and improved renal cortical blood flow, decreased cytotoxicity from hemoglobin associated proteinuria, and increased glomerular filtration rates can be seen. Although the overall number of patients requiring hemodialysis after standard CAB surgery is relatively low (1% to 5%), this remains a significant cause of morbidity following revascularization.

The effects of OPCAB on renal outcomes are somewhat variable throughout the literature, with some authors claiming that OPCAB may actually provide better renal protection than conventional on-pump techniques, particularly in patients with preoperative renal dysfunction.[45] Other studies demonstrated similar rates of renal injury in both cohorts.[46]

The STS defined renal failure as a twofold increase of serum creatinine, or an absolute creatinine above 2.0 mg/dL until 2009; the current definition of postoperative renal failure is a threefold increase or an absolute value greater than 4.0 mg/dL. Our initial rates of renal failure using STS database criteria are slightly higher than predicted, although only one patient required postoperative dialysis (Table 3). This patient had severe renal insufficiency prior to surgery and had been turned down by two programs for standard CAB for insufficient renal reserve. It is our practice to be aggressive in avoiding hypotension and minimizing vasopressors intraoperatively, maintaining an adequate hematocrit level and avoiding contrast-induced nephropathy by delaying surgery for at least 24 hours after catheterization. Trends in renal failure rates have been very positive in our series since these changes have been implemented.

Reoperation for Bleeding. It is not unexpected that a patient being admitted to the ICU after conventional CAB surgery has some degree of coagulopathy, and hypothermia can exacerbate this problem. Nevertheless, only a minority of patients will return to the operating room for mediastinal exploration. The latter should be considered for bleeding greater than 350 mL to 400 mL in the first two to three hours, or for bleeding greater than 200 mL per hour subsequent to that. Adequate heparin reversal, blood product administration to counteract thrombocytopenia and depletion of clotting factors, and restoration of normothermia must be established before a decision to reexplore is made.

By definition, MIDCAB obviates the need for bypass with its inherent alterations in the clotting profile, and subsequently one should have a much lower threshold for reexploration in this setting. Additionally, heparin dosing intraoperatively is a fraction of that needed for on-pump procedures, and heparin rebound is much less likely. If a patient has normal coagulation studies, ACT, and platelet count after MIDCAB, we consider a second look if the chest tube output is greater than 200 mL in the first hour after admission to the ICU. Potential areas of bleeding include port sites, anterior thoracotomy incision, internal mammary bed, the clipped distal end of the LIMA, and pulmonary parenchyma from adhesion takedown or direct lung injury.

We routinely reinsufflate the chest and reinspect these sites after thoracotomy closure and heparin reversal. As described previously, this is performed with a 5-mm camera through the most superior port site prior to leaving the operating room. Reexploration rates for bleeding in our MIDCAB group have been less than expected based on STS criteria (Table 3).

Blood Transfusion. Historically, the rate of perioperative blood transfusions in open heart surgery was as high as 50% to 70%. High rates of blood transfusions are likely multifactorial, and the contact of blood components with the artificial cardiopulmonary bypass circuit results in multiple changes to blood elements. Altered platelet function, activation of the clotting cascade, red cell hemolysis, clotting

Table 4. Blood Transfusions after MIDCAB

Parameter	STS 2011	SJMHS	O/E Ratio
Intraoperative blood use	34.8%	4.7%	0.1
Postoperative blood use	40.3%	8.4%	0.2

Abbreviations: STS, Society of Thoracic Surgeons; SJMHS, Saint Joseph Mercy Health System; O/E, observed/expected.

factor dilution, and excessive fibrinolysis all contribute to the coagulopathy associated with bypass surgery and extracorporeal support. These factors, exacerbated by hypothermia and the administration of high dose heparin, make some degree of bleeding inevitable after conventional CAB surgery.

Although intraoperative hemodilution can be protective, low hematocrit levels immediately following surgery can have undesirable rheologic effects necessitating transfusions. Blood transfusions can be both beneficial and harmful. The latter include immunomodulation, increased risk of infection, and transfusion-related acute lung injury (TRALI). Murphy et al. have delineated the adverse outcomes associated with transfusions and have not only shown an increase in infection rate, but also higher mortality, morbidity, LOS, and implicit hospital costs in transfused patients.[47] Although restrictive transfusion strategies have become more widespread, transfusion rates following on-pump surgical revascularization remain high.

Almost universally, transfusion rates following OPCAB are dramatically lower than after conventional CAB surgery. Compared to STS benchmarks, our MIDCAB transfusion rate was 8.4%, compared to a predicted 40.3% (Table 4).

Prolonged Ventilation. Postoperative pulmonary complications are the most frequent and significant contributor to morbidity, mortality, and costs associated with hospitalization after CAB operations. A path to early extubation is paramount in minimizing LOS, and arguably one of the most salient benefits of beating heart surgery is maintained pulmonary function.

Risk factors for pulmonary complications include:

- Advanced age
- Current smoker
- Chronic obstructive pulmonary disease (COPD) diagnosis
- Pleural effusions
- Abdominal distension
- Poor cardiac function

Lung changes associated with CPB may include:

- Increased microvascular permeability
- Increased pulmonary vascular resistance
- Increased shunt fraction
- Decreased vital capacity and FRC
- Decreased lung compliance

Table 5. Postoperative Length of Hospital Stay

Length of Stay (Days)	STS 2011	SJMHS
Mean	6.8	6.5
Median	6.0	5.0
Mode	N/A	4.0

Abbreviations: STS, Society of Thoracic Surgeons; SJMHS, Saint Joseph Mercy Health System.

The range of pulmonary dysfunction after cardiopulmonary bypass ranges from almost universal transient hypoxia to full-blown acute respiratory distress syndrome (ARDS), which is seen in 0.4% to 2% of patients. In a large cohort study, the use of CPB was an independent risk factor for postoperative intubation beyond 48 hours.[48] In addition, sternotomy produces significant pain, resulting in splinting and functional reduction of lung volumes.

In our experience, the avoidance of sternotomy and CPB in MIDCAB procedures has led to a significant decrease in the rate of prolonged ventilation (Table 3). Early in our series, most patients with reasonable cardiac and pulmonary reserve were extubated in the operating suite. However, initial reintubation rates secondary to inadequate analgesia approached 6%, which we deemed unacceptable. Subsequently, we have modified our algorithm such that a PCA is initiated upon admission to the ICU, and extubation is performed within 2 to 6 hours following operation if possible. Using this approach, we can manage any hemodynamic changes associated with the PCA early, while the patient remains intubated. It is rare to have a MIDCAB patient intubated beyond 6 hours.

Early extubation and transfer from the ICU have resulted in a shorter overall LOS compared to national averages (Table 5). Multiple patients turned down for standard revascularization underwent MIDCAB, and these outliers were included in our mean LOS. It can be seen, however, that the LOS mode was 2.5 days lower than this. Ventilator-associated pneumonia was virtually nonexistent.

Atrial Fibrillation. The incidence of postoperative atrial fibrillation in CAB patients ranges from 20% to 40%. Correlative risk factors include age older than 75 and the presence of COPD. It is unclear whether patients who develop postoperative atrial fibrillation have a predisposition toward this complication, or whether the inflammatory responses associated with CPB and pericardiotomy are likely culprits. Quite possibly it is a combination of both factors. The cost of postoperative atrial fibrillation can be high, including prolonged hospitalization, need for anticoagulation, and increased incidence of stroke. Fortunately, the majority of episodes are self-limited, lending credibility to the supposition that this complication is inflammation-mediated.

Interestingly, in our series, the risk of postoperative atrial fibrillation in MIDCAB patients was not lower than predicted by the STS model (Table 3), despite avoiding both sternotomy and CPB. In all cases, however, a pericardiotomy was performed, thus suggesting that a local inflammatory process secondary to irritation of the epicardium may be the culprit. Some authors have suggested a decreased incidence

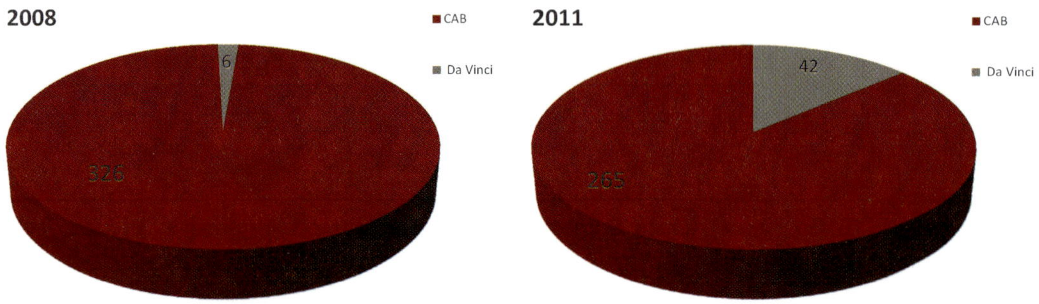

Figure 16. A comparison of conventional CAB and robotic MIDCAB at SJMHS in 2008 and 2011.

of atrial fibrillation in the OPCAB population,[49] although at our institution, rates have been identical for on-pump and OPCAB procedures.

Conclusion

Coronary artery bypass surgery with the use of CPB is the gold standard for surgical revascularization. However, even under ideal circumstances the perioperative mortality is up to 2%, and major adverse complications occur in 5% to 7% of patients. Any alternative strategy must compare with standard revascularization, and our results show that MIDCAB can be performed safely and effectively. Additionally, the potential to offer an arterial bypass to the anterior wall and septum to patients, who may otherwise have suboptimal alternatives, is appealing and satisfying.

At our institution, the frequency of robotic MIDCAB as a revascularization strategy has increased significantly since 2008 (Figure 16) and has proven to be an effective adjunct in the treatment of coronary artery disease.

References

1. Nabel EG, Braunwald E. A tale of coronary artery disease and myocardial infarction. *N Eng J Med*. 2012;366:54–63.

2. Roger VL, Go AS, Lloyd-Jones DM, et al. Heart disease and stroke statistics—2012 update: a report from the American Heart Association. *Circulation*. 2012;125:e2–e220.

3. Goetz RH, Rohman M, Haller JD, Dee R, Rosenak SS. Internal mammary-coronary artery anastomosis. A nonsuture method employing tantalum rings. *J Thorac Cardiovasc Surg*. 1961;41:378–86.

4. Favaloro RG. Saphenous vein autograft replacement of severe segmental coronary artery occlusion: operative technique. *Ann Thorac Surg*. 1968;5:334–9.

5. Greason KL, Schaff HV. Myocardial revascularization by coronary arterial bypass graft: past, present, and future. *Curr Prob Card*. 2011;36:325–68.

6. Stephenson L. *Cardiac Surgery in the Adult*. New York, NY: McGraw-Hill; 2008.

7. Puskas JD, Kilgo PD, Lattouf OM, et al. Off-pump coronary bypass provides reduced mortality and morbidity and equivalent 10-year survival. *Ann Thorac Surg.* 2008;86:1139–46; discussion 46.

8. Shroyer AL, Grover FL, Hattler B, et al. On-pump versus off-pump coronary-artery bypass surgery. *N Eng J Med.* 2009;361:1827–37.

9. Benetti FJ, Ballester C, Sani G, Doonstra P, Grandjean J. Video assisted coronary bypass surgery. *J Cardiac Surg.* 1995;10:620–5.

10. Reichenspurner H, Damiano RJ, Mack M, et al. Use of the voice-controlled and computer-assisted surgical system ZEUS for endoscopic coronary artery bypass grafting. *J Thorac Cardiovasc Surg.*1999;118:11–6.

11. Holzhey DM, Jacobs S, Walther T, Mochalski M, Mohr FW, Falk V. Cumulative sum failure analysis for eight surgeons performing minimally invasive direct coronary artery bypass. *J Thorac Cardiovasc Surg.* 2007;134:663–9.

12. Ben-Gal Y, Mohr R, Braunstein R, et al. Revascularization of left anterior descending artery with drug-eluting stents: comparison with minimally invasive direct coronary artery bypass surgery. *Ann Thorac Surg.* 2006;82:2067–71.

13. Cho KR, Kim JS, Choi JS, Kim KB. Serial angiographic follow-up of grafts one year and five years after coronary artery bypass surgery. *Eur J Cardio-Thorac.* 2006;29:511–6.

14. Tatoulis J, Buxton BF, Fuller JA. Patencies of 2127 arterial to coronary conduits over 15 years. *Ann Thorac Surg.* 2004;77:93–101.

15. Desai ND, Cohen EA, Naylor CD, Fremes SE. A randomized comparison of radial-artery and saphenous-vein coronary bypass grafts. *N Eng J Med.* 2004;351:2302–9.

16. Collins P, Webb CM, Chong CF, Moat NE. Radial artery versus saphenous vein patency randomized trial: five-year angiographic follow-up. *Circulation.* 2008;117:2859–64.

17. Achouh P, Isselmou KO, Boutekadjirt R, et al. Reappraisal of a 20-year experience with the radial artery as a conduit for coronary bypass grafting. *Eur J Cardio-Thorac.* 2012;41:87–92.

18. Hayward PA, Buxton BF. Contemporary coronary graft patency: 5-year observational data from a randomized trial of conduits. *Ann Thorac Surg.* 2007;84:795–9.

19. Grüntzig A. Transluminal dilatation of coronary-artery stenosis. *Lancet.* 1978;1:263.

20. Serruys PW, Unger F, Sousa JE, et al. Comparison of coronary-artery bypass surgery and stenting for the treatment of multivessel disease. *N Eng J Med.* 2001;344:1117–24.

21. SoS Investigators. Coronary artery bypass surgery versus percutaneous coronary intervention with stent implantation in patients with multivessel coronary artery disease (the Stent or Surgery trial): a randomised controlled trial. *Lancet.* 2002;360:965–70.

22. Hannan EL, Racz MJ, Walford G, et al. Long-term outcomes of coronary-artery bypass grafting versus stent implantation. *N Eng J Med.* 2005;352:2174–83.

23. Sousa JE, Costa MA, Abizaid AC, et al. Sustained suppression of neointimal proliferation by sirolimus-eluting stents: one-year angiographic and intravascular ultrasound follow-up. *Circulation.* 2001;104:2007–11.

24. Moses JW, Leon MB, Popma JJ, et al. Sirolimus-eluting stents versus standard stents in patients with stenosis in a native coronary artery. *N Eng J Med.* 2003;349:1315–23.

25. Serruys PW, Morice MC, Kappetein AP, et al. Percutaneous coronary intervention versus coronary-artery bypass grafting for severe coronary artery disease. *N Eng J Med.* 2009;360:961–72.

26. Levine GN, Bates ER, Blankenship JC, et al. 2011 ACCF/AHA/SCAI Guideline for Percutaneous Coronary Intervention: A report of the American College of Cardiology Foundation/American Heart Association task force on Practice Guidelines and the Society for Cardiovascular Angiography and Interventions. *J Am Coll Cardio.* 2011;58:e44–122.

27. Cohen DJ, Van Hout B, Serruys PW, et al. Quality of life after PCI with drug-eluting stents or coronary-artery bypass surgery. *N Eng J Med.* 2011;364:1016–26.

28. Park SJ, Kim YH, Park DW, et al. Randomized trial of stents versus bypass surgery for left main coronary artery disease. *N Eng J Med.* 2011;364:1718–27.

29. Hannan EL, Wu C, Walford G, et al. Drug-eluting stents vs. coronary-artery bypass grafting in multivessel coronary disease. *N Eng J Med.* 2008;358:331–41.

30. Shahian DM, O'Brien SM, Sheng S, et al. Predictors of long-term survival following coronary artery bypass grafting surgery: results from the Society of Thoracic Surgeons Adult Cardiac Surgery Database (The ASCERT Study). *Circulation.* 2012.

31. Wachter K. CABG Tops stents in high-risk patients. *ACS Surgery News.* 2012 March 2012;Sect. 20.

32. Kapoor JR, Gienger AL, Ardehali R, et al. Isolated disease of the proximal left anterior descending artery comparing the effectiveness of percutaneous coronary interventions and coronary artery bypass surgery. *J Am Coll Cardiol.* 2008;1:483–91.

33. Falk V, Jacobs S, Gummert J, Walther T. Robotic coronary artery bypass grafting (CABG)–the Leipzig experience. *Surg Clin North Am.* 2003;83:1381–6, ix.

34. Shennib H, Bastawisy A, McLoughlin J, Moll F. Robotic computer-assisted telemanipulation enhances coronary artery bypass. *J Thorac Cardiovasc Surg.* 1999;117:310–3.

35. Stahl KD, Boyd WD, Vassiliades TA, Karamanoukian HL. Hybrid robotic coronary artery surgery and angioplasty in multivessel coronary artery disease. *Ann Thorac Surg.* 2002;74:S1358–62.

36. Byrne JG, Leacche M, Vaughan DE, Zhao DX. Hybrid cardiovascular procedures. *JACC Cardiovasc Interv.* 2008;1:459–68.

37. Jaik NP, Umakanthan R, Leacche M, et al. Current status of hybrid coronary revascularization. *Expert Rev Cardiovasc Therapy.* 2011;9:1331–7.

38. Umakanthan R, Leacche M, Zhao DX, Gallion AH, Mishra PC, Byrne JG. Hybrid options for treating cardiac disease. *Semin Thorac Cardiovasc Surg.* 2011;23:274–80.

39. Magee MJ, Coombs LP, Peterson ED, Mack MJ. Patient selection and current practice strategy for off-pump coronary artery bypass surgery. *Circulation.* 2003;108 Suppl 1:II9–14.

40. Gummert JF, Funkat A, Krian A. Cardiac surgery in Germany during 2004: a report on behalf of the German Society for Thoracic and Cardiovascular Surgery. *Thorac Cardiovasc Surg.* 2005;53:391–9.

41. de Canniere D, Wimmer-Greinecker G, Cichon R, et al. Feasibility, safety, and efficacy of totally endoscopic coronary artery bypass grafting: multicenter European experience. *J Thorac Cardiovasc Surg.* 2007;134:710–6.

42. Patel NC, Deodhar AP, Grayson AD, et al. Neurological outcomes in coronary surgery: independent effect of avoiding cardiopulmonary bypass. *Ann Thorac Surg.* 2002;74:400-5; discussion 5–6.

43. Roach GW, Kanchuger M, Mangano CM, et al. Adverse cerebral outcomes after coronary bypass surgery. Multicenter Study of Perioperative Ischemia Research Group and the Ischemia Research and Education Foundation Investigators. *N Eng J Med.* 1996;335:1857–63.

44. Lev-Ran O, Braunstein R, Sharony R, et al. No-touch aorta off-pump coronary surgery: the effect on stroke. *J Thorac Cardiovasc Surg.* 2005;129:307–13.

45. Ooi JS, Abdul Rahman MR, Shah SA, Dimon MZ. Renal outcome following on- and off-pump coronary artery bypass graft surgery. *Asian Cardiovasc Thorac Ann.* 2008;16:468–72.

46. Di Mauro M, Gagliardi M, Iaco AL, et al. Does off-pump coronary surgery reduce postoperative acute renal failure? The importance of preoperative renal function. *Ann Thorac Surg*. 2007;84:1496–502.
47. Murphy GJ, Reeves BC, Rogers CA, Rizvi SI, Culliford L, Angelini GD. Increased mortality, postoperative morbidity, and cost after red blood cell transfusion in patients having cardiac surgery. *Circulation*. 2007;116:2544–52.
48. Reddy SL, Grayson AD, Griffiths EM, Pullan DM, Rashid A. Logistic risk model for prolonged ventilation after adult cardiac surgery. *Ann Thorac Surg*. 2007;84:528–36.
49. Athanasiou T, Aziz O, Mangoush O, et al. Do off-pump techniques reduce the incidence of postoperative atrial fibrillation in elderly patients undergoing coronary artery bypass grafting? *Ann Thorac Surg*. 2004;77:1567–74.

Chapter Four

Mitral Valve

Bobby K. Kong, MD; M. LaWaun Hance, PA-C;
Nicolas J. Mouawad, MD, MPH, MBA; Manak S. Sood, MD

History

In 1902, Sir Thomas Lauder Brunton of London first proposed treating the stenotic mitral valve surgically,[1] but it wasn't until May 20, 1923, that Dr. Elliott Cutler of Boston performed the first successful mitral valve operation. Using a tenotomy knife inserted through the left ventricular apex, he successfully performed a closed mitral valve commissurotomy on the beating heart of a 12-year-old patient dying from mitral stenosis. His patient lived for another 4.5 years before succumbing to her valvular disease.

The next era of mitral surgery began with the diligent efforts of Dr. Dwight Harken,[2] also of Boston, and Dr. Charles P. Bailey from Philadelphia, some 20 years later. Within 4 days of each other, they performed successful commissurotomies for mitral stenosis. Dr. Bailey, a charismatic salesman for ladies' girdles during his collegiate years, reported 810 cases of closed operations with a surprisingly low mortality rate of 8%. And thus, in an age where rheumatic disease was an epidemic, surgical mitral valve repair became a reality.

Paradoxically, the most common pathology amenable to reparative efforts currently is mitral insufficiency rather than stenosis. Although it can still be seen endemically in developing countries, the incidence of rheumatic fever has decreased significantly over recent decades with the discovery of antibiotics targeting the causative pathogen, group A *streptococcus.*

Dr. J. C. Davila proposed treating the insufficient valve with a "circumferential suture" in the 1950s. More sophisticated and reproducible techniques were subsequently championed over the next three decades, by pioneers such as Dr. D. C. McGoon of the Mayo Clinic, Dr. Carlo M. G. Duran from Spain, and most prominently Dr. Alain Carpentier of Paris.[3] In fact, Carpentier developed the first functional classification of mitral pathology, with type I being normal leaflets motion, type II involving excess leaflets motion, and type III describing the restricted leaflet motion.[3] This classification system has not only provided a common language for clinicians treating the mitral valve, but has also clarified the form and function of the mitral apparatus to guide therapy (Figure 1).

With regards to pathophysiology, anatomic and physiologic restoration of the mitral apparatus in the insufficient valve helps improve the volume overload and dilatation characteristic of this valvular cardiomyopathy.[4] In contrast, relief of mitral

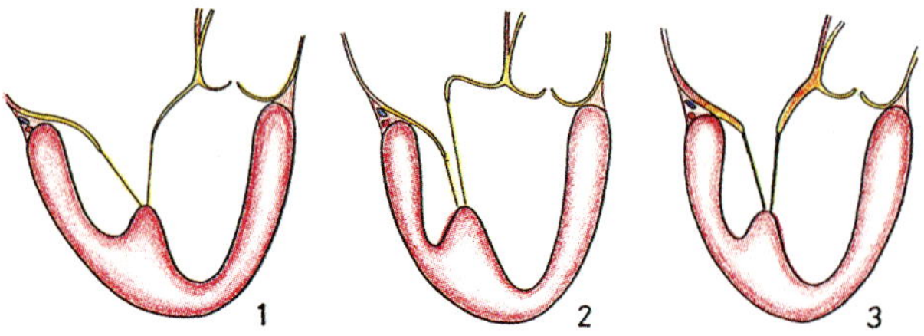

Figure 1. Carpentier's classification of mitral valve regurgitation according to leaflet motion. 1 = Normal. 2 = Excessive. 3 = Restricted. Credit: © 1989 Verlag R.S. Schulz.

stenosis corrects pulmonary venous outflow obstruction and resultant pulmonary hypertension. Both remedies not only prolong life, but also ameliorate the symptoms of congestive heart failure.

Prosthetic valves were introduced in 1952. The first ideation was a ball-cage valve that used a metal cage to house a moving silicone ball, analogous to a valve in a snorkel apparatus. Dr. Nina Braunwald is credited with performing the first successful mitral valve replacement in 1959.

Most current mechanical prostheses are based on a bi-leaflet tilting-disc design. Current valves have lifetime durability and acceptable rates of thrombotic and embolic complications, as long as the patient remains adequately anticoagulated; all mechanical valves require lifelong systemic anticoagulation to prevent thromboembolism. Warfarin is the mainstay of treatment in this regard. Its main downfall is the risk of associated significant bleeding complications that occur at a rate of 2–4% per patient year. This risk increases in the elderly population and is prohibitive in patients who are poorly compliant with medications, have an unsteady gait, or have a history of bleeding.

The first porcine valve, which has limited durability but obviates the need for anticoagulation, was available for implantation in 1969. The early enthusiasm for valve replacement likely delayed development strategies for valvular repair as they exist today. Numerous third-generation bovine pericardial and porcine bioprosthetic valves now exist, with an average durability of twelve years (shorter in younger patients and those on dialysis). These valves do not require systemic anticoagulation.

It must be remembered, however, that all artificial valves are considered "foreign objects" and are prone to infection, which, when present, is typically resistant to antibiotic therapy; an infected prosthetic valve usually mandates reoperation and replacement. Surgery in these patients is usually a formidable task and carries significant mortality and morbidity. In some regards, valve replacement substitutes one set of problems for another. Despite diligent efforts, the ideal artificial valve that is resistant to infection, is nonthrombogenic, and confers lifetime durability remains elusive.

The merits of mitral valve repair when compared to replacement become obvious with long-term follow-up. When native tissue is trimmed, folded, detached, and sutured to approach the form and function of a healthy valve, limited foreign material is introduced. Hence the thromboembolic and infectious potential approaches that of native tissue. In terms of durability, Dr. Alain Carpentier's pioneering work has shown a failure rate of only 1% with a 20-year follow-up when degenerative mitral valve is repaired. The Society of Thoracic Surgeons' (STS) database has also demonstrated a lower operative risk for repair (1.2%) compared to replacement (5.5%).

It is apparent that the paradigm regarding disease of the mitral valve is changing. Generally speaking, mitral valve repair is preferred over replacement whenever possible. While only half of repairable mitral valve tissue is repaired in the United States, tertiary hospitals report repair rates over 90%. This must be the gold standard for which any mitral valve surgeons strive.

Functional Anatomy

The mitral valve is the two-leaflet atrioventricular valve located at the junction between the left atrium and ventricle. The leaflets are described anatomically: the anterior leaflet is the larger of the two, is half-moon in shape, and its height and intertrigonal distance are used as reference for sizing an annular ring during repair. The posterior leaflet has less surface area and is more crescent-shaped. It has three scallops that have been classified by Dr. Carpentier as P1, P2, and P3. The scallops are located laterally, in the center, and medially, respectively. The anterior leaflet traverses approximately one-third of the annular circumference, whereas the posterior leaflet occupies the remaining two-thirds (Figure 2).

Functionally, the opening of the anterior leaflet provides the main orifice for blood flow. The leaflets are separated by two commissures—anterolateral and posteromedial. The anterior leaflet is supported by an average of 9 (range 5–13) primary chords along the free edge, while the posterior leaflet will typically have 14 chordae. These structures are analogous to the strings of a parachute and allow for ballooning of the leaflets so they can rise to the level of the mitral annulus during ventricular contraction. The chordae are then connected to papillary muscles arising from the ventricular wall. As a result, there is direct transmission of force between the ventricle and mitral leaflets.

With elongation or rupture, the leaflets will prolapse, resulting in poor apposition at the level of the annulus. This, in turn, will result in the leakage of blood into the left atrium. Eventually, this will impair pulmonary venous drainage, resulting in pulmonary hypertension. This pathophysiology can occur chronically or in the acute setting of a myocardial infarction involving the ventricular wall and papillary muscles.

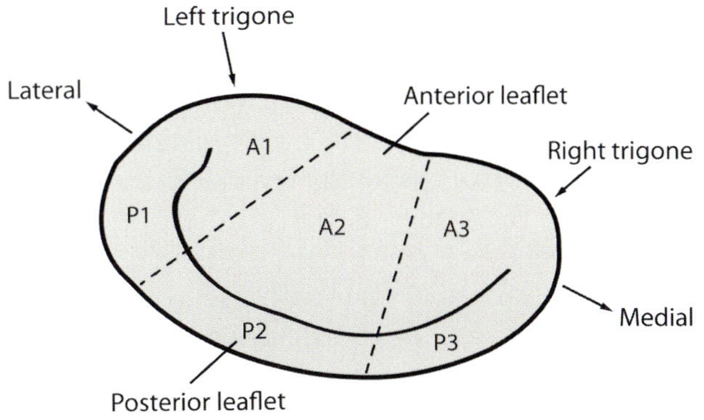

Figure 2. Nomenclature of the mitral valve leaflets as classified by Dr. Carpentier. © 2012 Spry Publishing.

Histologically, these structures have three layers. The

fibrosa is contiguous with the chordae tendineae, the *spongiosa* comprises the atrial surface, and a *fibroelastic layer* is prone to myxomatous changes that characterize the degenerative valve.

Conventional wisdom endorsed that leaflet movement was purely secondary to the hemodynamic changes in blood volume and mechanical ventricular contraction. It bears noting, interestingly, that leaflet tissue has contractile properties, is well innervated, and new data suggest that they may also be involved in moderating the appropriate valve closure.

The mitral annulus is a dynamic fibrous and muscular structure and is considered the "ring" that seats the mitral leaflets (Figure 2). Normally the annulus is kidney shaped, but can become distorted with ventricular dilatation resulting in poor leaflet coaptation. This structure moves in to the left atrium in diastole and toward the ventricular apex in systole.

Collagen-rich trigones serve as anchors for the anterior leaflet, which spans the distance between commissures supported by a relatively rigid fibrous band. The right fibrous trigone, or central fibrous body, is in direct continuity with the fibrous composition of the heart, which includes the aortic valve, the membranous septum, and the tricuspid valve. In fact, the annular segment supporting the anterior mitral leaflet extends in continuity with the left and noncoronary aortic valve leaflets. The left trigone is separated from the right by the intertrigonal space, which, in essence, defines the fibrous or anterior component of the mitral annulus. Classically, this is used as a measurement for valve sizing during replacement, although the septoposterior anterior leaflet dimension defines annular ring size during repair. In the setting of a dilated cardiomyopathy, the intertrigonal distance is less prone to enlargement than the posterior annulus.

The posterior two-thirds of the annulus are relatively devoid of fibrous tissue, and its muscular composition renders it pliable and amenable to annuloplasty repair. The posterior annulus conforms to the hemodynamic changes around the valve during the cardiac cycle. The mitral valve area ranges between 4 and 6 cm^2, and the usual annular diameter ranges between 5 and 11 cm^2, preserving a 3:4 ratio of the anterior-posterior to the commissural distance. Hemodynamic changes during the cardiac cycle will modify the configuration of the annulus by up to 40%, with the greatest size during late diastole and early systole (Figure 3).[7]

The chordae tendineae span the distance between the papillary heads and the leaflets themselves. These parachute-like structures prevent leaflet prolapse in systole (Figure 4). First-order chordae originate near the tips of the papillary muscles and insert on the leading edge of the leaflets; their function is to prevent prolapse of the respective leaflet tips. Second-order chordae originate in a similar manner. However, they insert a little further back on the leaflet, either on the rough zone or at the transition between the rough and membranous portions near the zone of coaptation. The secondary chordae stabilize the valve further, preserve the continuity between the valve and the ventricle, and augment ventricular performance in systole. Third-order chordae serve as scaffolding for nutrient vessels and originate from ventricular wall trabeculae. They typically insert at the base of the leaflets near the annular ring.

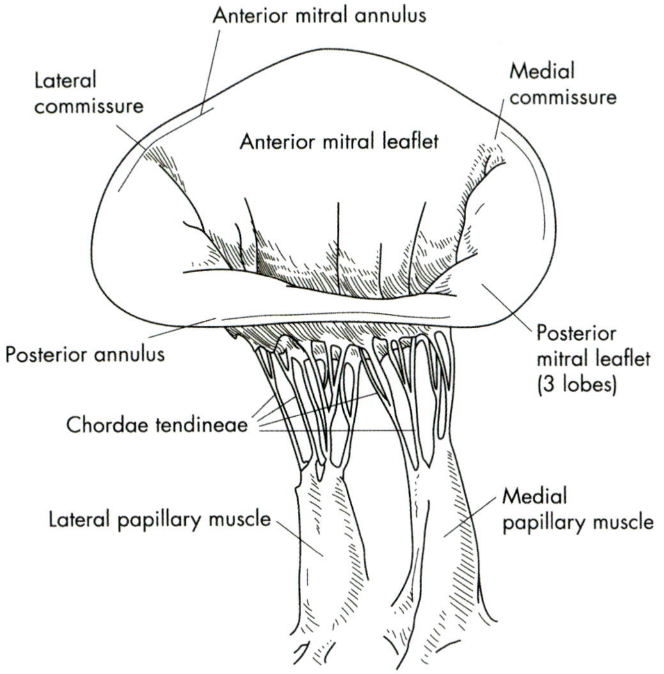

Figure 3. Vertically oriented myocardial fibers originating in the apex form two distinct muscular bands designated the anteromedial and posterolateral papillary muscles that, in turn, provide chordae tendineae to support both leaflets. The former is much larger and generally has one major head, whereas the latter may have multiple heads. Adapted from Otto: Valvular Heart Disease, Saunders 1999.

The left anterior descending artery and circumflex vessels supply the anterolateral papillary muscle, whereas its posteromedial counterpart derives its circulation from the posterior descending artery, which is typically off the right circulation in right dominant individuals. As expected, ischemia in the distribution of these feeding vessels can lead to papillary muscle dysfunction and mitral insufficiency in the acute setting.

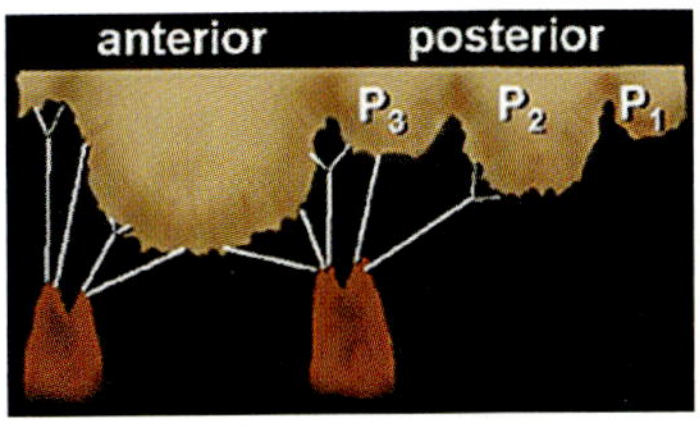

Figure 4. The mitral annulus is opened and viewed posteriorly. Note the three scallops of the posterior leaflet. Credit: Echo in Context Conference, Mitral Valve Anatomy.

Pathophysiology and Diagnosis

Mitral Stenosis

Causes

Mitral valve stenosis is most commonly a result of rheumatic fever, and although its incidence is increasingly rare in the Western hemisphere, it continues to be a common problem in developing countries. The peak incidence of rheumatic fever occurs between 5 and 15 years of age, and pharyngeal infection with

Lancefield group A β-hemolytic streptococci triggers the infectious process with a 2–4 week incubation period. Approximately 2% of the exposed population is susceptible to the more serious sequelae associated with this pathogen. With regard to valvular pathology, it is thought that an antibody-mediated cross-reactivity with valve tissue leads to the alteration in tissue mechanics with the mitral, aortic, tricuspid, and pulmonary valves being affected 70%, 40%, 10%, and 2% of the time, respectively.

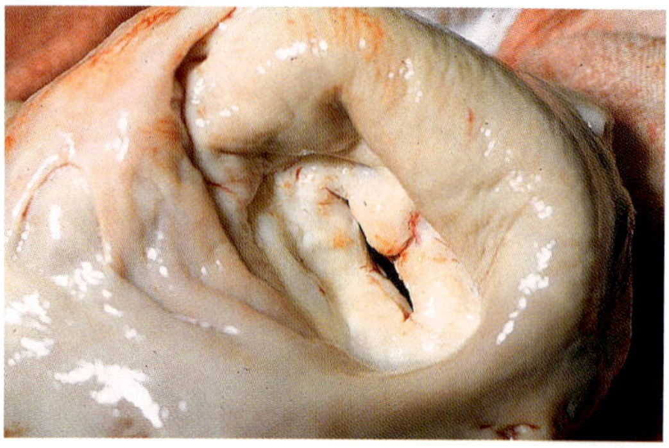

Figure 5. The main hemodynamic abnormality in mitral stenosis is related to elevated transvalvular gradients during diastole between the left atrium and ventricle. Significant stenosis exists if the valve orifice is < 1 cm^2/m^2 body surface area.

The initial pathology is one of valvular incompetence with stenosis developing years later. The classic findings are of chordal fusion and shortening, commissural fusion, and leaflet fibrosis. Other, less common causes of mitral stenosis include congenital abnormalities, mucopolysaccharidoses, endocardial fibroelastosis, malignant carcinoid, prolapsing left atrial myxoma, and iatrogenic disease resulting from improper placement of an undersized prosthetic valve (Figure 5).

Presentation and Diagnosis

Symptoms are generally insidious in onset, as mild to moderate stenosis is generally well compensated, although it may become manifest during periods of increased cardiac activity and exercise. Long-standing mitral stenosis will cause enlargement of the left atrium and increased left atrial pressures. More predictable symptoms develop when a low-output state or pulmonary hypertension has developed. With chronicity, irreversible severe pulmonary hypertension can be a preterminal finding.

Symptoms include dyspnea on exertion, fatigue, palpitations, cough, recurrent pulmonary infection, hemoptysis, and chest discomfort. Dilatation of the left atrium from a noncompliant valve predisposes to the development of atrial fibrillation. Slow flow of blood within this chamber and its appendage results in stasis and formation of intracardiac thrombus; cardioembolic complications are the mode of presentation for up to 20% of patients with mitral stenosis. It should also be noted that the enlarged left atrium might actually cause mechanical compression of nearby structures, possibly presenting as hoarseness (recurrent laryngeal nerve), dysphagia (esophagus), and bronchial obstruction (Figure 6). Although uncommon, pulmonary venous congestion from long-standing stenosis can cause pulmonary varices with patients presenting with hemoptysis.

Long-standing elevation of pressures in the pulmonary bed (>60 mmHg) will be reflected on the right side of the heart, with subsequent right heart failure, tricus-

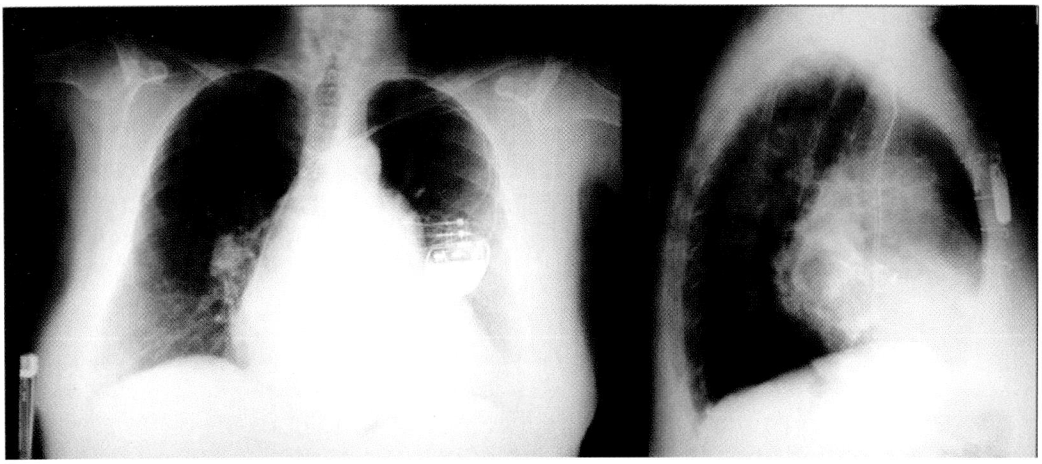

Figure 6. Radiographic findings suggestive of mitral stenosis include enlargement of the left atrium as manifest by a double contour of the right heart border and elevation of the left main stem bronchus. With advanced disease, plain films will show prominence of the pulmonary vasculature and pleural effusions.

pid regurgitation, hepatic and mesenteric venous congestion, ascites, and peripheral edema. Cardiac cachexia and generalized wasting are preterminal findings.

A physical exam can reveal the characteristic malar flush. A low volume pulse is generally palpated, and a tapping, undisplaced apex beat is felt. Additionally, one may appreciate a right ventricular heave along the left sternal border and a prominent presystolic murmur will be heard, with auscultation at the apex that correlates with closing of the mitral leaflets. Other auscultatory findings include a disproportionately loud S_1, an opening snap, and a rumbling mid-systolic murmur best heard during expiration with the patient lying on their left side. A pre-systolic murmur can be soft and easily missed. Signs and stigmata of right heart failure include ascites, liver enlargement, pedal edema, and a characteristic "butterfly" rash on both cheeks.

Echocardiography is the standard diagnostic modality for evaluation of the mitral valve. Transthoracic (surface) echo will provide information regarding anatomy, cross-sectional area, atrial and ventricular dimensions, and gradients across the mitral valve, seen best in parasternal long-axis views (Figure 7). Right-sided findings of tricuspid insufficiency, diminished ventricular contractility, and elevated estimated pulmonary pressures are consistent with mitral stenosis.

Given the posterior location of the mitral apparatus, transesophageal echocardiogram (TEE) is more accurate in documenting valvular pathology. Three-dimensional TEE further delineates the mitral valve morphology and is becoming the most valuable preoperative test for mitral valve repair (Figure 8).

Cardiac catheterization is not necessary for the diagnosis of mitral stenosis, but should be obtained if an operation is being considered in an effort to define coronary anatomy in patients older than forty years of age. Right-sided catheterization should also be performed to measure atrial, ventricular, and pulmonary pressures.

If severe pulmonary hypertension is documented, gauging reversibility after administration of vasoactive drugs such as adenosine and inhaled nitric oxide will provide insight regarding the patient's operative risk and long-term prognosis.

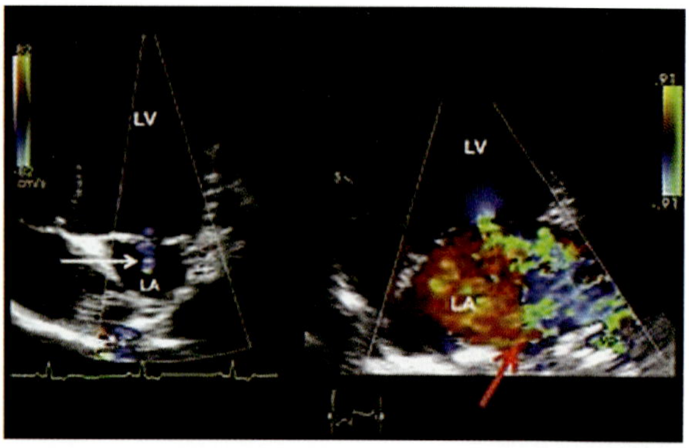

Figure 7. The parasternal long-axis view is best for viewing prolapsed segments, whereas the short axis provides excellent visualization of the papillary anatomy and subvalvular apparatus. Overall, TEE is more definitive in analysis of the mitral valve.

Mitral Insufficiency

Mitral insufficiency, also described pathophysiologically as mitral regurgitation, has a myriad of causes. The etiologies are best divided into four groups: degenerative or myxomatous, rheumatic, ischemic, and infectious.

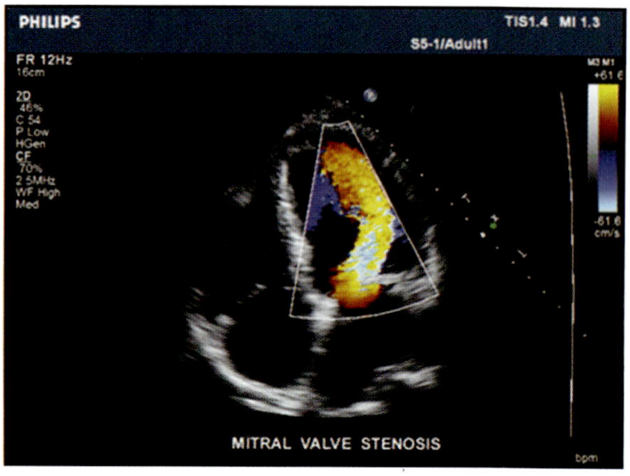

Figure 8. Three-dimensional TEE.

Causes

Degenerative. Degenerative mitral valve disease is, by far, the most common cause of mitral insufficiency, affecting more than 2 million people in the United States alone. This disease process is characterized by myxomatous degeneration involving the leaflets, chordae, and annulus. There is no genetic predisposition to this disease, although its etiology remains unclear.

Anatomic findings include chordal elongation and rupture, thickened and enlarged leaflets with excess tissue, and annular dilatation. Prolapse of the middle scallop (P2) of the posterior leaflet is the most common cause (60%) of myxomatous mitral regurgitation, although any anatomic or functional alteration of either leaflet can result in a leaky valve. Returning the diseased valve to normal anatomic and geometric ratios will restore competency of the valve.

Rheumatic. As noted previously, rheumatic heart disease, as qualified by the Jones' criteria, typically results in mitral stenosis. However, combined stenosis and insufficiency are possible in this setting. Although the sine qua non of rheumatic disease (leaflet fibrosis, calcification, and contracture) is invariably present, chordal shortening and commissural fusion can cause a restrictive valvular leak.

Ischemic Mitral Disease. Ischemic mitral disease can be subdivided temporally as acute and chronic. Acute mitral valve insufficiency is most often a result of papillary muscle dysfunction from occlusion of the nutrient coronary artery; the anterolateral papillary muscle derives its blood supply from the left anterior descending or circumflex systems, whereas the posteromedial muscle is right coronary dependent in 80–90% of patients.

Ischemia can cause direct papillary dysfunction or, alternatively, decrease contractility of the left ventricular free wall at its site of attachment. Infarction can result in scarring, elongation, and dyskinesia of the papillary muscle.

Frank rupture of the papillary head can be seen with an ischemic insult, resulting in untethering of supporting chordae originating at this site. This results in a flail segment and often torrential regurgitation in the acute setting, constituting a true surgical emergency, often necessitating expeditious replacement of the mitral valve in these critically ill patients, often with shock and pulmonary edema.

Chronic mitral insufficiency is characterized by long-term fibrotic changes and thinning of the papillary muscles and ventricular wall. Undesirable ventricular remodeling results in dilated cardiomyopathy and annular dilatation. Volume overload from insufficiency is a self-propagating phenomenon, and further dilatation perpetuates a downward spiral as chamber size increases and contractility declines.

Endocarditis. Like other valves of the heart, the mitral valve is not immune to systemic infection and sequelae such as endocarditis. A diseased valve with primary mitral pathology is fertile soil for infection. However, 30% of mitral endocarditis occurs in valves with no identifiable underlying pathology. Pathogens are typically streptococcal and staphylococcal species, and resultant valvular destruction is characterized by leaflet perforation, ulceration, and perivalvular abscesses. Antibiotics are first-line therapy, but indications for early surgical intervention include:

- refractory congestive heart failure
- sepsis
- shock
- repeat embolization
- annular abscess
- large vegetation size (1.5 cm)
- persistent bacteremia despite 4–6 weeks of antibiotics

Presentation and Diagnosis

Symptoms of mitral insufficiency typically parallel those of stenosis but are more insidious in their development; even moderate-severe to severe mitral insufficiency may have a prolonged asymptomatic period. Symptoms, when present, are secondary to elevated left atrial and pulmonary artery pressures, increased pulmonary vascular resistance, and increased right heart pressures. Patient complaints include dyspnea with exertion and in advanced stages at rest, paroxysmal nocturnal dyspnea, palpitations from atrial fibrillation when present, and, rarely, hemoptysis. Once symptomatic, yearly mortality increases and this is an absolute indication for intervention.

Echocardiography is the diagnostic modality of choice. Doppler imaging demonstrates a high-velocity signal best seen in the 4-chamber apical view. Grading the degree of insufficiency is based on the size and extent of the color-flow Doppler signal into the left atrium (LA):

- Mild: proximal 1/3 LA
- Moderate: filling to mid-cavity
- Severe: filling of posterior 1/3 LA with reversal of flow into pulmonary veins.

A more precise quantification of degree of insufficiency by echocardiogram can be made using regurgitant volume (RV), regurgitant fraction (RF), effective regurgitant orifice (ERO), and jet area (Table 1).

It is not uncommon to diagnose mitral insufficiency incidentally upon cardiac catheterization (Figure 9). A grading system has been developed to estimate severity after injection of the left ventricle (LV):

1+ trace contrast in left atrium
2+ contrast opacifies entire LA and clears within 2–3 beats
3+ contrast opacifies LA and LV equally
4+ frank reversal of contrast into pulmonary veins

Table 1. Quantification of Degree of Mitral Insufficiency by Echocardiogram

Grade	RV (mL)	RF (%)	ERO (mm^2)	Jet Area (%)
1	<30	<20	<20	<20
2	30–44	30–39	20–29	20–29
3	45–59	40–49	30–39	30–39
4	>60	>50	>40	>40

Medical Management of Mitral Valve Disease

Mild cases of mitral insufficiency usually do not require treatment and should be followed serially by echocardiography. Moderate insufficiency is usually asymptomatic and can be treated medically with afterload reduction and fluid and sodium restrictions. Target pressures include maintaining a systolic value of 110–120 mmHg, although in elderly patients this may result in relative hypotension, dizziness, fatigue, and presyncope. Diuretic therapy, ACE inhibitors, and pure vasodilators such as hydralazine may help to accomplish this goal.

The mainstay of medical management for acute mitral insufficiency in the ICU setting, especially in the hemodynamically unstable patient, is also predicated on afterload reduction, either chemically or mechanically. Sodium nitroprusside is the vasodilator of choice and can be used in conjunction with an intra-aortic balloon

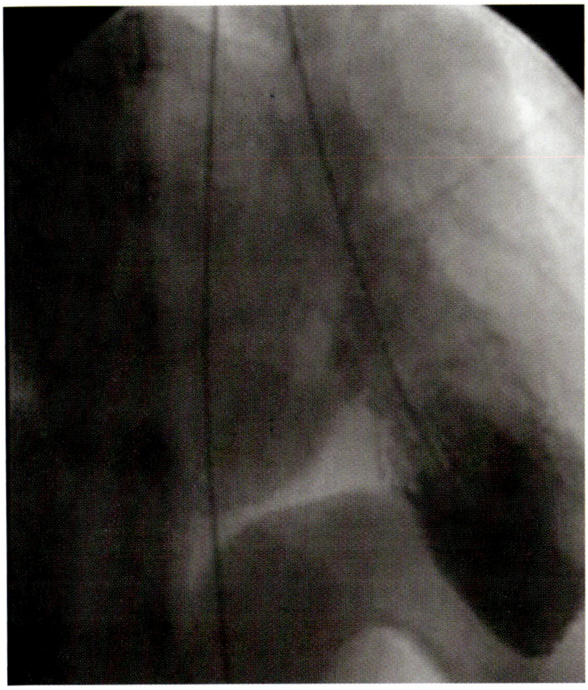

Figure 9. Mitral insufficiency shown during cardiac catheterization.

pump (IABP) or left ventricular assist device for maximum benefit in cases of cardiogenic shock.

Surgical Management of Mitral Valve Disease

All symptomatic patients with severe or moderately severe mitral regurgitation (MR) with a regurgitant volume greater than 45 mL should undergo mitral valve surgery, unless their life expectancy from other illness would act as a contraindication to surgery. In this cohort, without intervention, the clinical course is somewhat predictable with progressive insufficiency, ventricular dilatation, heart failure, and decreased quality of life as inevitable endpoints. There is actually a survival advantage to surgical intervention for the symptomatic patient with mitral insufficiency.

In the past, asymptomatic patients had been treated medically. Referring physicians were reluctant to recommend early surgical intervention given the morbidity and invasive nature of the operation, somewhat protracted recovery, and inherent downside of a prosthesis with valve replacement.

However, as experience has accrued and the potential for repair approaches 85–90%, consideration must be given to early and aggressive surgical intervention in the asymptomatic patient with moderate to severe insufficiency (regurgitant volume ≥45 cc). Successful repair presents as low risk for endocarditis, does not require anticoagulation, and carries a lower risk of operative mortality (<1%) in experienced centers and patients who are good surgical candidates. A minimally invasive robotic approach also allows for rapid recovery and early return to normal life for appropriate candidates.

With this new paradigm of reduced risk and added benefit, many cardiologists are now favoring early mitral valve repair with the following inclusion criteria for patients who are asymptomatic:

- Decreased left ventricular function or left ventricular dilation (left ventricular end diastolic dimension [LVED] <60%; left ventricular end-systolic diameter [LVESD] >45 mm).
- Preserved left ventricular function, but with new onset atrial fibrillation or pulmonary hypertension at rest (systolic pulmonary artery pressure at rest >50 mmHg).
- Preserved left ventricular function in a patient with flail mitral valve leaflets and LVESD greater than 40 mmHg who has a low operative risk and high likelihood of durable repair.
- Can consider repair for patients with preserved left ventricular function, left atrial dilation (volume ≥60 cc/m^2), and systolic pulmonary artery pressure greater than 60 mmHg during exercise who have low operative risk and high likelihood of durable repair.
- Effective regurgitant orifice (ERO) >40 mm^2.

Obviously, the treatment algorithm must be individualized, and a thorough and detailed discussion must occur between the primary care physician, cardiologist, surgeon, and patient.

Mitral Valve Repair vs. Replacement: A Word about Timing

Once the determination has been made that surgical intervention for mitral valve disease is inevitable, timing of the intervention must be decided and feasibility of repair must be assessed. Repair has been shown to have multiple benefits over replacement, including preservation of left ventricular function, lack of need for anticoagulation, reduced need for reoperation, and restoration of normal life expectancy. For these reasons, the timing of the operation in the setting of a repairable valve should not be postponed until left ventricular geometry or function begins to suffer. Such a delay actually reduces the maximum benefit achievable with a well-timed repair. As a result, the current recommendation is that the onset of any symptoms heralds the need for intervention in the setting of a repairable valve.

Valve Replacement

Valve replacement is most often required for acute mechanical regurgitation caused by ischemia (papillary muscle rupture), for severe post-inflammatory fibrotic or calcific changes, and for valve leaflet destruction caused by bacterial endocarditis. For patients in whom valve repair is unlikely, timing of the elective intervention is somewhat less pressing, simply because there is no perfect valve substitute yet available. Waiting for increasing symptoms is more acceptable than in the repairable valve; deterioration of the left ventricular function, though, has been roundly denounced as resulting in a wait that is too long for any intervention, regardless of how imperfect valve substitutes may be.

Choice of valve prosthesis is based on a number of factors germane to all valve replacement decisions:

- What is the patient's life expectancy?
- What is the patient's level of tolerance or acceptance of anticoagulation?
- What is the patient's level of tolerance or acceptance of reoperation?

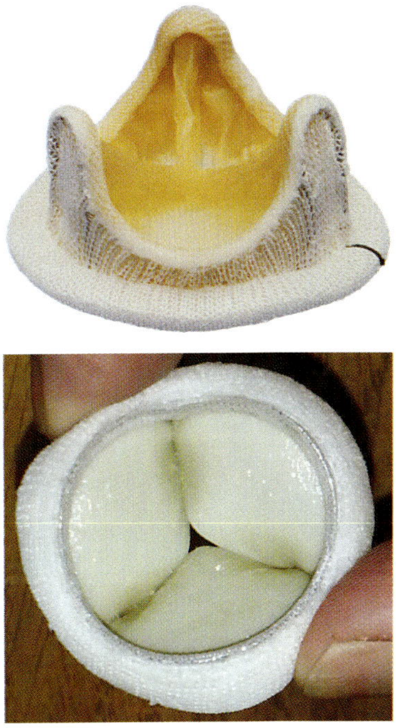

Figure 10. Porcine valve prostheses.

In general, tissue valve substitutes (xenografts) are reserved for patients who are thought to be in the final decades of their life due to the limited structural longevity of the tissue (12–15 years maximum for currently available valves), or patients for whom anticoagulation is not an option. Porcine valve prostheses are constructed of glutaraldehyde-preserved pig aortic valve leaflets sewn to a Dacron-covered, flexible titanium strut (Figure 10). Bovine pericardial valve substitutes are constructed of glutaraldehyde-preserved cow pericardium that has been cut in a trefoil design and also sewn to a Dacron-covered, flexible titanium strut (Figure 11). The primary benefit of tissue valves is the ability to limit reliance on anticoagulation. However, the incidence of atrial fibrillation in mitral patients often diminishes this advantage.

Mechanical valve substitutes have evolved from a caged-ball design to single or bi-leaflet rotating or tilting discs, with occasional variations on those themes (Figure 12). Many attempts have been made to create the perfect valve substitute. This valve replacement would combine durability without the need for anticoagulation. Unfortunately, this solution remains elusive, further stimulating the pursuit to perfect mitral valve repair techniques.

Robotic Mitral Valve Surgery

Evolution of Minimally Invasive and Robotic Surgery

In recent decades an abundance of enthusiasm has developed for "minimally invasive operations" in all areas of surgery, much of this driven by patients. Everyone agrees that a well-performed operation is a very effective treatment; however, all surgeries are inherently invasive. It is common sense that if an operation can achieve a similar outcome, but is performed through a less-invasive approach with improved cosmetic appearance and less discomfort, this would be strongly preferred.

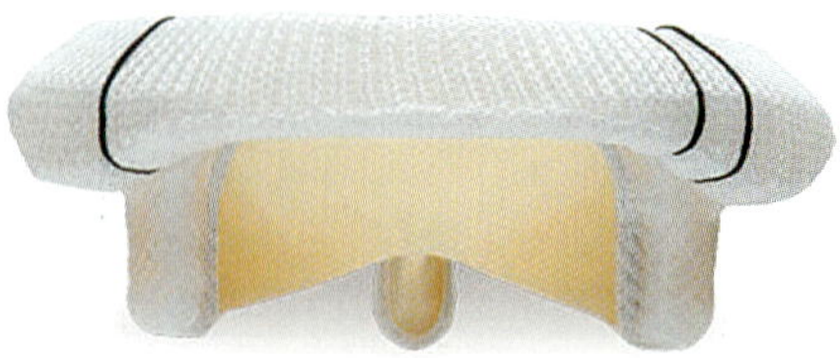

Figure 11. Bovine pericardial valve substitute.

In 1997, Dr. Delos Cosgrove of the Cleveland Clinic conducted an international telesymposium that demonstrated repairing or replacing the aortic or mitral valve through a 10 cm mid-line partial sternotomy. The sternum is divided from the sternal notch to the 4th intercostal space on the right side (Figure 13). Cardiopulmonary bypass is conducted by direct aortic and vena cava cannulation through the same incision. The mitral valve is exposed through a combined incision through the dome of the left atrium and atrial septum (Figure 14). The operation is carried out through direct vision and "standard" surgical instruments.

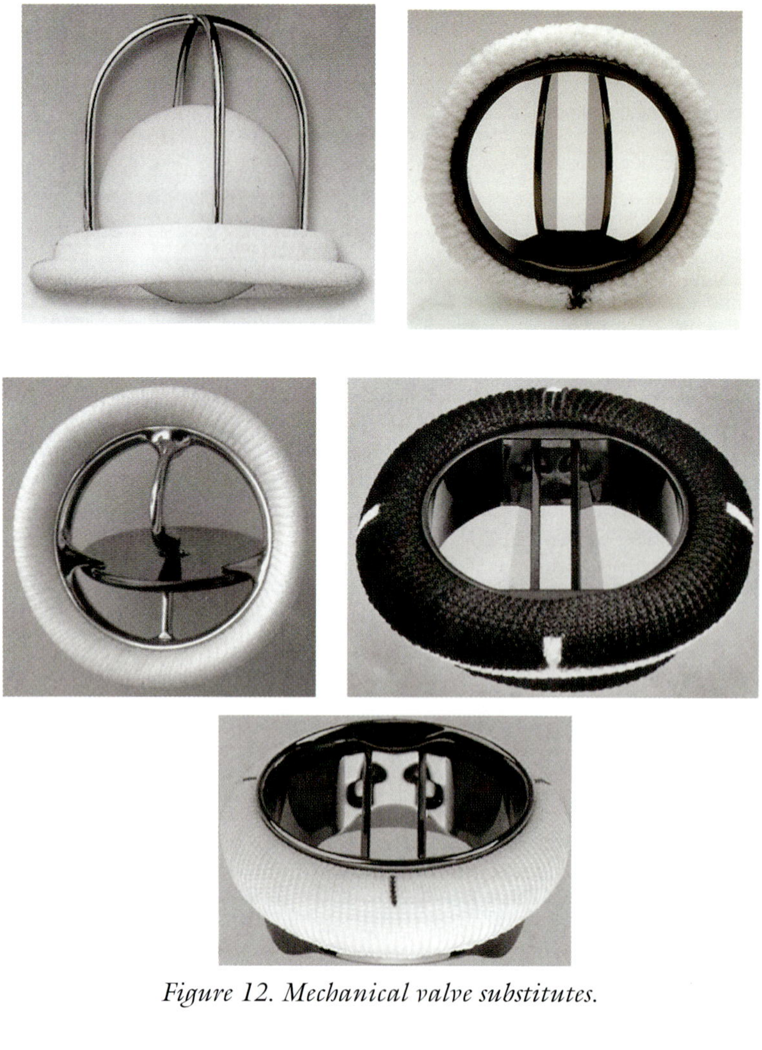

Figure 12. Mechanical valve substitutes.

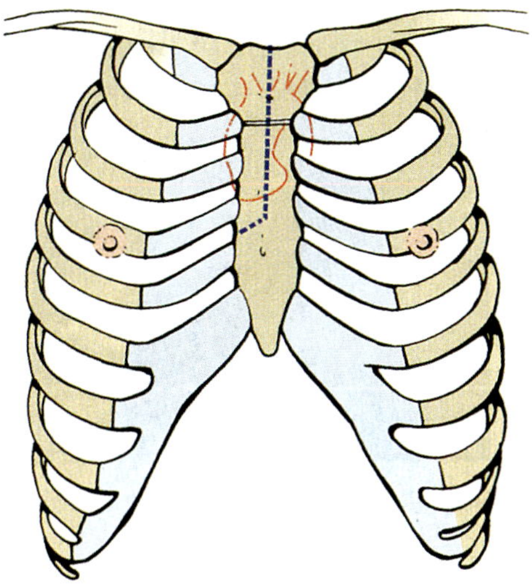

Figure 13. The hemisternotomy used for minimally invasive mitral and aortic valve surgery. Credit: McGraw-Hill Companies, Inc.

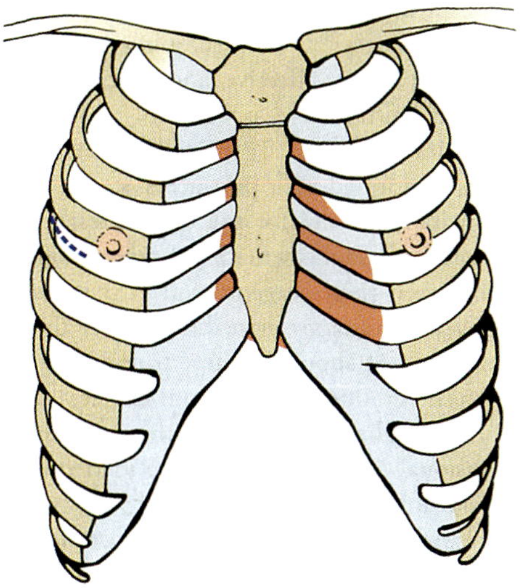

Figure 14. The minithoracotomy used for minimally invasive mitral valve surgery. Credit: McGraw-Hill Companies, Inc.

Dr. Cosgrove reported 50 such partial sternotomy aortic valve replacements, with a mortality of 2%. Since 1997, the majority of my isolated aortic valve replacements have been done in this manner with results similar to the full sternotomy. This allows for a shorter incision and improved sternal stability when compared to a full sternotomy.

Evolution in minimally invasive mitral valve surgery, however, is quite a different story. While the aortic valve lies a short distance underneath the sternum and a partial sternotomy provides adequate exposure, the mitral valve rests close to the center of the heart. It can be difficult to visualize even through a full sternotomy. Oftentimes, significant retraction on the heart is required for adequate exposure, and this distorts the valve from its natural state. Repair of the mitral valve through partial sternotomy is feasible, but exposure of the valve is difficult.

The concept of closed-chest heart surgery with cardiopulmonary bypass, cardioplegia, and video-assisted visualization was suggested in 1993 by W. S. Peters.[5] In 1996, the Stanford group reported closed-chest cardiopulmonary bypass with antegrade cardioplegic-induced cardiac arrest in 4 dogs (stopping the heart is not a must, but it facilitates the operation by offering a still field). The animal was cannulated via the femoral vein and artery for the in-flow and out-flow of blood to and from the heart-lung machine. The aorta was occluded by a balloon positioned in the ascending aorta. Diastolic cardiac arrest was induced via antegrade blood cardioplegia (Figure 15). The dogs' left internal mammary arteries were harvested via a thoracope and anastomosed onto the left anterior descending coronary artery.[6] These innovative instruments were made by Heart Port Inc., Redwood City, California, and positioned by fluoroscopy. This procedure laid the foundation for the "minimally invasive" and robotic-assisted mitral valve operation; the basic arrangement is still being widely used clinically 20 years later.

In March 1996, Drs. Carpentier and Loulmet reported the first successful mitral valve repair through a 4 × 5 cm mini-thoracotomy on a 30-year-old female with rheumatic mitral insufficiency and stenosis. The operation was aided by video transmission and peripheral cardiopulmonary bypass. They hypothesized that this new approach would result in reduced perioperative disability and reduced cost.[7] In 1997, Dr. Friedrich W. Mohr of the University of Leipzig reported that 24 patients underwent minimally invasive mitral valve repair using a similar approach, but with the Heart Port catheters positioned by TEE. One patient had moderate mitral insufficiency and required valve replacement, and one patient had retrograde aortic dissection. A year later, Dr. Mohr reported eight successful mitral repairs with help of a voice-controlled "robotic camera mount" (AESOP 2000; Computer Motion, Santa Barbara, California) and a 3-D video scope (Carl Zeiss). Superior visualization of the mitral was reported.[8]

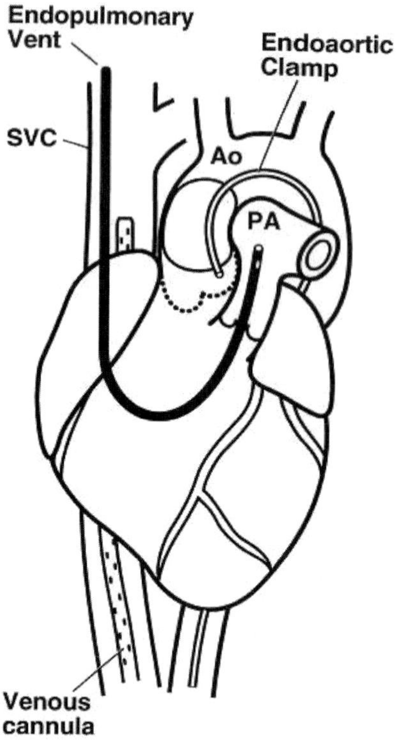

Figure 15. The model of cardiopulmonary bypass with an inferior vena cava cannula and occlusion of the ascending aorta with an endo-aortic balloon.[6]

Dr. Hugo Vanermen of Onze-Lieve-Vrouw Hospital in Aalst, Belgium, takes credit for perfecting the nonrobotic, non–rib-spreading minithoracotomy mitral valve repair operation. Not spreading or resecting the ribs allows patients to experience significantly reduced pain. Long, single-shafted instruments made by CardioVations® (previously Heart Port) (Figure 16) are being used, which allow for operations in the center of the heart through a 5 × 2 cm skin incision (Figure 17). Between 1997 and November 2000, 175 patients underwent port-access mitral valve repair, with a hospital mortality rate of 1.1%.[9] This researcher spent a week with Dr. Vanermen about ten years ago and revisited him three years ago in order to observe his work and learn this operation—the technique was swift with great results. By 2007, at least 978 such operations have been done in Aalst. Dr. Vanermen dissects the femoral artery and vein only anteriorly. By avoiding circumferential dissecting and clamping the femoral vessels, he reported a 1% vascular complication.[12] This technique is being used at Saint Joseph Mercy Hospital for our minimally invasive mitral valve operations.

My mentor, Dr. C. Hargrove, of Presbyterian Hospital University of Pennsylvania, has also done more than 1,000 Belgium-style minimally invasive mitral repairs in the past 10 years. He came to St. Joseph Mercy Hospital three years ago to help me initiate my "minimally invasive" mitral valve operation, and for that I am indebted to him.

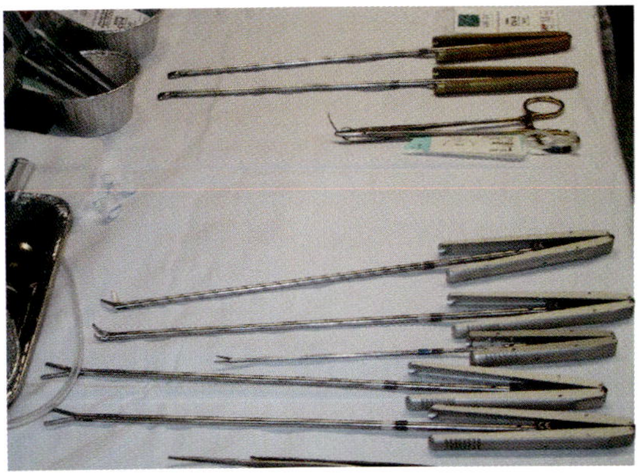

Figure 16. Long, single-shafted instruments manufactured by CardioVations®.

Although operating with a long-shafted instrument via a small incision has been perfected in Belgium, it is still technically demanding; Dr. Vanermen once stated that this amounts to "transferring the pain from the patient to the surgeon." Fifteen years ago, this prompted Professor Carpentier, the father of mitral valve surgery, to explore doing heart operations with an earlier version of the da Vinci Robotic System. This computer system translates the movement of the surgeon's hands to the tiny 2 cm robotic hands, which are placed inside the patient's body—in this case the left atrium—through 12 mm ports. The robotic hands mimic the movements of human hands. The da Vinci robot does not perform the operation; rather, it is the human who drives the machine to perform the operation through a console. Visibility of the mitral valve is unparalleled through the 3-D robotic camera placed inside the left chest. After doing many hundreds of mitral operations in the last twenty some years, I have never seen the mitral as clearly and as undistorted as through the 3-D da Vinci robotic camera. In 1998, after 10 months of active work to adapt this system to intracardiac surgery, Dr. Carpentier and Dr. Loulmet reported the first successful intra-cardiac robotic operation on a 52-year-old woman with an aneurysm and atrial septal defect.[10]

Two years later, Dr. W. R. Chitwood, of East Carolina University, performed the first robotic mitral valve repair in the United States.[11] Robotic mitral valve pioneers

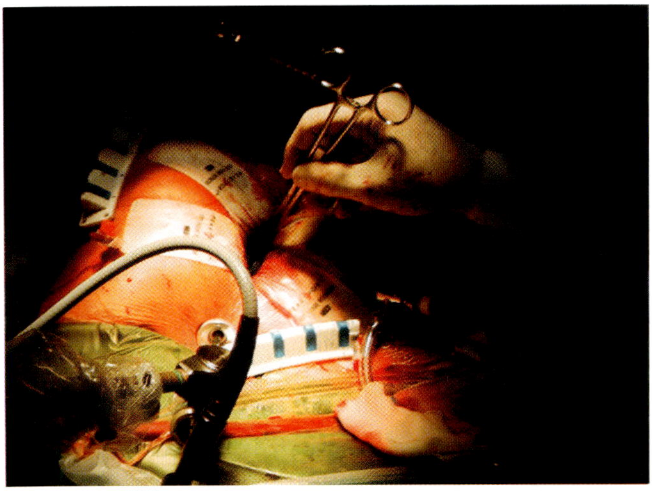

Figure 17. Non-rib-spreading mini right thoracotomy incision.

such as Dr. W. R. Chitwood, Dr. D. Murphy, Dr. M. J. Smith, Dr. M. Gillinov, and Dr. T. Mihaljevic have collectively performed thousands of these robotic-assisted minimally invasive mitral valve repair or replacement operations.

In 2011, Dr. W. R. Chitwood reported his ten years of experience with 540 patients (454 patients with isolated mitral valve repair and 86 patients with robotic mitral valve repair along with cryoablation for atrial fibrillation). These surgeries comprised consecutive mitral valve repairs including concomitant atrial fibrillation cryoablation. He used an 8-cm argon-cooled flexible probe by Medtronic to reproduce the Cox maze III lesion pattern. His positive results were: 30 day mortality (0.4%), myocardial infarction (0.7%), stroke (0.6%), bleeding requiring reoperation (2.4%), blood or blood product transfusion (29%), renal insufficiency (1.1%), femoral complication (0%), hospital length of stay (5.6 +/– 4 days), and repair failure (2.8%).[13]

Dr. Suri of the Mayo Clinic compared 202 patients who underwent conventional sternotomy or minimally invasive robotic-assisted mitral valve repair. One year after operation, the robotic repaired group (n = 36) had less fatigue and chest pain compared to the sternotomy group (n = 28). Approximately half of the patients in the robotic group returned to work in one month, while about half of the patients of the conventional group returned to work in two months.[14]

Dr. T. Mihaljevic compared the outcome of 759 patients with degenerative mitral valve disease with posterior leaflet prolapse who underwent mitral valve surgery in Cleveland Clinic from January 2006 to January 2009, utilizing different surgical incisions. The 759 patients were grouped as such: complete sternotomy (n = 114), partial sternotomy (n = 270), right mini-anterolateral thoracotomy (n = 114), and robotic approach (n = 261). There were no in-hospital deaths. The quality of mitral valve repair was similar. Despite the robotic group's longer cardiopulmonary bypass time (42 minutes more than full sternotomy) and longer myocardial ischemic time (26 minutes longer than full sternotomy), neurologic, pulmonary, and renal complications were similar among all groups. The robotic group had the shortest hospital stay (median of 4.2 days).[15]

Dr. Allen Raczkowski of the University of Arizona performed the first robotic mitral valve repair with the beating heart. This eliminates the need for aortic cross clamping, endo-aortic balloon or cardioplegia, and there is no ischemic time for the heart. After three years of experience with nonrobotic, non–rib-spreading mini-right thoracotomy mitral valve repair, I (BK) had the privilege of having Dr. Raczkowski visit in order to help me get started with robotic mitral valve repair. With the robot as an extra tool, dexterity and visualization for mitral operation are significantly improved.

Robotic mitral valve repair is a technically demanding operation and, therefore, this technique should be acquired in stages. Surgeons should be experienced with mitral valve repair through traditional sternotomy, with consistent outcome, before progressing to "smaller" rib-spreading right thoracotomy employing the endo-aortic balloon (or the long shafted "Chitwood" clamp), long single-shafted instruments, and femoral artery and vein cannulation. The final stage advances to operating through a 3 cm–4 cm non–rib-spreading right thoracotomy with assistance of a video scope or a robot. Information from the Society of Thoracic Surgeons (STS) national database from 2010 and 2011 reveals 12% of mitral valves repaired in United States were performed with robotic assistance.

Patient Benefits

- Sternotomy is avoided. Therefore, the risk of deep sternal wound infection is eliminated.
- Rib-spreading incision is avoided and results in decreased postoperative pain.[14]
- Improved cosmesis
- Shorter hospital stay and faster recovery[16,15]
- Quicker return to normal activity[14]
- Quicker return to work[14]

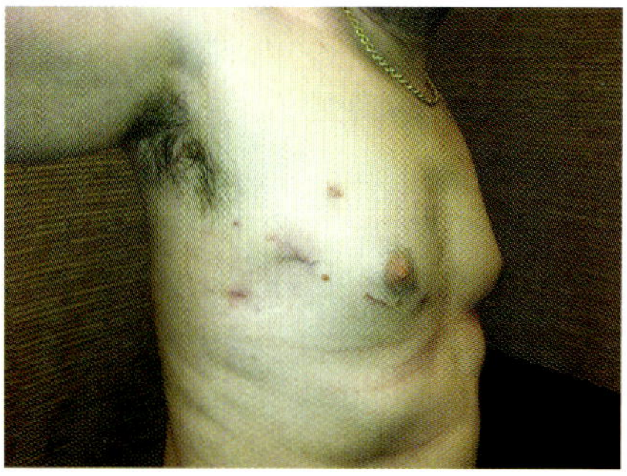

Figure 18. Patient one month after robotic mitral valve repair.

Patient Selection

Ideal patients are those who are:

- Relatively slim (BMI <30 kg/m^2)
- <70 years old
- Need isolated mitral valve operation (concomitant coronary bypass or aortic replacement will need sternotomy)
- No previous cardiac or thoracic operation

This surgery is not recommended for patients with:

- Femoral artery <6 mm
- Aortal iliac occlusive disease
- Mobile plaque in aorta
- Mitral annulus calcification
- Morbid obesity
- Right pleural adhesion
- History of pericarditis
- Cardiomyopathy
- Pulmonary hypertension

Preoperative Testing

- Transesophageal echocardiogram, preferable 3-D TEE (Figure 19).
- CT scan of chest, abdomen, and pelvic area with and without contrast with 3-D reconstruction of the right chest.
- Cardiac catheterization for patients >40 years old.
- Pulmonary function testing to assess tolerance of single-lung ventilation during the surgery.

Operation

Robotic mitral valve repair is done with general anesthesia utilizing a double lumen endotracheal tube. After induction of general anesthesia, a retrograde cardioplegia catheter and an 18 Fr superior vena cava venous catheter are placed percutaneously through the internal jugular vein by anesthesiologists (Figure 20).

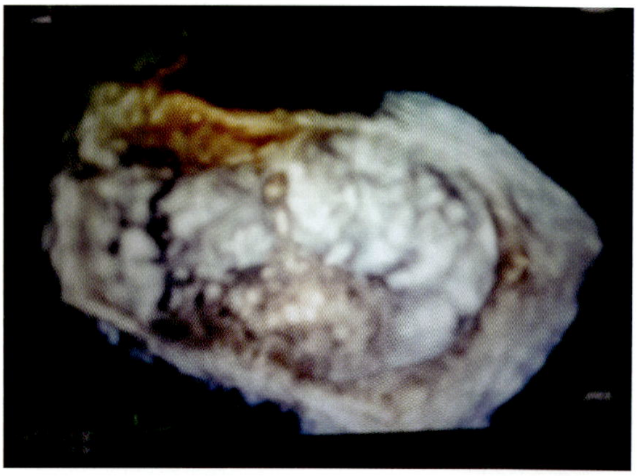

Figure 19. 3-D TEE image of a mitral valve with prolapse and a rupture chord of the middle scallop of the posterior leaflet.

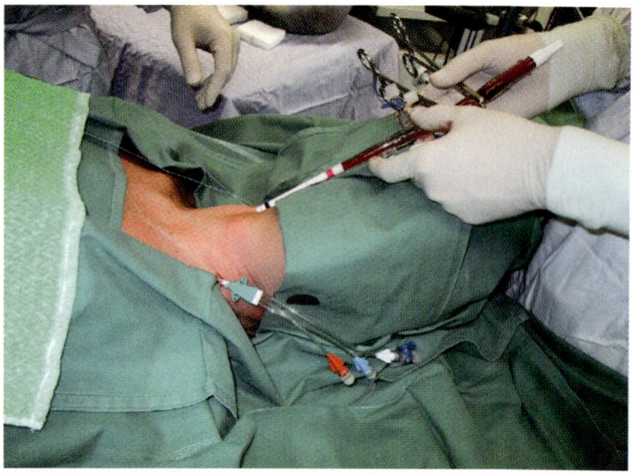

Figure 20. Placement of a superior vena cava venous catheter.

The patient's femoral artery and vein are dissected out anteriorly through a 3 cm incision as described by Dr. Vanermen.[12] After heparin is given, the inferior vena cava outflow (to the heart-lung machine) catheter (usually 25 Fr) and the femoral in-flow (from the heart-lung machine) catheter (usually 23 Fr) are inserted under TEE guidance. In the right chest, a 12 mm incision is made just lateral to the nipple in men and more laterally in the inframammary crease in women. This is for the da Vinci camera port to be inserted into the 4th intercostal space (Figure 21). A 3–4 cm incision is made lateral to the camera port in the 4th interspace to serve as the "working" port through which sutures, mitral annuloplasty rings, or the mitral valve prosthesis are passed into the left atrium. A 10 mm incision is made three finger-breadths to the left of the working port through the 3rd intercostal space for the introduction of the left "arm" port of the robot. Another 8 mm incision is made three finger-breadths to the right and posterior to the working port (usually on the level of the anterior-axillary line) to access the 5th or the 6th interspace for the introduction of the right "arm" of the robot. Doctors Mihaljevic and Chitwood prefer the 5th intercostal space for the robotic right arm, feeling it may decrease the risk of left atrial tear, while other surgeons prefer the traditional 6th intercostal space.[13] Lastly, a 10 mm incision is made close to the right parasternal area at the 4th or 5th intercostal space for the introduction of the robotic dynamic left atrial retractor (while remaining cognizant of the position of the right internal mammary artery or vein).

The da Vinci robot is now positioned. Correct positioning of the robotic "spine" and arms is extremely important in order to avoid "external conflict" of the robotic arms. The mid-point or "spine" of the robot should be in line with the robotic camera and at a right angle to the patient's body. The robot should be at a distance from the patient so that its camera arm has a full range of motion. Lastly, the "elbows" for the robotic arms should be aligned so that the arm "number" is facing forward.

At this point, cardiopulmonary bypass is initiated, and good decompression of the right atrium is ensured. Vacuum-assisted suction on the venous line is often required. The robot is then "docked." The pericardium is opened longitudinally 3–4 cm anterior to the phrenic nerve from the aortic root close to the diaphragm. Diastolic cardiac arrest is induced. This is accomplished by infusing a high-potassium cardioplegic solution into the aortic root or coronary sinus after the ascending aorta is occluded with the endo-aortic balloon positioned in mid-ascending aorta (similar to the occlusion balloon used on dogs in the experiment twenty years ago by the Stanford group) under TEE guidance. After the left atriotomy air enters the chamber and TEE is no longer available, direct inspection of the aortic root distended by the balloon via the robotic camera is helpful to ensure the proper position of the endo-aortic balloon.

With the assistant surgeon stationed on the patient's right side, the primary surgeon controls the robotic arms through the da Vinci console a few feet away. The assistant and primary surgeons should have a direct line of vision for communication. Earbuds or headphones are also helpful for communication.

With the robot driven by the surgeon, a lateral left atriotomy is made, and superior exposure of the mitral valve is achieved by fine adjustments of the robotic dynamic left atrial retractor. The diseased mitral valve is inspected, analyzed, and repaired. Due to the superior lighting and magnification, along with the fact that

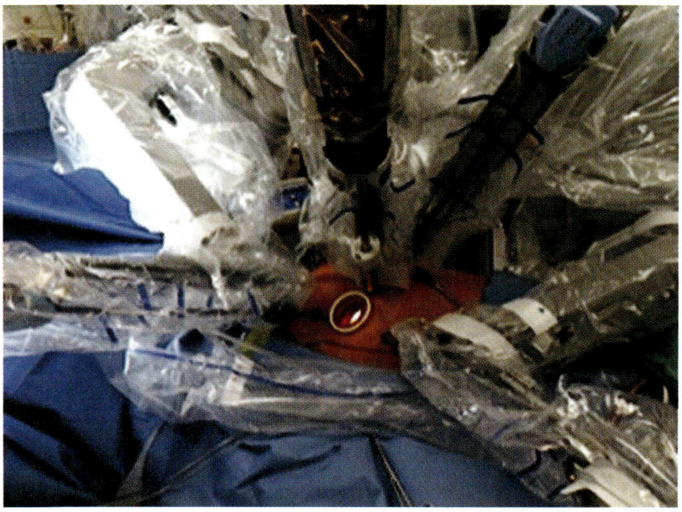

Figure 21. A working port in the 4th intercostal space. The left and right robotic arms are bottom left and right in the picture, respectively. The large structure center top is the 3-D camera. To the immediate right of the camera is the left atrial retractor.

the mitral valve is in a more relaxed state and is being viewed at a less tangential angle, repair technique utilizing neo-chord is aided. Triangular resection of the posterior leaflet of the mitral valve, as described by researchers at the Mayo Clinic, is frequently utilized (Figure 22).

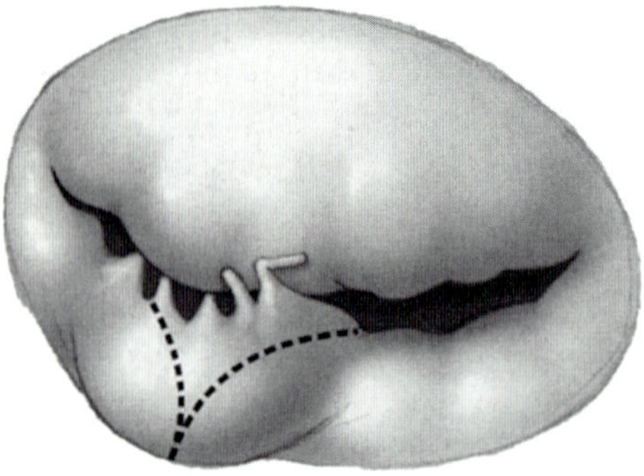

Figure 22. Triangular resection of the posterior leaflet of the mitral valve.

Complete mitral valve annuloplasty ring or partial ring can be anchored with interrupted sutures on the annulus, as described by Dr. Carpentier. It can also be anchored with running techniques, as described by Dr. Gerald Lawrie of Houston, Texas, or with a running horizontal mattress. After the mitral valve repair, the left atriotomy is closed and the aortic occlusion balloon is deflated and pulled back from the ascending aorta. Spontaneous cardiac contraction follows. The two robotic arms, atrial retractor, and camera are removed. The da Vinci is "undocked" and the patient is weaned from cardiopulmonary bypass. After the mitral valve competency is confirmed by the TEE and hemostasis in the chest wall is meticulously achieved (visualization can be aided with a 5 mm thoracoscope), the femoral arterial and venous cannulae are removed and heparin is reversed. We usually place a single 24 Fr tube in the dependent position of the right chest and selectively place a drain in the oblique sinus. After the chest and groin wounds are closed, the operation is completed.

Postoperative Care

Postoperative care in the surgical intensive care unit is usually not significantly different than for patients undergoing traditional mitral valve operation. Despite a longer cardiopulmonary bypass time, there appears to be fewer occurrences of coagulopathy and bleeding. Since no bone is divided, this less invasive surgical approach appears to result in decreased inflammatory response and coagulopathy. Unilateral pulmonary edema/ARDS (Figure 23) of a yet unknown cause has been reported. We have also experienced this in one of our patients, who was managed successfully by staying on the "dry" side and was extubated on postoperative day three.

Discussion

In the treatment of mitral valve disease, repair techniques have supplanted replacement strategies in the management of degenerative disease, thereby achieving better survival and excellent durability. Carpentier and others have provided exceptional results with up to 20 years of follow-up helping to establish repair as the gold standard when approaching mitral insufficiency.[26] The literature is replete with studies showing a demonstrable benefit from preserving the native valve

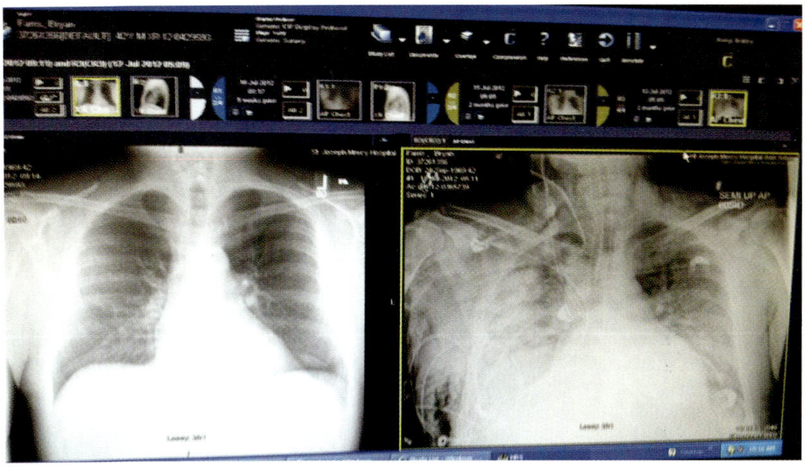

Figure 23. The image on the right shows a right-side pulmonary edema. The image on the left shows full resolution of the edema.

whenever possible. Repaired patients have less risk of endocarditis and operative mortality. They have superior preservation of left ventricular function, are relieved from anticoagulation beyond an ASA-a-day, and the results are often more durable than a bio-prosthetic valve. Almost uniformly, outcomes are superior in the repair cohort.[22] The STS national database for 2010 and 2011 reflects an overall 30-days mortality for mitral valve replacement (N = 11002) of 5.5% while for MV repair (N = 14622) of 1.2%.

Advances in techniques of cardiopulmonary bypass and video-telemetric surgery have paved the way for minimally invasive mitral valve operations using a robotic approach. Qualified centers with highly trained surgical teams can reproduce conventional repair techniques even with complex valve pathology.

Critics of the robotic approach cite prolonged operative times as a limiting factor in applying this technology. Although there is a steep learning curve, the experienced operator will invariably see a progressive decline in cross-clamp and bypass times. At this juncture, this has not translated to increased complications. On the contrary, shorter hospitalization, less pain, and earlier return to work are observed. As experience accrues and advancement in robotic instruments occur, repair and overall operative times will eventually approach those of a traditional sternotomy.

Reports have confirmed that the principles of open repair can be reliably reproduced with high success rates and low mortality in experienced centers. This may pave the way for earlier intervention in mitral valve disease, even in asymptomatic patients. This leads to the prevention of the development of cardiomyopathy and pulmonary hypertension, as well as promotion and anticipated regression of LV volume and function as early as one month following surgery.[19] In fact, one can expect to see close to normal survival rates with an aggressive approach to repairing the mitral valve.[23,24]

Prior studies have definitively shown the substantial benefits of mitral valve repair using a minimally invasive approach, including shorter time to extubation and improved respiratory mechanics, decreased postoperative pain, shorter length of hospitalization, fewer transfusion requirements, and excellent operative outcomes.[25] In fact, when compared to the STS database, patients enrolled in multicenter trials had significantly lower mortality, fewer neurologic complications (especially with a transthoracic cross-clamping technique), and fewer reoperations.[18,20]

In addition to the aforementioned perioperative benefits, several series have delineated the advantages of a robotic approach using quality of life indices. This is especially relevant in the asymptomatic patient with moderate to severe regurgitation (3+), when considering an invasive procedure with obvious functional limitations, albeit transient, using proactive criteria.

Suri et al. have demonstrated that not only does a robotic approach provide for excellent functional recovery early after mitral valve repair, this benefit translates to improved performance, decreased fatigue, less postoperative pain, and earlier return to work when compared to conventional surgery.[14] The median time to return to work was 33 days for the robotic group compared to 54 days for the patient undergoing sternotomy in this series.

Timing of the surgery is paramount in the treatment of mitral insufficiency, and indications for intervention continue to evolve. Referring physicians are beginning to realize the benefits of early referral and intervention, especially if there is a high likelihood of repair using a minimally invasive approach. Several authors have reported decreased survival, increased incidence of atrial fibrillation, more symptoms of congestive heart failure, and an overall reduction in quality of life in those patients whose surgery is deferred in favor of expectant management.[27,28]

Delaying surgery not only impacts long-term survival by development of sometimes irreversible cardiomyopathy, pulmonary hypertension, cardiorenal syndrome, and hepatic dysfunction from right heart failure, but also reduces the feasibility of repair at the time of operation. Operative risk will also increase and sometimes, sadly, get to the point of being prohibitive. Surgeons at the East Carolina Heart Institute, under the direction of Dr. Randolph Chitwood, have reported repair rates of 97%, 96%, 89%, and 76% for New York Heart Association (NYHA) class I, II, III, and IV, respectively.[18]

In summary, robotic repair of the degenerative mitral valve has proven to be an excellent option conferring better outcomes and earlier functional recovery. Experienced centers can ensure high repair rates regardless of valve pathology. An aggressive approach to the leaky valve may improve both survival and outcomes. A minimally invasive approach should allow this option to become available to more asymptomatic patients with moderate to severe insufficiency (3+).

References

1. Brunton L. Preliminary note on the possibility of treating mitral stenosis by surgical methods. *Lancet.* 1902;159(4093):352.

2. Harken DE, Ellis LB, Ware PF, et al. The surgical treatment of mitral stenosis. I. valvuloplasty. *NEJM.* 1948;239:801.

3. Carpentier A. Cardiac valve surgery: the "French correction." *J Thorac and Cardiovasc Surg.* 1983;86:323.

4. Duran CG, Pamar JL, Revulta JM, et al. Conservative operation for mitral insufficiency. critical analysis supported by postoperative hemodynamic studies of 72 patients. *J Thorac and Cardiovasc Surg.* 1980;79:326.

5. Peters WS. Minimally invasive surgery by cardioscopy. *Aust J Thorac Cardiovasc Surg.* 1993;2:152–154.

6. Stevens OH, Burdon TA, Siegel L, et al. Port-access coronary artery bypass with cardioplegia arrest: acute and chronic canine studies. *Ann Thorac Surg.* 1996;62:435–440.

7. Carpentier A, Loulmet D, Carpentier A, et al. Open heart operation under videosurgery and minithoracotomy. first case (mitral valvuloplasty) operated with success. *C R Acad Sci III* 1996 Mar;319(3):219–23.

8. Falk V, Walther T, Autschbach R, Diegeler A, Battellini R, Mohr FW. Robot-assisted minimally invasive solo mitral valve operation. *J Thorac Cardiovasc Surg.* 1998;115: 470–471.

9. Schroeyers P, Wellens F, De Geest R, et al. Minimally invasive video-assisted mitral valve surgery: our lessons after a 4-year experience. *Ann Thorac Surg.* 2001;72:S1050–S1054.

10. Carpentier A, Loulmet D, Aupecle B, et al. Computer assisted open heart surgery. first case operated on with success. *C R Acad Sci III.* 1998 May;321(5):437–42.

11. Chitwood WR Jr, Nifong LW, Elbeery JE, et al. Robotic mitral valve repair: trapezoidal resection and prosthetic annuloplasty with the da Vinci surgical system. *J Thorac Cardiovasc Surg.* 2000;120:1171–1172.

12. Jeanmart H, Casselman FP, De Grieck Y, et al. Avoiding vascular complications during minimally invasive, totally endoscopic intracardiac surgery. *J Thorac Cardiovasc Surg.* 2007;133:1066–1070.

13. Nifong W, Rodriguez E, Chitwood WR Jr. 540 consecutive robotic mitral valve repairs including concomitant atrial fibrillation cryoablation. *Ann Thorac Surg.* 2012; 94:38–43.

14. Suri RM, Antiel RM, Burkhart HM, et al. Quality of life after early mitral valve repair using conventional and robotic approaches. *Ann Thorac Surg.* 2012;93:761–769.

15. Mihaljevic T, Jarrett CM, Gillinov AM, et al. Robotic repair of posterior mitral valve prolapse versus conventional approaches: potential realized. *J Thorac Cardiovasc Surg.* 2011;141:72–80.

16. Smith JM, Mihaljevic T, Murphy D. *da Vinci Mitral Valve Repair Procedure Guide.* Intuitive Surgical Inc.

17. Suri RM, Burkhardt HM, Daly RC, et al. Robotic mitral repair for all prolapse subsets using techniques identical to open valvuloplasty: establishing the benchmark against which percutaneous interventions should be judged. *J Thorac Cardiovasc Surg.* 2011;142: 970–979.

18. Stevens LM, Rodriguez E, Lehr EJ, et al. Impact of timing and surgical approach on outcomes after mitral valve regurgitant operations. *Ann Thorac Surg.* 2012;93: 1462–1468.

19. Suri RK, Burkhardt HM, Rehfeldt KH, et al. Robotic mitral repair for all categories of leaflet prolapse: improving patient appeal and advancing standard of care. *Mayo Clinic Proc.* 2011;89(9):838–844.

20. Nifong LW, Chitwood R, Pappas PS, Smith CR, Argenziano M, Starnes VA, Shah PM, for the Multi-center Mitral Repair Group. Robotic mitral valve surgery: a United States multicenter trial. *J Thorac Cariovasc Surg.* 2005;129:1395–1404.

21. Enriquez-Sarano M, Sundt TM III. Early surgery is recommended for mitral regurgitation. *Circulation.* 2010;121(6):804–811.

22. Shuhaiber J, Anderson RJ. Meta-analysis of clinical outcomes following surgical mitral valve repair or replacement. *Eur J Cardiothorac Surg.* 2007;31:267–75.

23. Suri RM, Schaff HV, Dearani JA, et al. Recovery of left ventricular function after surgical correction of mitral valve regurgitation caused by leaflet prolapse. *J Thorac Cardiovasc Surg.* 2009;137(5):1071–1076.

24. Suri RM, Schaff HV, Dearani JA, et al. Survival advantage and improved durability of mitral repair for leaflet prolapse subsets in the current era. *Ann Thorac Surg.* 2006; 82(3):819–826.

25. Svensson LG, Atik FA, Cosgrove DM, et al. Minimally invasive versus conventional mitral valve surgery: a propensity matched comparison. *J Thorac Cardiovasc Surg.* 2010; 139(4):926–932.

26. Braunberger E, Deloache A, Berebi A, et al. Very long-term results (more than 20 years) of valve repair with Carpentier's techniques in non-rheumatic mitral valve insufficiency. *Circulation.* 2001;104:1–8.

27. Enriquez-Sarano M, Averinos JF, Messika-Zeitoun D, et al. Quantitative determinants of the outcome of asymptomatic mitral regurgitation. *N Engl J Med.* 2005;352: 875–83.

28. Kang DH, Kim JH, Rim JH, et al. Comparison of early surgery versus conventional treatment in asymptomatic severe mitral regurgitation. *Circulation.* 2009;119:797–804.

Chapter Five

The Mediastinum

Thomas A. Stark, MD; Ajay Gupta, MD; Vita V. McCabe, MD

Surgical Evolution

Advances in mediastinal surgery of the adult have paralleled advances in understanding lung physiology, improved radiographic imaging with computerized tomography, single-lung ventilation anesthesia techniques, as well as the use of gas insufflation techniques in the chest and current day perioperative care. In the modern era, minimally invasive techniques using robotic platforms allow patients to enter and leave a hospital within a few days, returning to their activities of daily living with minimal morbidity and virtually no long-term consequences of thoracic surgical procedures.

The median sternotomy was first described in 1897 to facilitate access to the mediastinum. Surgical excision of mediastinal lesions was performed with regularity. Prior to the turn of the twentieth century, there were no reported cases of cure for primary malignancy of the mediastinum. In 1901, a spindle cell sarcoma was successfully removed from behind the sternum. Hans Jacobeus in Stockholm, Sweden, first described thoracoscopy in 1910 when he employed a cystoscope to lyse pleural adhesions to facilitate collapsed-lung infusion of chemotherapy for the treatment of tuberculosis.

During the 1950s and 60s, these techniques were expanded to include biopsy of pleural and peripheral lung lesions. Mediastinoscopy was developed to improve ergonomics and facilitate easier visualization.[1] Mediastinoscopy was particularly useful in the staging of tumors in the chest and mediastinum and allowed tissue to be obtained for biopsy. The mechanics of mediastinoscopy, however, limited the surgeon's ability to resect most tumors for cure. The applications of thoracoscopy expanded rapidly during the late 1980s and 1990s, following the advent of video optics. Video-assisted thoracoscopic surgery (VATS) allowed the surgeon and assistant a clear view of the surgical field and enabled technical maneuvers similar to open surgery. VATS has advantages over open surgery as it offers fewer respiratory complications, smaller incisions, improved cosmesis, decreased length of hospital stay, and less pain in the immediate postoperative period. VATS has largely replaced many open procedures for non-cardiac operations in the chest. It is safe, effective, and, in many applications, superior to open surgery.[2,3,4]

The da Vinci Robotic System has been safely used to resect tumors in the mediastinum.[5] This system offers advantages over traditional VATS, including improved surgeon ergonomics, binocular optics with magnification, and articulated instrumentation that more closely replicates traditional surgical movements. This allows smaller more difficult areas to be reached and dissected with greater precision. The da Vinci Robotic System has also been shown to hasten the learning curve for surgeons adopting minimally invasive procedures.[6] There are relatively few contraindications to performing VATS or robotic procedures in the chest. These include inability to tolerate single-lung ventilation, severe pulmonary hypertension, severe coagulopathy, and pleural symphysis.

Anatomy

The mediastinum is the central compartment of the thoracic cavity. Classically, the mediastinum is divided into compartments based on radiographic landmarks. The superior compartment extends from the thoracic inlet inferiorly to the superior border of the pericardial sac and the inferior edge of the manubrium. The anterior compartment lies anterior to the pericardium. The middle mediastinum is divided from the posterior mediastinum by a line that extends inferiorly from the tracheal bifurcation to the diaphragm. Shields proposed a three-compartment system based on the anatomic contents: the *anterior compartment* is bounded posteriorly by the great vessels and the pericardium; the *middle compartment* lies between the anterior mediastinum and the anterior border of the thoracic vertebral bodies; and the *posterior compartment* includes everything along the thoracic vertebrae.[7] Each compartment of the mediastinum has characteristic benign and malignant tumors as well as cysts, dependent upon the structures that it incorporates (Table 1).

The superior border of the mediastinum is at the thoracic inlet and extends inferiorly to the diaphragm. The anterior to posterior borders are the sternum and the pleural surface overlying the vertebral column, respectively. The lateral borders are the left and right pleura. Contents include the heart, great vessels, phrenic and vagus nerves, lymph nodes, thoracic duct, thymus, esophagus, trachea, and main stem bronchi. The mediastinum does not have a dedicated serosal lining and receives contact from surrounding compartments. Free fluid or air in the mediastinum is never physiologic. Therefore, infection disseminates rapidly and, if not recognized promptly, progresses to severe sepsis and death.

The combination of rigid superior, anterior, and posterior borders relative to compliant lateral and inferior borders has unique clinical implications. That is to say, the range of clinical presentation is extremely broad. For instance, small tumors may present with significant compressive symptoms in some scenarios, while large neoplasms are often discovered incidentally on imaging studies only, such as computerized tomography (CT) scans or magnetic resonance imaging (MRI).

Symptoms encompass an expansive array of presentations, from vague constitutional changes to highly specific paraneoplastic syndromes. It is not uncommon to encounter hoarseness, stridor, dysphagia, dyspnea, chest pain, back pain, palpitations, cough, Horner's syndrome, diaphragmatic paralysis, or, less commonly, chylothorax. Compression of the superior vena cava (SVC) causes a defined constellation of symptoms referred to as SVC syndrome. This syndrome is characterized by facial flushing; edema of the face, neck, and arms; headache; light-headedness;

Table 1. Compartments of the Mediastinum and Most Common Abnormalities

Anterior	Middle	Posterior
Substernal thyroid	Bronchogenic cysts	***Benign***
Lymphoma	Enteric cysts	Neurofibroma
Metastatic cancer to the lymph nodes	Pericardial cysts	Heurilemoma
	Granulmonatous disease	Ganglioneuroma
Thymoma	Metastatic cancer to lymph nodes	Chemodectoma
Thymic carcinoma		Enteric cysts
Thymic cysts		Bronchogenic cysts
Thymic hyperplasia		
Neuroendocrine tumors of the thymus		***Malignant***
		Neuroblastoma
Germ cell tumors		Neuorosarcoma
Seminoma		Ganglioneuroblastoma
Non-Seminoma		Sympathicoblastoma
Choriocarcimona		Malignant peripheral nerve sheath tumor
Embrymonal		
Teratoma		
		Can Be Benign or Malignant
		Pheochromcytoma
		Paraganglioma

dyspnea; and venous engorgement. When an SVC syndrome presents acutely, this constitutes a medical emergency.

The Anterior Mediastinum

Solid masses in the anterior mediastinum warrant careful evaluation. Injudicious use of biopsies may cause dissemination of a potentially curable cancer, as in the case of thymoma. In addition, surgical resection may expose the patient to unnecessary operative risks, as in the case of lymphoma. Fine needle aspiration has a minor role in the workup of anterior mediastinal masses, because the results are usually nondiagnostic and may seed malignancy into unwanted areas. Once a solid anterior mediastinal mass is identified, typically via CT scanning, the decision about whether to proceed with core biopsy or excision of the mass and surrounding tissue is best directed with thoracic surgical consultation from the beginning stages of the workup. If core biopsies are indicated, optimally there is direct communication between the thoracic surgeon and interventional radiologist or other subspecialist(s). Preoperative evaluation may include measurement of serum beta-human chorionic gonadotropin (β-hCG), alpha-fetoprotein (αFP), lactate dehydrogenase (LDH), and/or testicular examination with ultrasound examination when there is clinical suspicion of germ-cell tumors. When myasthenia gravis is suspected, a diagnostic evaluation may include a Tensilon test, serum anti-acetylcholine-receptor antibody assay, and/or single-fiber electromyography.

Thymoma is the most common primary mediastinal mass, representing approximately 25–30% of all neoplasms.[8] Most thymomas occur in the fourth decade of life. About half of patients with thymoma present with symptoms. These are typically local symptoms such as cough, dyspnea, chest pain, and, less commonly, limb swelling or superior vena cava syndrome. Constitutional symptoms may also be present such as fever, fatigue, and weight loss. Paraneoplastic syndromes can occur in association with thymoma. These include myasthenia gravis, pure red cell aplasia, rheumatoid arthritis, systemic lupus erythematosus, ulcerative colitis, and other cytopenias or rheumatologic disorders.

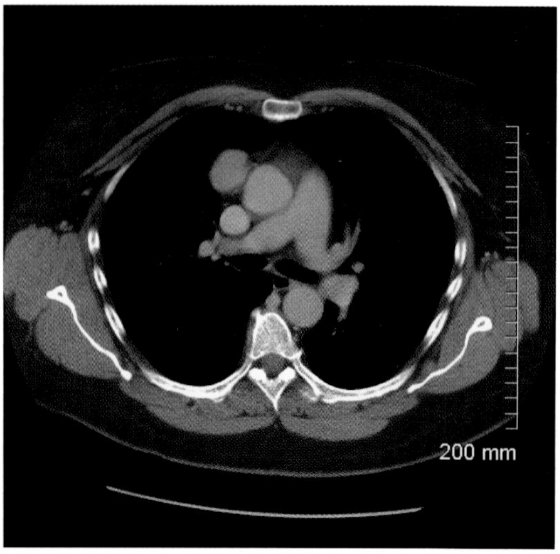

Figure 1. CT of anterior mediastinal mass consistent with thymoma.

The diagnosis of thymoma is suspected largely on CT imaging (Figure 1). In some situations when the CT is equivocal, MRI is sometimes helpful in determining solid versus cystic masses. Fluorine-18 fluorodeoxyglucose (FDG) positron emission tomography (PET) can be a useful tool in distinguishing thymic hyperplasia (lower uptake, more homogenous) from carcinoma.[9] FDG-PET is also highly sensitive in identifying residual, recurrent, or ectopic tissue.[10]

Many staging and classification systems have been developed, though few have offered accurate prognostic information. Current staging of thymic masses is based on a system devised by Masaoka and colleagues in 1981.[11] Masaoka staging is a system based on tumor invasion combining gross inspection at the time of surgery as well as histologic evaluation (Table 2a). The World Health Organization (WHO) histological classification system (Table 2b) has also been adopted. Yet the value of its prognostic information still remains the subject of debate.[12]

Table 2a. Modified Masaoka Staging for Thymoma

Masaoka Stage	Disease Extent
I	Macroscopic and microscopic encapsulation
IIA	Microscopic transcapsular invasion
IIB	Macroscopic invasion into mediastinal fat or adherent to but not through the mediastinal pleura
III	Invasion into surrounding organs
IVA	Pleural or pericardial dissemination
IVB	Lymphogenous or hematogenous metastases

Table 2b. WHO Classification of Thymoma

WHO Classification	Histology
Type A	Spindle cell; medullary
Type AB	Mixed
Type B1	Lymphocyte-rich; lymphocytic; predominantly cortical
Type B2	Cortical
Type B3	Well-differentiated thymic carcinoma; epithelial; squamoid
Type C	Thymic carcinoma

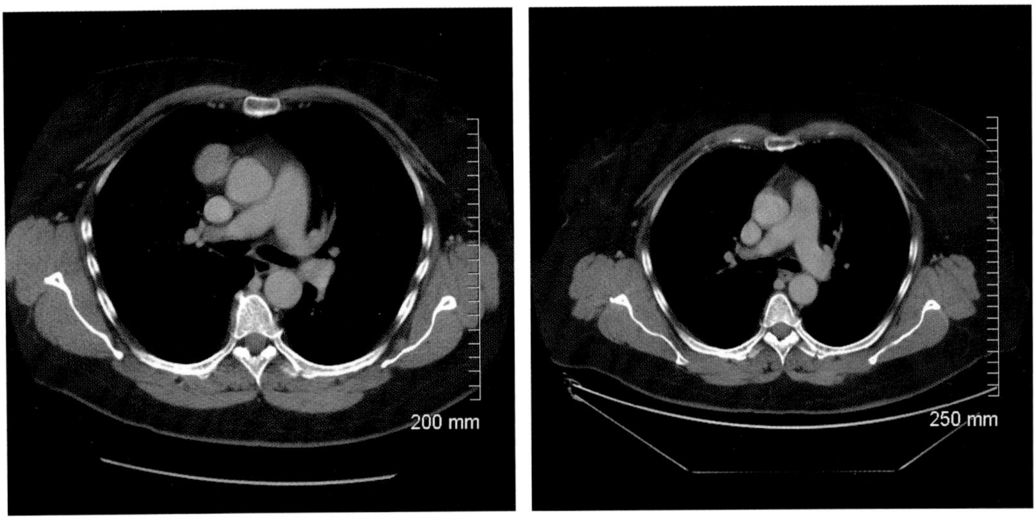

Figure 2. Pre- (left) *and post-resection* (right) *CT of Masaoka stage 1 thymoma via right robotic technique.*

An isolated, well-circumscribed mass in the anterior mediastinum suspicious for thymoma should prompt surgical removal (Figures 2, 3a, 3b). This eliminates the possibility of disrupting the capsule of a thymoma and negating a potential cure. For Masaoka stage I tumors, surgical resection alone is sufficient. Consideration of adjuvant radiation for resected stage II tumors should be given when there is histologic evidence of extracapsular invasion. For Masaoka stage III and IV tumors, multimodality treatment strategies continue to be the topic of ongoing investigation. The National Comprehensive Cancer Network® guidelines are an excellent reference for the workup and management of thymomas, as well as thymic carcinomas and other cancers. These guidelines are the result of 21 leading cancer centers' expert opinions and summary statements of evidence-based data.[13]

Other masses of the thymus include benign thymic hyperplasia (Figure 4), thymic cysts (Figure 5), thymolipoma, small cell carcinoma of the thymus and neuroendocrine tumors of the thymus. Thymic hyperplasia and thymolipoma are often associated with paraneoplastic syndromes, and resection is typically curative. Neuroendocrine tumors and small cell carcinoma of the thymus are aggressive cancers

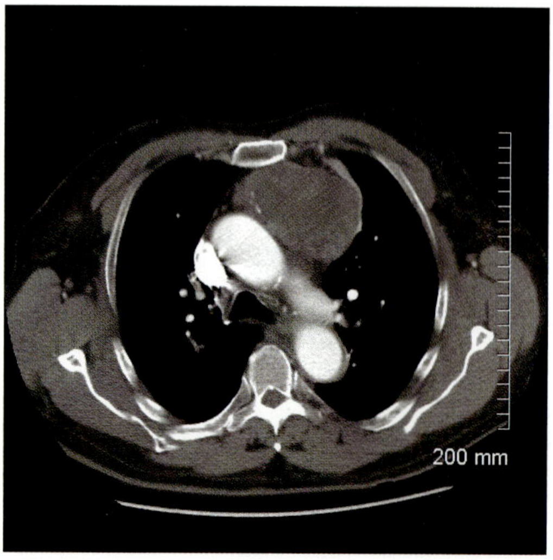

Figure 3a. CT of Masaoka stage IIA thymoma. Required sternotomy for resection.

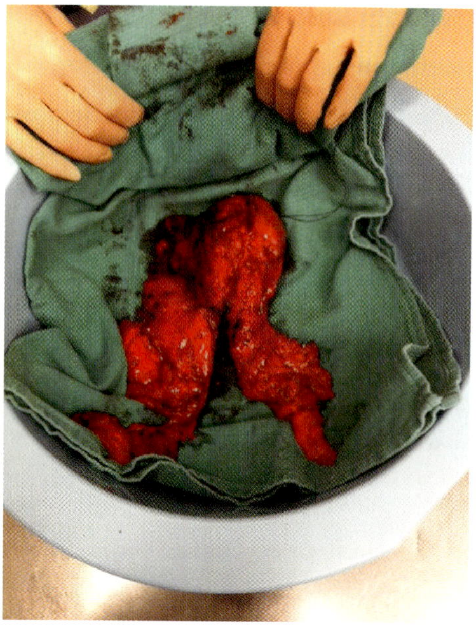

Figure 3b. Corresponding photo of the gross specimen. Thymoma measured 9.5 cm × 8.5 cm × 5.5 cm, thymus gland measured 28.5 cm × 12.5 cm × 6.5 cm and weighed 393 grams.

with low survivability, though surgery can be curative if the tumors are small and confined to the thymus.[14]

Myasthenia gravis (MG) occurs in association with thymoma. Myasthenia gravis is an autoimmune neuromuscular disorder in which autoantibodies are produced against the nicotinic acetylcholine receptors. Patients present with weakness and rapid voluntary muscle fatiguability. Ocular muscles are often involved, manifesting diplopia as the most common initial symptom and rendering ptosis on examination. The incidence of myasthenia is 3 to 4 per million per year and is twice as high in women. Approximately 10% of patients with MG have thymomas, whereas 30% of patients with a thymoma will have clinical evidence of MG. Surgical resection of the thymus in myasthenia gravis can be indicated with or without the presence of thymoma. For patients offered thymectomy, 35% experienced complete remission and 33% experienced significant improvement, where only 7.6% and 17%, respectively, were found in medically managed controls.[15] Resection of thymoma in patients with MG is best approached in a multidisciplinary fashion, including a neurologist and thoracic surgeon, as these patients may require IVIG or plasmapheresis preoperatively. Obtaining baseline pulmonary function testing and monitoring the postoperative pulmonary reserve, narcotics, and myasthenic medications must be done with great attention to detail to minimize morbidity.

Lymphoma is the most common mediastinal mass among adult patients younger than 40. It frequently presents with B-type symptoms: fever, chills, night sweats, and malaise. Both Hodgkin's and non-Hodgkin's lymphoma can present with mediastinal masses. When palpable, extrathoracic lymphadenopathy should be biopsied first. When lymphadenopathy is isolated in the mediastinum, image guided multiple ***core*** biopsies can be performed. If this does not provide adequate

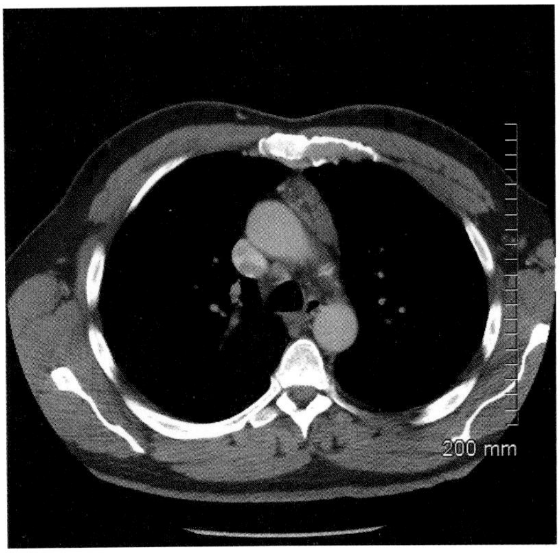

Figure 4. CT of thymic hyperplasia.

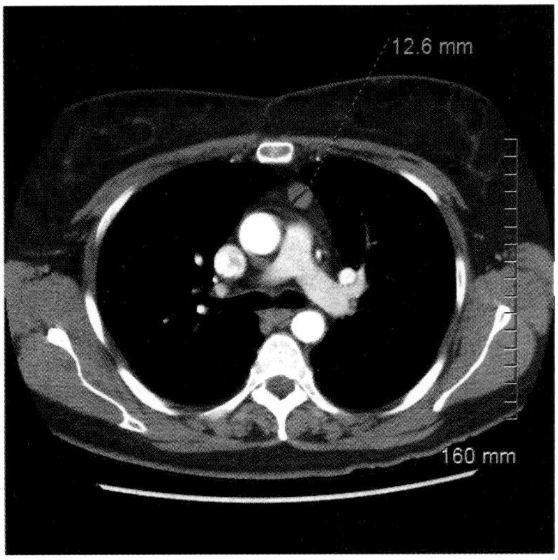

Figure 5. CT of thymic cyst.

tissue, a surgical approach with mediastinoscopy, anterior mediastinotomy, or VATS is required to establish the diagnosis. Combination chemotherapy regimens, with or without radiation, are the mainstays of treatment.

The mediastinum is the most common extragonadal location of *primary germ-cell tumors.* Malignant germ-cell tumors occur almost exclusively in men.[16] The peak incidence occurs in the third decade. Most patients with malignant germ-cell tumors present with symptoms. CT imaging demonstrates characteristic, though nonspecific, findings of a heterogeneous mass with areas of calcification, necrosis, and often hemorrhage.[17] Malignant germ-cell tumors are classified as either seminomatous or non-seminomatous. The diagnosis can be suggested with serum LDH, αFP, and β-hCG and confirmed with needle biopsy. Seminomas are *not* associated with elevated αFP, whereas non-seminomas have high levels of αFP and β-hCG. The primary treatment for seminomas includes radiation. Non-seminomas require chemotherapy *and* radiation. Surgery is reserved for patients who normalize their serum markers after chemoradiotherapy but have a residual mediastinal mass. Benign teratomas are the only germ-cell tumor that occurs with equal frequency in men and women. Surgical resection should be offered for symptomatic lesions.

Thyroid masses in the mediastinum most frequently extend from a cervical goiter or represent primary mediastinal thyroid tissue. Signs and symptoms include stridor, hoarseness, dysphagia, and other locally compressive symptoms. It is rare for tumors other than thyroid masses to demonstrate tracheal deviation on chest x-ray.[7] The most common pathology is benign multinodular goiter. Primary thyroid carcinomas and lymphomas can also occur. Unlike in the easily accessible cervical thyroid, fine needle aspiration (FNA) is not indicated prior to surgical resection as it can lead to bleeding and other complications. If surgical risk is low, CT imaging is usually adequate for the diagnosis of substernal thyroid, and its presence usually warrants resection if the benefit of such surgery outweighs the potential harm.

A transverse collar incision usually provides sufficient access to most substernal goiters since the blood supply almost always arises from the inferior thyroid vessels. When this exposure is not adequate, a partial sternotomy is classically performed. Combined open cervical and mediastinal robotic procedures have been performed with excellent results. Complete mediastinal aberrant thyroid, also termed primary intrathoracic goiter, is encountered in less than 1% of all surgically resected goiters.[18] These lesions gain their blood supply from thoracic vessels and thus preclude safe removal through the neck. Surgical removal with VATS or robotic-assisted techniques can be performed safely and effectively, and thus avoids the morbidity associated with thoracotomy or median sternotomy.[19]

There are multiple experiences using VATS and robotic approaches to the anterior mediastinum.[20] Our single institution experience has included more than 30 minimally invasive approaches to the anterior mediastinum using a VATS or da Vinci platform with no mortality and minimal morbidity. The typical length of stay has been 2 to 3 days. The robotic approach to the anterior mediastinum in our practice has been typically through the right hemithorax with 4 ports. On occasion, a bilateral approach is utilized, if additional left sided visualization is required. The right chest offers the advantage of being larger and thus allows more working room and better visualization. There have been reports of lethal cardiac injuries through left-sided approaches. Therefore, we do not utilize a solely left-sided technique, nor do we advocate this. There are centers in Europe that approach the anterior mediastinum through the left and have done so in larger series with no adverse complications.[21]

Our practice is to place an arterial line preoperatively. General anesthesia is induced via placement of a double lumen endotracheal tube, which is positioned bronchoscopically. A Foley catheter is then placed. The patient's right lateral torso is positioned at the right edge of the operating table. The patient has a pressure bag infuser placed vertically beneath the right hemithorax, which is inflated maximally. The right arm is held in a foam cradle posteriorly in order to expose the lateral hemithorax. We place our ports in the third, fifth, seventh, and eighth interspaces in the right hemithorax (Figure 6). The third and seventh interspace ports are 8 mm da Vinci ports available for a hook cautery and

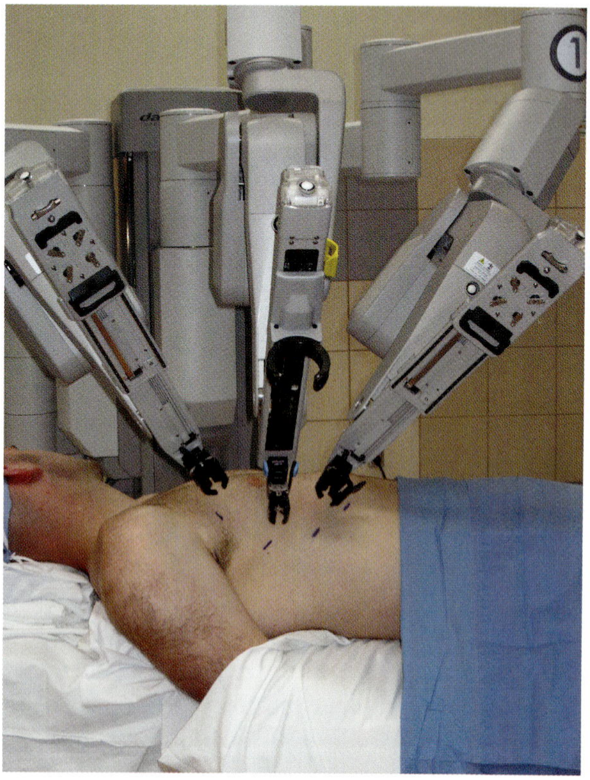

Figure 6. Setup and positioning for anterior mediastinal mass resection.

Cadiere forceps. The fifth interspace port is for the 30 degree angled camera, and the eighth interspace port is a 5 mm or 12 mm assistant port for suction and retraction, based on the surgeon's preference. Insufflation of CO_2 gas to a pressure of 6–10 mmHg can be helpful, as well, as long as hemodynamic stability is maintained.

Dissection for an anterior mediastinal exoneration or thymectomy for thymoma typically proceeds from inferior to superior, with specific attention given to the phrenic nerve and its course. No undue tension is placed on the phrenic nerve, and electrocautery in this area is avoided. Clips can be placed medial to the nerve for guidance of postoperative radiation, should it be required. A "no touch" technique is used when a thymoma, in particular, is being resected to avoid tumor cell spillage. In addition, great effort is taken to inspect the pleural space for any drop metastases.

The dissection proceeds inferiorly to superiorly with inclusion of the pericardiophrenic fat as well as the adipose tissue around the upper poles of the thymus, which are teased down from the neck. Care is also taken to doubly clip all larger venous branches from the innominate vein in the mediastinum. Smaller vessels are typically controlled with cautery. In myasthenia gravis, it is critical to remove every gram of thymus, as even a small amount left behind can affect the patient's remission rate. Once the thymus with the tumor has been detached, it is placed into an Endobag and removed through a port, which is typically extended to 2 cm in size with cautery of the intercostal muscles on either side. We prefer removal through the fifth or seventh interspace, as the rib space is wider at this point. The hemithorax is copiously irrigated with sterile water, a chest tube is placed, the CO_2 insufflation is evacuated, and re-expansion of the lung is directly visualized. The port sites are closed, and the patient is extubated in the operating room suite.

The Middle Mediastinum

Solid masses in the middle mediastinum are rarely primary cancers. Metastases to the subcarinal lymph nodes from head and neck, lung, and esophageal cancers make up a large portion of tumors found here. Lymphomas, granulomatous infections such as histoplasmosis and coccidiomycosis, as well as sarcoidosis represent the remainder of commonly encountered solid lesions in the middle mediastinum.

Unlike the anterior and posterior compartments, surgical resection of solid lesions in the middle mediastinum is rarely indicated as a primary treatment modality. Endobronchial ultrasound-guided transbronchial needle aspiration (EBUS-TBNA) and endoscopic ultrasound-guided fine needle aspiration (EUS-FNA) are capable of safely diagnosing and staging most solid lesions in the middle mediastinum and are largely becoming the initial modality of choice. EBUS-TBNA and EUS-FNA are performed with local anesthesia and sedation in an outpatient setting. For lesions in certain paraesophageal and subcarinal stations, however, mediastinoscopy is still required and carries low morbidity.[22] When these techniques fail to provide adequate tissue, VATS or, very rarely, a right thoracotomy may be required.

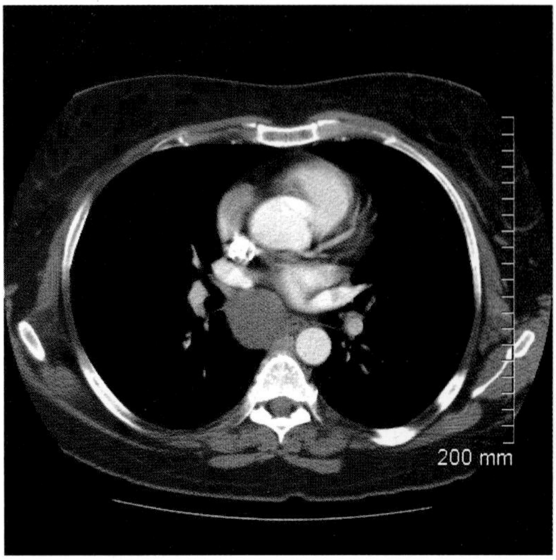

Figure 7. CT of incidental finding of middle mediastinal bronchogenic cyst.

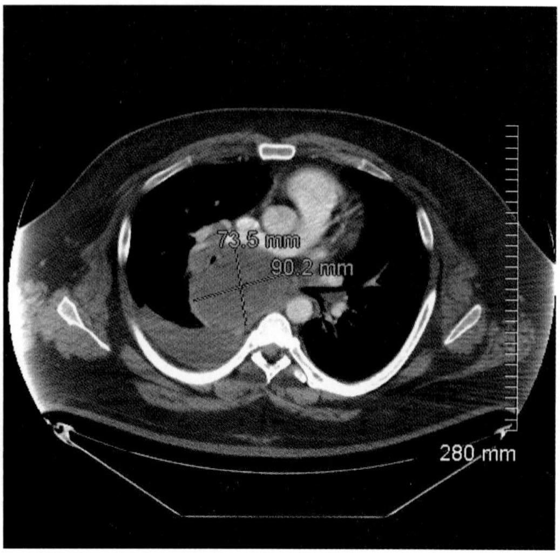

Figure 8. CT of infected middle mediastinal bronchogenic cyst after Wang needle biopsy.

Cystic lesions occur throughout the mediastinum. The majority are found in the middle mediastinum. Cysts represent between 13 and 30% of all mediastinal masses.[23] Their appearance on imaging is a dense, often calcified, outer capsule with a homogenous, fluid-filled center. Mediastinal cysts are defined by their histology rather than their location. The most common are bronchogenic cysts followed by esophageal duplication cysts and neuroenteric cysts. Pericardial, thymic, and thoracic duct cysts are rare.

The diagnosis of a mediastinal cyst is typically made on CT imaging (Figure 7). A barium esophogram, upper endoscopy, or bronchoscopy should be considered if there is concern for communication with the foregut or tracheobroncheal tree. Surgery is reserved for symptomatic lesions. However, some physicians advocate for surgery prior to the onset of symptoms, as asymptomatic patients may have better outcomes, especially with the low morbidity of resection using minimally invasive techniques. As a general guideline, cystic lesions of the mediastinum should not be biopsied bronchoscopically or via endoscopic ultrasound guidance as they may become infected and cause grave morbidity and potential mortality to the patient (Figure 8). Many of these lesions can be approached via minimally invasive techniques with a VATS or robotic platform for complete or near total excision to minimize the morbidity for the patient. The workup, operative approach, and positioning are variable depending on the location of the cyst. Typically a minimally invasive resection includes two 8 mm robotic ports and two 12 mm ports as well as single-lung ventilation as described above. Conversion rates to thoracotomy are low. The postoperative hospital stay is typically 1–2 days, and morbidity is minimal.[20]

Our approach has been via an over-rotated lateral decubitus position (Figure 9). A 30-degree thoracoscope is positioned in the mid axillary line eighth interspace, a hook cautery in the sixth interspace anterior axillary line, and a Cadiere forceps in the posterior auscultory triangle after the da Vinci Robotic System has been docked. An assistant port can be placed in the seventh interspace more anteriorly if needed for suction, clips, or staplers, as required. Gas insufflation is established to a pressure of 6–10 mmHg after initiation of single-lung ventilation to facilitate downward retraction of the lung. The inferior pulmonary ligament is mobilized to the level of the pulmonary vein. The pleura overlying the cystic mass is then opened. Typically, we do not recommend aspiration of the cystic mass unless it is so tense it cannot be grasped, in which case a 21 gauge aspirating needle is used to remove 10–20 cc of fluid. The Cadiere is then placed over the needle entrance point to prevent further spillage. The cystic mass is mobilized to its base. It is important to have no suction within the bronchus, as this can distort the membranous portion and cause potential cautery injuries during dissection. Once the base of the cyst is localized and dissected, an articulating stapler, 45 mm in length and 3.5 mm in diameter, is passed across the base, and the cyst is ligated and divided. The cyst is then placed into an Endobag and removed. After irrigation, a chest tube is placed through the most inferior port. The robotic system is undocked. The lung is reexpanded under direct visualization, port sites are closed, and the patient is extubated in the operating suite. In our experience, the patients are discharged on postoperative day 2 pending chest tube removal and acceptable pain control. The exception to the above scenario has been in patients with infected mediastinal cysts. Management of infected cysts is far more complex and beyond the scope of this discussion.

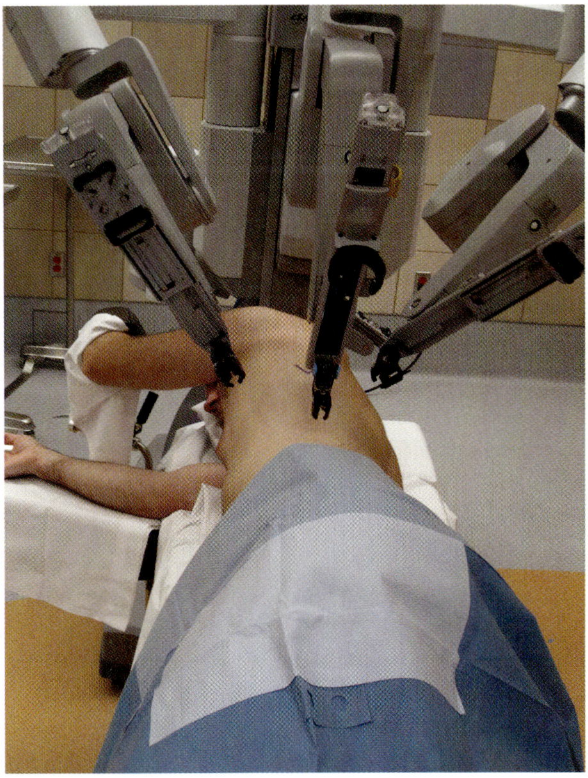

Figure 9. Setup and positioning for middle and posterior mediastinal mass resection.

The Posterior Mediastinum

Primary tumors of the posterior mediastinum are rarely malignant in adults and seldom present with symptoms. In children, however, up to 60% of posterior mediastinal tumors are malignant.[24] In adults, these lesions most commonly originate from the nerve sheath, whereas in pediatric neoplasms, ganglionic morphologies predominate. Patients with von Recklinghausen's neurofibromatosis may present with multiple cancers and tend to have a poor prognosis.

In general, CT imaging is typically sufficient for preoperative evaluation (Figure 10). When suspicion of pheochromocytoma

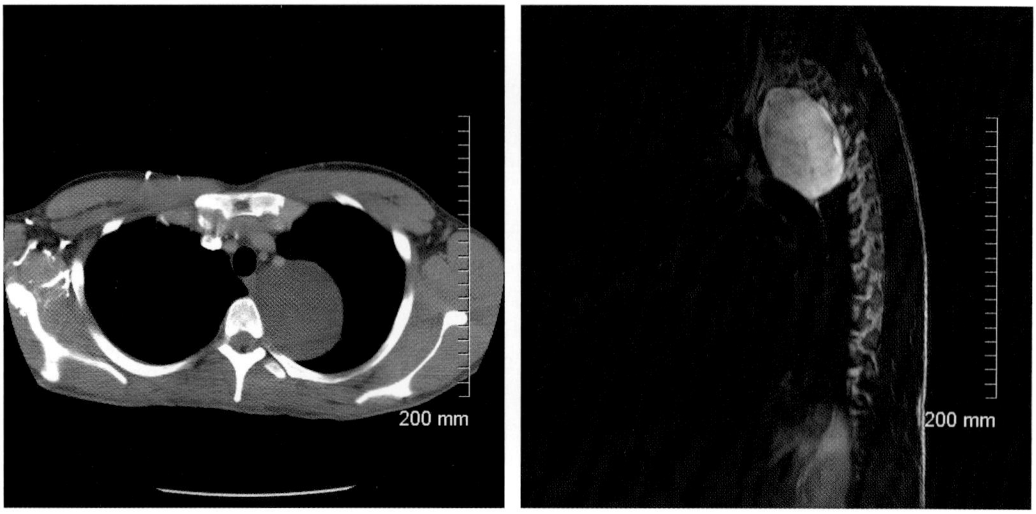

Figure 10. CT (left) *and MRI* (right) *of posterior mediastinal tumor (7.5 cm × 7.5 cm × 2.0 cm, 172 gm ganglioneuroma, removed via da Vinci robotic resection).*

exists, consideration should be made to perform an assessment of catecholamine metabolites. I^{131} meta-iodobenzylguanidine (MIBG) scintigraphy may also be a useful adjunct for pheochromocytoma evaluation.

When a CT scan demonstrates a posterior mediastinal mass and there is extension into the neural foramina, this is termed a *dumbbell tumor.* Suspicion of this problem should prompt a preoperative MRI. Once confirmed, a combined thoracic and neurosurgical approach should be employed. Dumbbell tumors add technical complexity to surgical resection, though intraspinal extension does not worsen the prognosis.[25]

Complete surgical resection is the preferred treatment for both benign and malignant neoplasms of the posterior mediastinum. This is curative for stage I and II cancers. For stage III and IV cancers, a multimodality treatment strategy with chemo/radiotherapy, either neoadjuvantly or adjuvantly, is recommended.

The standard surgical approach is through a posterolateral thoracotomy, though VATS and robotic surgery in the posterior mediastinum can be performed safely. In some reported cases, the added dexterity afforded to the robotic surgeon has allowed tumors not accessible to conventional VATS to be resected with minimally invasive robotic techniques.[26] Median hospital lengths of stay in some current series are as short as 1 day.[27] Our experience with minimally invasive excision of posterior mediastinal tumors has been favorable. Our single institution experience has performed over 5 posterior mediastinal tumor excisions robotically with no mortality or morbidity. The length of stay was approximately 2 days.

The positioning of the patient is similar to that of a middle mediastinal cystic mass resection (Figure 9). When combined with neurosurgery, the intraspinous component is performed first. The patient's endotracheal tube is exchanged for a double lumen tube and the patient is repositioned. Single-lung and intrathoracic CO_2 gas insufflation is employed as described above. Clips are used at all the nerve roots and for larger vessels. Each of our cases utilized an assistant port.

Summary

Solid masses of the anterior mediastinum warrant careful evaluation. Fine needle aspiration has little role unless metastatic cancer is suspected in paratracheal lymph nodes. Thymoma is the most common primary solid mediastinal mass, representing approximately 25–30% of all neoplasms, and often requires excision with en bloc thymectomy for diagnosis and treatment. Minimally invasive thymectomy via VATS or robotic techniques is becoming less controversial, though large series with long-term data are not available in the setting of early stage thymoma. Minimally invasive VATS and robotic techniques for biopsy of anterior mediastinal masses are important tools in the armamentarium for diagnoses and treatment along with mediastinoscopy, endobronchial ultrasound guided bronchoscopy, standard bronchoscopy, and electromagnetic navigation guided bronchoscopy.

It is advantageous to have thoracic surgical input for guidance regarding the necessity and type of biopsy for anterior mediastinal masses. Injudicious use of certain modalities can lead to morbidity from procedures that were, from the onset, likely to be nondiagnostic, and seeding of tumors can occur if performed incorrectly. More advanced neoplasms require multidisciplinary strategies.

Middle mediastinal masses, when solid, rarely require resection as the primary treatment modality. Endobronchial ultrasound-guided transbronchial needle aspiration and endoscopic ultrasound-guided fine needle aspiration are capable of safely diagnosing and staging most solid lesions in the middle mediastinum and are largely becoming the initial modality of choice. They are performed with local anesthesia and minimal sedation in an outpatient setting. Mediastinoscopy is still required for some lesions to establish diagnosis. Cystic lesions in the middle mediastinum should, in general, *not* be needle biopsied as they can become infected. If symptomatic or large, resection is indicated and can often be performed using minimally invasive techniques via VATS or robotic assistance in experienced centers, with little or no morbidity or mortality and low conversion rates to thoracotomy.

Posterior mediastinal masses in adults are typically benign incidental findings. These tumors can have an intraspinous component (the dumbbell tumor). Posterior mediastinal tumors are best referred for surgical evaluation and opinion as to the risk versus benefit of a watchful waiting strategy versus operative excision.

Minimally invasive and robotic surgery continues to evolve. The goal of our era as physicians and surgeons is to maximize diagnostic and oncologic resection abilities, while minimizing recovery time and the physical insult to the human being. This allows our patients to tolerate multimodality therapies with ease, recover faster, and preserve their quality of life without the consequences that patients historically have suffered with traditional open approaches via thoracotomy and/or sternotomy.

References

1. Carlens D. Mediastinoscopy: a method for inspection and tissue biopsy in the superior mediastinum. *Dis Chest.* 1956;36(10):343–52.
2. Hazelrig S., Nunchuck S, LoCicero J. Video Assisted Thoracic Surgery Study Group data. *Ann Thorac Surg.* 1993 Nov;56(5):1039–43.
3. Swanson SJ, Meyers BF, Gunnarsson CL, et al. Video-assisted thoracoscopic lobectomy is less costly and morbid than open lobectomy: a retrospective multiinstitutional database analysis. *Ann Thorac Surg.* 2012 Apr;93(4):1027–37.
4. Scott W, Allen M, Darling G, et al. Video-assisted thoracic surgery versus open lobectomy for lung cancer: a secondary analysis of data from the American College of Surgeons Oncology Group Z0030 randomized clinical trial. *J Cardiovasc Surg.* 2010;139 (4):976–81.
5. Augustin F, Schmid T, Bodner J. (2006). The robotic approach for mediastinal lesions. *Int J Med Robot.* 2006;2(3):262–70.
6. Kajiwara N, Taira M, Yoshida K, et al. Early experience using the da Vinci Surgical System for the treatment of mediastinal tumors. *Gen Thorac Cardiovasc Surg.* 2011;59(10): 693–8.
7. Shields TW. Primary tumors and cysts of the mediastinum. In: *General Thoracic Surgery.* Philadelphia, PA: Lea & Febiger; 1972.
8. Whooley BP, Urschel JD, Antkowiak JG, Takita H. Primary tumors of the mediastinum. *J Surg Oncol.* 1999 Feb;70(2):95–99.
9. Ferdinand B, Gupta P, Kramer E. Spectrum of thymic uptake at 18F-FDG PET. *Radiographics.* 2004;24(6):1611–6.
10. El-Bawaba H, Al-Sugaira A, Rafaya M, Hajjarb W, Mahdya M, Al-Kattana K. Role of flourine-18 fluorodeoxyglucose positron emission tomography in thymic pathology. *Eur J Cardiothor Surg.* 2007;31(4):731–6.
11. Masaoka A, Monden Y, Nakahara K. Follow-up study of thymomas with special reference to their clinical stages. *Cancer.* 1981;48:2485–92.
12. Kim D, Yang W, Choi S, Kim K, Chung K. Prognostic and clinical relevance of the World Health Organization schema for the classification of thymic epithelial tumors: a clinicopathologic study of 108 patients and literature review. *Chest.* 2005;127(3):755–61.
13. National Comprehensive Cancer Network. NCCN guidelines for treatment of cancer by site. Retrieved July 12, 2012, from http://www.nccn.org/professionals/physician_gls/f_guidelines.asp#site.
14. Galanis E, Frytak S, Lloyd R. Extrapulmonary small cell carcinoma. *Cancer.* 1997; 79(9):1729–36.
15. Buckingham JM, Howard Jr FM, Bernatz PE, et al. The value of thymectomy in myasthenia gravis: a computer-assisted matched study. *Ann Surg.* 1976;184(4):453–58.
16. Moran C, Suster S. Primary germ cell tumors of the mediastinum: analysis of 322 cases with special emphasis on teratomatous lesions and a proposal for histopathologic classification and clinical staging. *Cancer.* 1997;80(4):681–90.
17. Strollo D, Rosado de Christenson M, Jett J. Primary mediastinal tumors. Part I: tumors of the anterior mediastinum. *Chest.* 1997;112(2):511–22.
18. Katlic MR, Wang CA, Grillo HC. Substernal goiter. *Ann Thorac Surg.* 1985 Apr; 39(4):391–99.
19. Grondin S. Buenaventura P, Luketich J. Thoracoscopic resection of an ectopic intrathoracic goiter. *Ann Thorac Surg.* 2001 May;71(5):1697–98.

20. Weissenbachaer A, Boner J. Robotic surgery of the mediastinum. In: Mineo TC, Ferguson MK, eds. *Thoracic Surgery Clinics: Technical Advances in Mediastinal Surgery.* Philadelphia, PA: W. B. Saunders; 2010: vol. 20, 331–338.

21. Ruckert JC, Swierzy M, Ismail M. Comparison of robotic and nonrobotic thoracoscopic thymectomy: a cohort study. *J Thorac Cardiovasc Surg.* 2011 Mar;141(3):673–77.

22. Cerfolio R, Bryant A, Eloubeidi M, et al. The true false negative rate of esophageal and endobronchial ultrasound in the staging of mediastinal lymph nodes in patients with non-small cell lung cancer. *Ann Thorac Surg.* 2010;90(2):427–34.

23. Takeda S, Miyoshi S, Minami M, Ohta M, Masaoka A, Matsuda H. Clinical spectrum of mediastinal cysts. *Chest.* 2003;124(1):125–32.

24. King D, Groner J, Teich S. Mediastinal cysts and tumors. In: Zeigler M, Azizkhan RG, Weber TR, *Operative Pediatric Surgery.* New York, NY: McGraw-Hill; 2003:407–419.

25. Carlsen N, Christensen I, Schroeder H, et al. Prognostic factors in neuroblastomas treated in Denmark from 1943 to 1980: a statistical estimate of prognosis based on 253 cases. *Cancer.* 1986;58:2726–35.

Chapter Six

Lung Cancer

Christina L. Harsant, MD; Vita V. McCabe, MD; Ajay Gupta, MD

Epidemiology and Screening for Lung Cancer

Lung cancer is the most lethal cancer in the United States. According to statistics from the National Cancer Institute Surveillance Epidemiology and End Results (SEER) Program, there will be an estimated 226,160 new diagnoses with 160,340 deaths due to lung cancer in 2012.[1] By examining recent trends, approximately 6.99% or 1 in 14 of the contemporary population will be diagnosed with lung cancer during their lifetime.[1]

Unfortunately, an estimated 85–90% of all lung cancer cases are attributable to cigarette smoking or secondhand smoke.[2] Despite advances in imaging, the majority of lung cancer cases present at an advanced stage, where tumor resection is not beneficial. Considering all patients diagnosed with lung cancer, overall 5-year survival remains only 15% from the time of diagnosis.[1] Fifteen percent of all lung cancer patients present with disease confined to their primary tumor and 22% with spread limited to regional lymph nodes, resulting in 5-year survival rates for these two groups of 52.2% and 25.1%, respectively.[1]

Lung cancer is broadly divided into two major categories—small cell and non–small cell lung cancer (NSCLC), with the latter representing greater than 85% of all lung cancers. Surgical therapy has a central role in the treatment of early-stage NSCLC. Thus, this type of cancer treatment is the focus of the following discussion. It is in this group of patients that surgical resection is of greatest benefit.

Survival rates are significantly improved when lung cancers are diagnosed at early stages. As a result, screening to increase the number of patients diagnosed at an early stage is reasonable. Data from both the National Lung Screening Trial (NLST) and the International Early Lung Cancer Action Program (I-ELCAP) have demonstrated decreased mortality in patients who underwent low-dose helical computerized tomography (CT) scanning. Both screening protocols, however, were targeted at higher-risk individuals. Therefore, current National Comprehensive Cancer Network (NCCN) screening guidelines recommend baseline low-dose computed tomography (LDCT) imaging of the chest for high-risk individuals with no symptoms suggestive of lung cancer. High-risk individuals are defined as:

- older than 50 years of age,
- *and* those with a greater than 20-pack per year history of smoking,
- *and* those with one additional risk factor such as COPD, family or personal history of lung cancer, or occupational exposure.

Additionally, individuals with the following criteria are also considered high risk:

- aged 55–74 years,
- *and* those who have a greater than 30-pack per year history of smoking,
- *or* less than 15 years of smoking cessation.

If no lung nodules are detected on initial baseline imaging, repeat LDCT should occur on an annual basis for at least three years. The total duration for the highest-risk patients is yet to be determined. Once a nodule is detected, specific algorithms are in place dependent upon the size and characteristics of the nodule. These algorithms include recommendations for further diagnostic workup if needed, as well as subsequent screening.[2] At present, insurance companies have not adopted payment strategies for LDCT lung cancer screening programs nationally despite endorsement by multiple expert panels such as the American College of Chest Physicians, American Society of Clinical Oncology, American Thoracic Society, and the American Lung Association, among others.

Lung Cancer Presentation and Diagnosis

Asymptomatic patients may present for evaluation of a pulmonary nodule from an incidental finding on chest imaging or from results of screening protocols. Symptomatic patients may complain of cough, wheezing, hemoptysis, shortness of breath, or chest wall pain. Symptoms suggestive of advanced tumors include dysphagia, hoarseness, recurrent pneumonia, lung abscess, and weight loss. Paraneoplastic syndromes are present in a minority of patients and may include symptoms associated with hypercalcemia, syndrome of inappropriate antidiuretic hormone (SIADH), Cushing's syndrome, and/or Lambert-Eaton syndrome. Central nervous system complaints, such as headache or visual changes, should be noted. Bone pain can be suggestive of metastatic disease.

The imaging workup begins with CT of the chest and should include the upper abdomen, to the level of the adrenal glands. Important characteristics to note on CT imaging include the size of the nodule, its location with regard to the hilum and anatomic lobes, invasion beyond the lung including pleural and mediastinal surface, the presence of a pleural and/or pericardial effusion, lymphadenopathy, and evidence of suspicious liver or adrenal metastases. Any change in the size of a nodule is important if past serial imaging is available and should be retrospectively reviewed.

Tissue diagnosis is the next objective. This is accomplished via a variety of techniques, customarily guided by the location of the lesion. Peripheral lesions may be accessed via CT-guided percutaneous biopsy. More centrally located lesions, or those in close approximation to a sizable bronchus, may be reached with a bronchoscope. Advanced, real-time image-guided techniques for bronchoscopic biopsy are available, such as the superDimension inReach System (Figure 1). Such systems employ electromagnetic navigation linked to the patient's CT scan to guide placement of the bronchoscope within reach of the nodule for more accurate biopsy. In addition, minimally invasive surgical biopsies can be performed with intraoperative

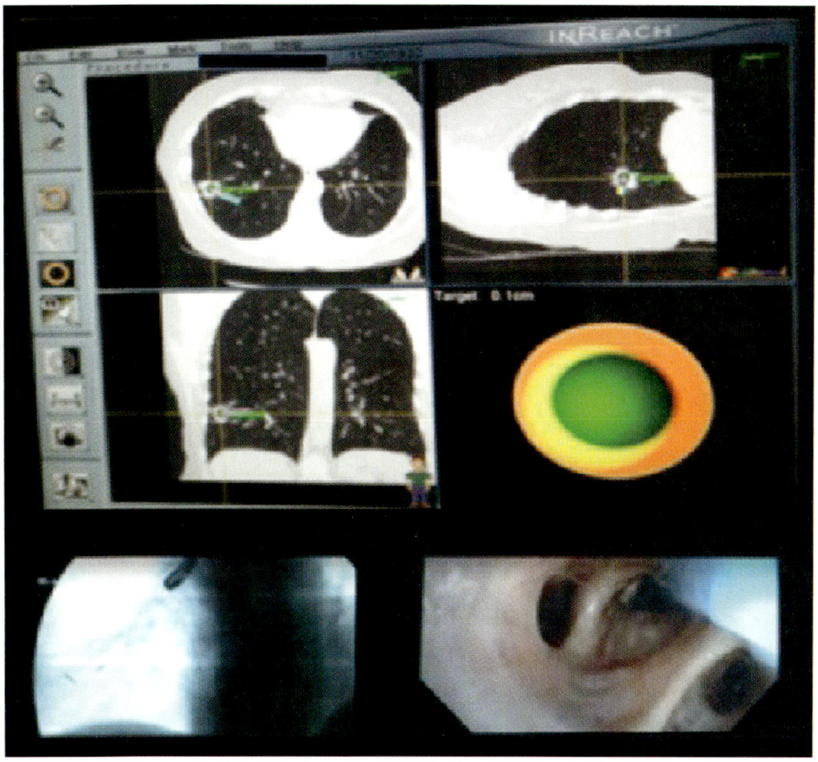

Figure 1. superDimension™ inReach guided placement of fiducials. The left lower image is the corresponding fluoroscopy image and the right lower is the bronchoscopic view.

analysis of the tissue with immediate definitive surgical treatment during the same anesthetic.

Clinical Staging and Preoperative Assessment

The work of a multidisciplinary team is beneficial in the diagnosis, staging, and development of a treatment strategy for lung cancer patients. Team members include thoracic surgeons, pulmonologists, interventional radiologists, medical and radiation oncologists, and nurse navigators, as well as research coordinators. Their cooperative work is essential in the clinical staging of the patient with NSCLC.

The characteristics of the nodule represent the first component of clinical lung cancer staging. Standard TNM staging, as agreed upon by the *American Joint Commission on Cancer*, 7th edition, is outlined in Table 1. Detailed and careful clinical staging is performed, as this determines whether surgical resection is offered. Computerized tomography–positron emission tomography scan and pulmonary function testing are obtained as part of the clinical staging that may include a brain MRI for cases in which advanced disease is suspected. The National Comprehensive Cancer Network® guidelines are an excellent reference for the workup and

Table 1. TNM Staging According to *AJCC* 7/e (with stages offered primary surgical resection highlighted in gray)

T	N	M	Stage
1: does not invade the main bronchus			
a: <2 cm	0	0	IA
b: 2–3 cm	0	0	
Either of above	1	0	IIA
	2	0	IIIA
	3	0	IIIB
	any	1	IV
2: involving any of the following: • main bronchus >2 cm from the carina • atelectasis/obstructive pneumonitis extending to the hilar region, but *not* the entire lung			
a: 3–5 cm	0	0	IB
	1	0	IIA
	2	0	IIIA
	3	0	IIIB
b: 5–7 cm	0	0	IIA
	1	0	IIB
	2	0	IIIA
	3	0	IIIB
Either of above	any	1	IV
3: >7 cm or involves	0	0	IIB
• main bronchus <2 cm from carina	1	0	IIIA
• chest wall	2	0	IIIA
• phrenic nerve	3	0	IIIB
• diaphragm	any	1	IV
• pericardium			
• multiple nodules in a single lobe			
• atelectasis/obstructive pneumonitis of the entire lung			
4: involvement of *any* of the following:	0	0	IIIA
• trachea or carina	1	0	IIIA
• nodules in separate lobes	2	0	IIIB
• mediastinum, heart, or great vessels	3	0	IIIB
• recurrent laryngeal nerve	any	1	IV
• esophagus			
• vertebral bodies			

N

- **0:** no regional nodal involvement
- **1:** *ipsilateral* intrapulmonary, peribronchial, hilar (stations 10–14)
- **2:** *ipsilateral* mediastinal or subcarinal (stations 1–9)
- **3:** *contralateral* mediastinal or hilar nodes *or* ipsilanteral supraclavicular or scalene nodes

M

- 0: no distant metastasis
- 1: distant metastasis (includes malignant pleural effusion)

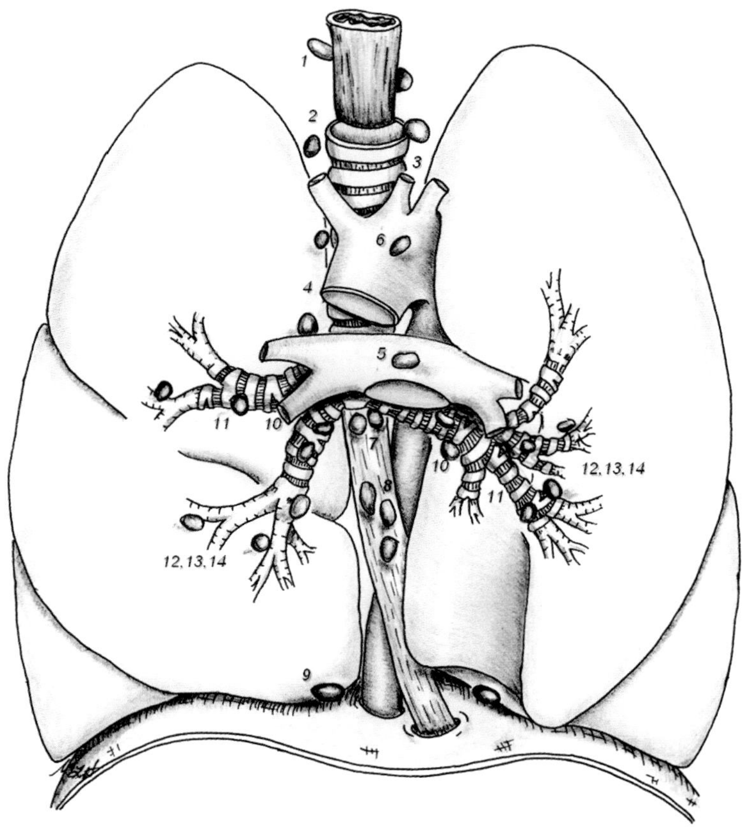

Figure 2. Regional lymph nodes, numbered by station. Note: Stations 5 and 6 are located in a plane ventral to this image with subaortic and para-aortic nodes (5) located lateral to the ligamentum arteriosum and the anterior mediastinal nodes (6) located anterior to the ligamentum arteriosum. Station 1 are the highest mediastinal nodes, located cranial to the image shown. Credit: LaWaun Hance.

management of NSCLC based on an alliance of 21 leading cancer centers' expert opinions and summary statement of evidence-based data.[2]

Continuing with the TNM staging, nodal status is the next component. Preoperative imaging may identify enlarged lymph nodes suspected of harboring malignancy. These are defined as hilar or mediastinal lymph nodes greater than 10 mm in short axis on CT imaging. Pulmonary lymph nodes are classified by stations, according to anatomic location (Figure 2).

Various techniques are employed in lymph node sampling, when indicated, and are dependent upon the location of interest. Endobronchial ultrasound (EBUS)–guided fine needle aspiration can be performed as an outpatient procedure. Mediastinoscopy is another outpatient procedure that allows for larger sample procurement, though it requires a general anesthetic. For this procedure, a small incision is made above the sternal notch and a plane is developed anterior to the trachea and great vessels where a mediastinoscope can be inserted to visualize and guide sampling and/or removal of lymph nodes. For left-sided tumors, the aortic arch poses an obstacle for the sampling of stations 5 and 6 (aortopulmonary window lymph nodes) via a mediastinoscope and these are therefore not reachable via EBUS either. Aortopulmonary (AP) window lymph nodes classically were sampled via a modified Chamberlain procedure with a small incision made on the anterior chest wall in the left second intercostal space, allowing direct access to the aortopulmonary window. This procedure often resulted in significant pain. Many institutions now perform AP window lymph node sampling via left video-assisted thoracoscopic techniques, which offers the advantage of additional evaluation of the pleural cavity and less pain for the patient.

The PET scan and brain MRI imaging complete the evaluation for metastatic disease, which is commonly clinically silent in patients with NSCLC. Clinical staging can now be determined. Ideally, if there is evidence of metastatic disease, such as adrenal or liver metastases, this should be confirmed by biopsy.

Finally, pretreatment pulmonary function assessment is essential. This provides not only a baseline evaluation of the patient's pulmonary status, but also assesses their fitness to tolerate a major operation and provides predictions for postoperative pulmonary function following a proposed resection. If the patient is to undergo radiation therapy as a primary modality, it is also an important pretreatment reference point. Surgical evaluation of pulmonary function should include specific attention to the patient's FEV1 ratio and diffusing capacity factor of the lung for carbon monoxide (DLCO), as well as changes following the use of bronchodilators if the patient suffers from bronchospastic disease. Calculations of postoperative predicted FEV1 and DLCO are helpful risk stratification tools. For higher-risk patients, defined as those with postoperative predicted FEV1 $<40\%$ and/or DLCO $<40\%$, additional cardiopulmonary exercise testing should be obtained to estimate a VO_2 max to further determine the patient's candidacy for surgery.[3] A patient with VO_2 of max <10 or <15, combined with a postoperative predicted DLCO and FEV1 $<40\%$, is considered to have relatively prohibitive surgical risk.[3]

Stage-Specific Treatment of Non–Small Cell Lung Cancer

Patients with clinical stages I and II NSCLC are recommended for curative surgical resection[2] provided they are of acceptable operative risk. Since cardiac disease is often comorbid with pulmonary disease, cardiovascular evaluation is often necessary prior to proceeding with surgical resection. Stage II disease requires adjuvant chemotherapy for highest cure rates. Multimodality protocols, using radiation and chemotherapy, exist for patients with stage IIIA disease in an effort to downstage the patient, making them resectable.[2] Stage IV disease is typically treated with palliative chemotherapy, depending on the patient's performance status and desire to seek treatment. Palliative radiation therapy also plays a role in stage IV disease to decrease pain from metastases, treat brain metastases, or relieve obstruction from tumor invasion within the thoracic cavity.

For patients with early stage tumors but comorbidities or functional status that precludes pulmonary resection, advances in radiation therapy offer hope for curative treatment. Stereotactic radiosurgery, such as CyberKnife®, is an image-guided, robotic-assisted method for the precise delivery of radiation treatment. Pulmonary tumors pose the added difficulty of being in constant motion due to the patient's respirations. Systems such as CyberKnife are ideal for these patients. Preoperative CT imaging is utilized to pinpoint the exact location of the patient's tumor. Gold markers, called fiducials, can then be placed, either via an image-guided percutaneous approach or bronchoscopic procedure. The CyberKnife system combines sensors with the CT imaging to not only locate the tumor, but to track its constant movement with respiration during treatment sessions. The robotic arm and patient-positioning couch adjust to deliver precise radiation beams to the tumor, minimizing effects on adjacent tissues. Two-year survival and local control rates for patients with stage IA tumors are reported as 90% and 95%, respectively, after stereotactic radiosurgical treatment.[4]

The NCCN guidelines delineate treatment regimens for advanced, metastatic, and recurrent disease.[2] Platinum-based chemotherapy regimens are chosen for systemic therapy for advanced or metastatic disease. Intrathoracic irradiation may be used concurrently for locally advanced tumors. Advances in the understanding of tumor biology have paralleled development of targeted therapies according to expression of various receptors by the individual tumor. Pathologic analysis of an adenocarcinoma variant NSCLC should thus include molecular analysis for the expression of epidermal growth factor receptor (EGFR) mutation and anaplastic lymphoma kinase (ALK) positivity. Monoclonal antibody treatment with erlotinib or crizotinib is included as a first line therapy for tumors expressing the EGFR or ALK receptors, respectively. Bevacizumab, targeted at the vascular endothelial growth factor (VEGF) receptor, may also be used in combination with traditional chemotherapy agents.

Surgical Treatment for Non–Small Cell Lung Cancer

The lungs are paired organs in which the primary function is gas exchange. The right lung has three lobes—upper, middle, and lower. The left lung has an upper and lower lobe. The right lung is larger than the left lung. Each lobar bronchus subdivides further into the main unit of the lung known as the bronchopulmonary segment. Individual bronchopulmonary segments are enveloped in connective tissue that is continuous with the visceral pleura and is served by an individual segmental bronchus, artery, and vein. There are 18 bronchopulmonary segments, as listed in Figure 3.

Historically, pneumonectomy was thought to be required for all tumors. The first successful procedure of this type was completed by Graham and Singer in 1933.[5] As early as the 1940s, techniques for the resection of pulmonary lobes and anatomic segmentectomies were developed. Lobectomy, as opposed to pneumonectomy, became the standard oncologic procedure for appropriately located and sized tumors. Lobectomy is recommended over segmentectomy or wedge resection for patients fit to tolerate this anatomic resection due to better survival statistics. Total thoracic mediastinal lymph node dissection is also an integral component of surgical treatment of NSCLC.

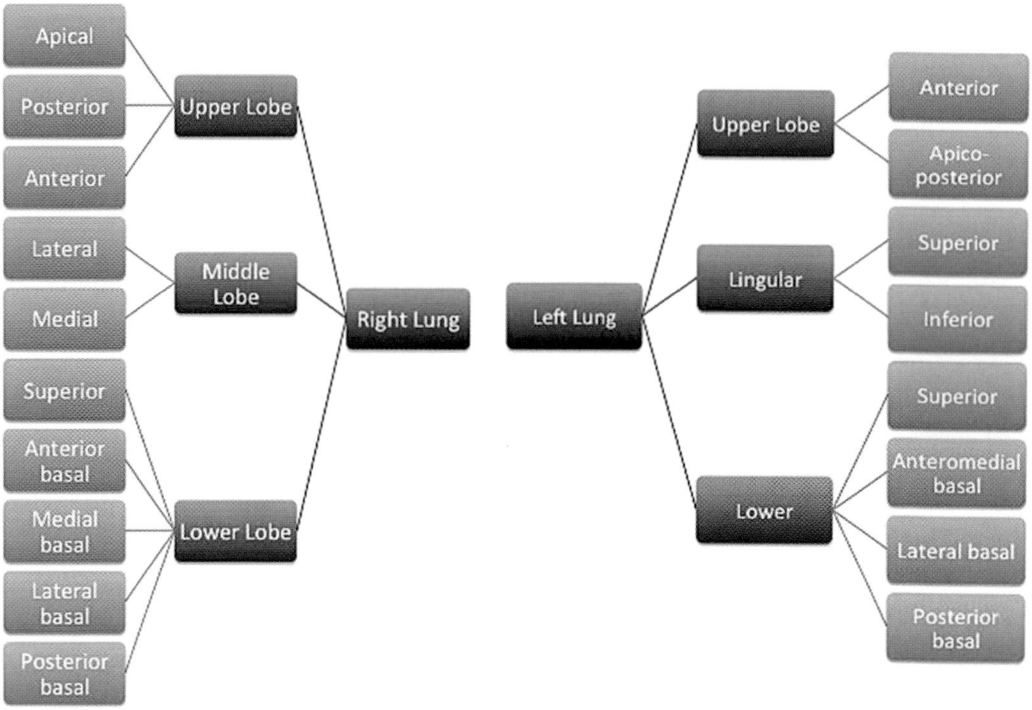

Figure 3. Organization of the bronchopulmonary segments.

Traditionally, lobectomy has required a thoracotomy, which causes significant postoperative pain and is directly attributable to respiratory complications such as pneumonia. Video-assisted thoracoscopic surgery (VATS) had been used for the treatment of benign and infectious disease, as well as diagnostic evaluation of the pleura. It was a natural extension for VATS to be utilized for excisional wedge resection of tumors. However, it soon became clear that formal lobectomy with adequate lymph node dissection is feasible as well. Subgroup analysis of results from the American College of Surgeons Oncology Group Z30 (ACOSOG Z30)[6] trial showed a similar number of lymph nodes could be harvested via a VATS lobectomy as compared to an open thoracotomy.

Further work by Denlinger and colleagues showed that while fewer total number of nodes were sampled with VATS lobectomy, there was no difference in 2-year survival between the VATS and open thoracotomy groups (83% vs. 81% $p = 0.4$).[7] VATS lobectomy became the standard approach for patients with peripheral, early stage cancers.[2] Furthermore, it was demonstrated that patients who needed adjuvant chemotherapy after surgery could receive this treatment at higher rates following VATS versus thoracotomy.[8] Data have shown the oncologic equivalency in outcomes in regard to number of lymph nodes recovered and survival following resection with VATS lobectomy in comparison to open lobectomy.[6] In addition, multiple series have demonstrated an advantage in decreased morbidity with VATS lobectomy, specifically due to decreased postoperative pain and time to return of normal function and improved postoperative pulmonary function.[9] VATS lobec-

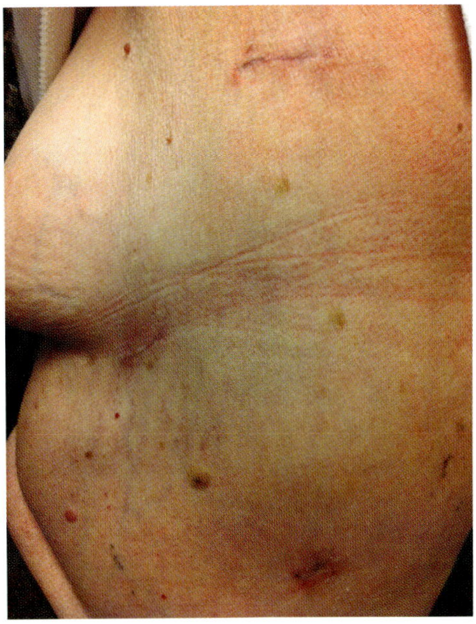

Figure 4. Three small incisions on a patient who underwent a VATS left lower lobectomy.

tomy has also been shown to be cost effective, with decreased length of hospital stays with comparable or even decreased upfront cost to hospitals performing a high volume of VATS cases.[10] Despite these benefits, just over 30% of lobectomies are performed via VATS techniques, according to data from the Society of Thoracic Surgeons database. Since this technique has been adopted as the standard of care for earlier stage tumors, the number of lobectomies performed in this fashion will likely demonstrate a continued increase over the upcoming years.

For a lobectomy via open thoracotomy or VATS approach, general anesthesia with single-lung ventilation is utilized. The patient is placed in a lateral decubitus position with the operative table flexed to maximally open the intercostal spaces. For an open approach, a 10 cm or greater posterolateral thoracotomy incision is made along the direction of the rib space, just inferior to the tip of the scapula. Conversely, VATS lobectomy utilizes two 1 cm incisions and one 3 cm access incision through which the specimen is removed (Figure 4). VATS techniques do not spread the ribs, thereby limiting postoperative pain syndromes, which in post-thoractomy patients can be seen in upwards of 30% of patients.[11] Tumors greater than 6 cm are technically challenging using the VATS approach.

The basic principles for lobectomy are the same whether utilizing an open thoracotomy or a minimally invasive approach. The pulmonary artery, vein, and bronchus supplying the lobe for resection must be dissected and individually ligated and divided. Dissection of the pulmonary artery is particularly delicate as it is more fragile than the corresponding vein. The order in which the artery, vein, and bronchus are dissected and divided is dependent upon surgeon preference and individual anatomic constraints. Vessel loops or ligatures may be used to encircle the structures to aid in the gentle handling of each. Stapling is the most secure method for division and closure of the bronchus and is typically used for the vascular structures as well. Finally, division of the lobe with staplers from the remaining lung is achieved by completing the fissure. Advances in minimally invasive surgical equipment, such as articulating staplers, slide-action instruments, and energy devices, have made VATS lobectomy technically easier and more feasible.

Disadvantages to VATS lobectomy include the two-dimensional view with impairment of depth perception, awkward or unfamiliar viewing and working angles, and concern for the ability to swiftly control sudden significant bleeding. Contrary to this final concern, McKenna and coworkers have shown via a case series of 1,100 VATS lobectomies that these procedures sustain a safe and acceptable blood loss and exhibit no difference in the requirement for re-exploration for bleeding, as compared to open lobectomy.[12] The risk of recurrence at incision sites with VATS lobectomy has also been raised as a concern. However, McKenna's large series again demonstrated a minimal risk, as specimens are typically removed in occlusive bags to prevent tumor spillage and port-site seeding.[11]

Robotic-Assisted VATS Lobectomy

Robotic-assisted VATS techniques provide new dimension to the well-established minimally invasive lobectomy techniques. Completely portal robotic lobectomy with 4 arms (termed CPRL-4) has been reported with safe and oncologically sound results in a study of over 100 patients.[13] Our preference is a 3-arm approach with an assistant working through a traditional thoracoscopic port.

Basic requirements for the operation are similar to those for a traditional VATS setup, including a double-lumen endotracheal tube, large bore intravenous access, and cardiopulmonary monitoring. The patient is then placed in the lateral decubitus position, with the arm held anteriorly and cephalad to expose the posterolateral chest wall. Initial access is obtained at the anterior axillary line in the inframammary fold with a 5 mm incision. The chest is entered and a 30 degree thoracoscope is utilized. Carbon dioxide insufflation to a pressure of 6–10 mmHg is helpful in expediting compression of the lung. Additional ports are placed under direct visualization and the initial site is upsized to a robotic 8 mm port. Another 5 mm robotic port is placed within the posterior auscultatory triangle at the approximate tip of the superior segment of the lower lobe. A 10 mm port, which will serve as the camera port, is placed in the 10th intercostal space along the posterior axillary line. Finally, an accessory port is positioned at a convenient location between the inframammary and posterior axillary ports (often, this is the second port within the 10th intercostal space). The robot is docked over the patient's shoulder and a 30 degree camera, angled downward, is introduced (Figure 5). Monopolar or bipolar electrocautery is placed in the robotic right hand and a thoracic grasper in the left. The inferior pulmonary ligament is divided to the level of the inferior pulmonary vein. Lymph nodes from levels 8 and 9 are collected.

Attention is now turned to the hilar dissection. The pulmonary vein and artery branches are dissected and individually transected with a stapling device (Figure 6). Lymph nodes from stations 10 and 11 are generally procured during this portion of the dissection. Division of the bronchus and fissure completes the lobectomy, again performed with a stapling device. Attention is then returned to completion of the lymph node dissection. Stations 2, 4, and 7 lymph nodes are collected for right-sided pulmonary resections. Stations 5, 6, and 7 lymph nodes are collected for left-sided resections. The specimen is placed in an occlusive bag and removed through the assistant port. A single, 28 Fr chest tube is placed through the camera port site and the lung is re-expanded under direct visualization.

The maintenance of a near bloodless field afforded by meticulous dissection is one area where robotic assistance shows particular merit. Dylewski and colleagues have demonstrated a series of 200 robotic lobectomies with a median blood loss of

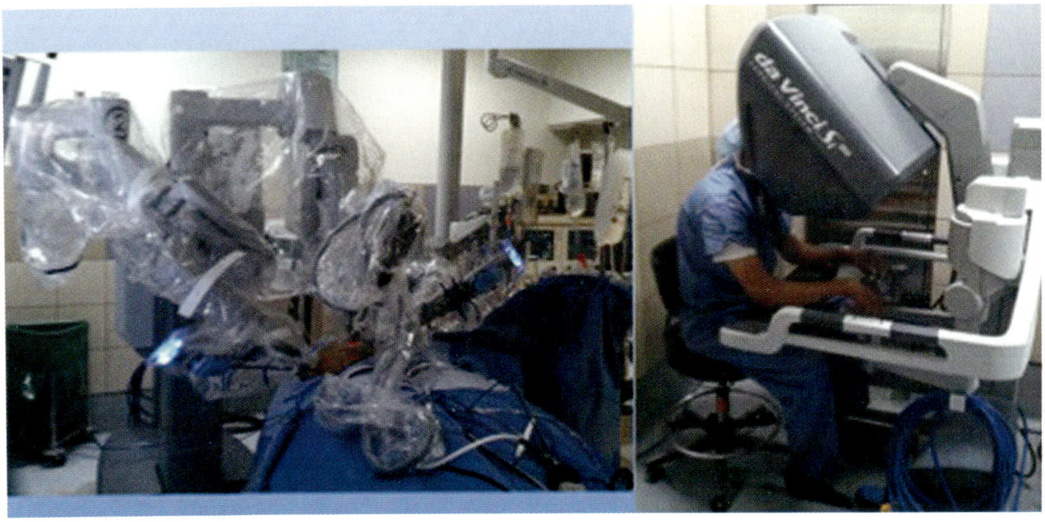

Figure 5. The surgical robot is docked for a right upper lobectomy. The patient is in the left lateral decubitus position with the robot docked over the right shoulder. The surgeon is operating from the console.

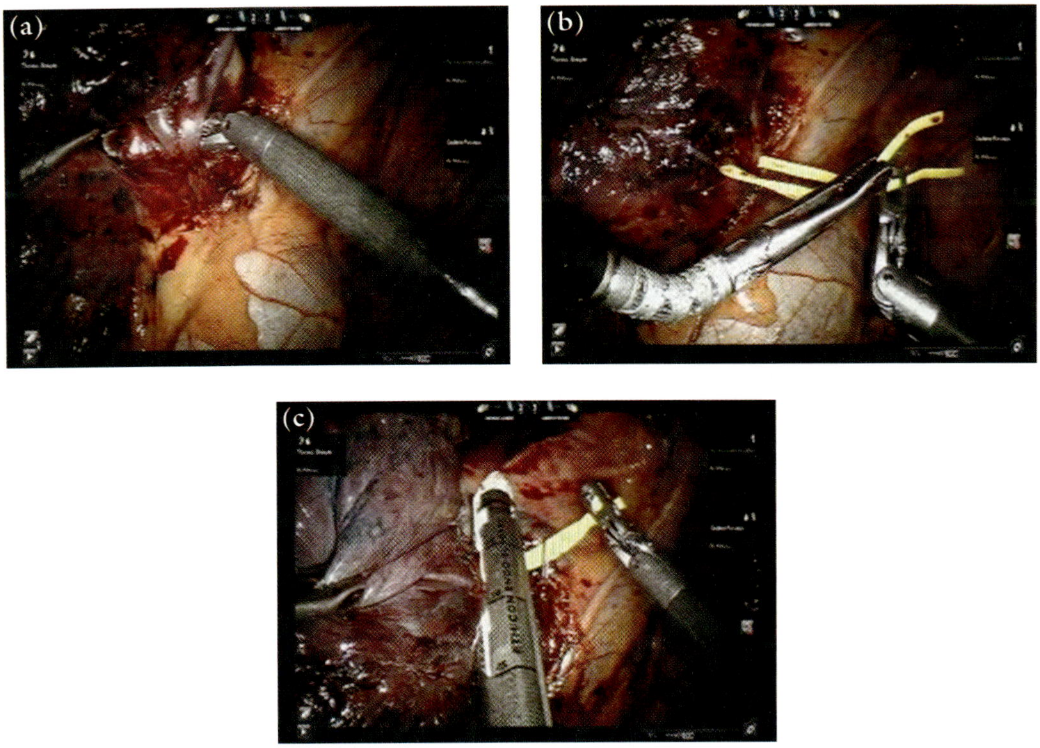

Figure 6. The pulmonary vasculature is (a) dissected, (b) isolated, and (c) divided with a stapler during a robotic-assisted lobectomy.

Table 2. Summary of 5-Year Survival Statistics for Non–Small Cell Lung Cancer

Stage	Overall	Following Best Treatment
IA	50%	60–80%
IB	43%	
IIA	36%	25–50%
IIB	25%	
IIIA	15%	10–40%
IIIB	7%	<5%
IV	2%	<5%

70 ml and 1% rate of bleeding that required transfusion.[14] The transfusion rate in the largest VATS series to date is 4.1%.[11]

Since robotic lobectomy is a relatively new technique, long-term survival data are currently being collected. The overall 5-year survival rates for all patients diagnosed with stages I and II NSCLC range from 25% to 50%.[15] Survival rates are improved following appropriate, stage-specific therapy, as outlined in Table 2. Superior survival observed in patients following surgical resection is admittedly biased by the selection of patients with an overall clinical status and performance level appropriate to tolerate pulmonary resection. Nonetheless, survival is significantly improved following VATS lobectomy. Survival rates for stages IA, IB, and II disease following VATS lobectomy are reported as 89%, 69%, and 48%, respectively.[16] Thus far, analysis of 325 robotic lobectomies shows equivalent 5-year survival to VATS lobectomy.[17] Minimally invasive lobectomy provides an adequate oncologic resection while minimizing morbidity, improving quality of life, and maximizing the patient's ability to tolerate multimodality therapies.

References

1. National Cancer Institute, Surveillance Epidemiology and End Results. SEER Stat Facts Sheets: Lung and Bronchus. Retrieved from http://seer.cancer.gov/statfacts/html/lungb.html.

2. National Comprehensive Cancer Network. NCCN Clinical Practice Guidelines in Oncology. Non–Small Cell Lung Cancer. 2012. Version 3.2-12. Retrieved from nccn.org.

3. Scott WJ, Howington J, Feigenberg S, Movsas B, Pisters K; American College of Chest Physicians. Treatment of non–small cell lung cancer stage I and stage II: ACCP evidence-based clinical practice guidelines (2nd edition). *Chest* 2007 Sept;132(3 Suppl):234S–242S.

4. Vahdat S, Oermann EK, Collins SP, Yu X, et al. CyberKnife radiosurgery for inoperable stage IA non–small cell lung cancer: 18F-fluorodeoxyglucose positron emission tomography/computed tomography serial tumor response assessment. *J Hematol Oncol.* 2010 Feb 4;3:6.

5. Horn L, Johnson D, Evarts A. Graham and the first pneumonectomy for lung cancer. *J Clin Oncol.* 2008;26(19):3268–75.

6. Scott WJ, Allen MS, Darling G, et al. Video-assisted thoracic surgery versus open lobectomy for lung cancer: A secondary analysis of data from the American College of Surgeons Oncology Group Z0030 randomized clinical trial. *J Thorac Cardiovasc Surg.* 2010 April;139(4):976–83.

7. Denlinger CE, Fernandez F, Meyers BF, et al. Lymph node evaluation in video-assisted thoracoscopic lobectomy versus lobectomy by thoracotomy. *Ann Thorac Surg.* 2010;89:1730–5; discussion 1736.

8. Nicastri DG, Wisnivesky JP, Litle VR, et al. Thoracoscopic lobectomy: report on safety, discharge independence, pain, and chemotherapy tolerance. *J Thorac Cardiovasc Surg.* 2008;135(3):642–47.

9. Whitson BA, Groth SS, Duval SJ, Swanson SJ, Maddaus MA. Surgery for early-stage non–small cell lung cancer: a systematic review of the video-assisted thoracoscopic surgery versus thoracotomy approaches to lobectomy. *Ann Thorac Surg.* 2008 Dec;86(6):2008–16; discussion 2016–8.

10. Swanson SJ, Meyeers BF, Bunnarsson CL, et al. Video-assisted thoracoscopic lobectomy is less costly and morbid than open lobectomy: a retrospective multi-institutional database analysis. *Ann Thorac Surg* 2012;93:1027–32.

11. Dajczman E, Gordon A, Kreisman H, Wolkove N. Long-term post-thoracotomy pain. *Chest.* 1991;99:270–74.

12. McKenna RJ, Houck W, Fuller CB. Video-assisted thoracic surgery lobectomy: experience with 1,100 cases. *Ann Thorac Surg.* 2006;81:421–6.

13. Cerfolio RJ, Bryant AS, Skylizard L, Minnich DJ. Initial consecutive experience of completely portal robotic pulmonary resection with 4 arms. *J Thorac Cardiovasc Surg.* 2011;142(4):740–6.

14. Dylewski MR, Ohaeto AC, Pereira JF. Pulmonary resection using a total endoscopic robotic video-assisted approach. *Semin Thorac Cardiovasc Surg.* 2011 Spring; 23(1):36–42.

15. Goldstraw P, Crowley J, Chansky K, et al. The IASLC lung cancer staging project: proposals for the revision of the TNM stage groupings in the forthcoming (seventh) edition of the TNM classification of malignant tumours. *J Thorac Oncol.* 2007;2:706–714.

16. Yamamoto K, Ohsumi A, Kojima F, et al. Long-term survival after video-assisted thoracic surgery lobectomy for primary lung cancer. *Ann Thorac Surg.* 2010 Feb;89(2): 353–9.

17. Park BJ, Melfi F, Mussi A, et al. Robotic lobectomy for non-small cell lung cancer (NSCLC): long-term oncologic results. *J Thorac Cardiovasc Surg.* 2012 Feb;143(2): 383–9.

Chapter Seven

Esophageal Myotomy

Christina L. Harsant, MD; Vita V. McCabe, MD; Ajay Gupta, MD

Initial Diagnosis

Surgical access to the esophagus has historically been a difficult task, accompanied by significant morbidity. In addition to advances in the treatment of lung cancer, robotic surgery has made it possible for health-care professionals to tackle achalasia in an efficient manner. Achalasia, a benign motility disorder of the esophagus, represents an area where surgical intervention has been shown to be superior to medical management. The morbidity associated with surgical treatment has been significantly decreased with the introduction of minimally invasive procedures.

Normal esophageal motility is dependent upon coordinated contraction and relaxation along the body of the esophagus and relaxation of the lower esophageal sphincter to allow passage of a food bolus into the stomach. Achalasia is defined by two components: incomplete relaxation of the lower esophageal sphincter (LES) and aperistalsis of the body of the esophagus. Subsequent dilation of the body of the esophagus with ineffective or incomplete emptying is also present. This idiopathic condition affects approximately 6 in 100,000 individuals.[1] Achalasia is attributed to dysfunction of Auerbach's plexus in which a lymphocytic infiltration is noted. An autoimmune cause, while postulated, has not been definitively demonstrated.

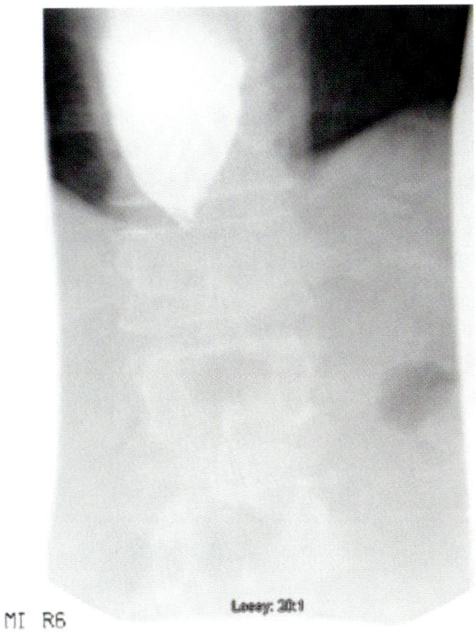

Figure 1. Barium esophagram of a patient with achalasia, displaying narrowing at the gastroesophageal junction.

Patients with achalasia typically present with complaints of dysphagia. This is often accompanied by regurgitation and reflux-like symptoms due to the incomplete clearance of ingested material from the esophagus. Chest pain is also common. Other symptoms include aspiration, weight loss, and worsening with cold liquids and stressful situations. Evaluation should be initiated with a barium esophagram. This study typically reveals a classic "bird's beak" tapering of the distal esophagus as well as a dilated and sometimes tortuous esophagus (Figure 1). In advanced cases, the esophagram can demonstrate a "sigmoid" shape.

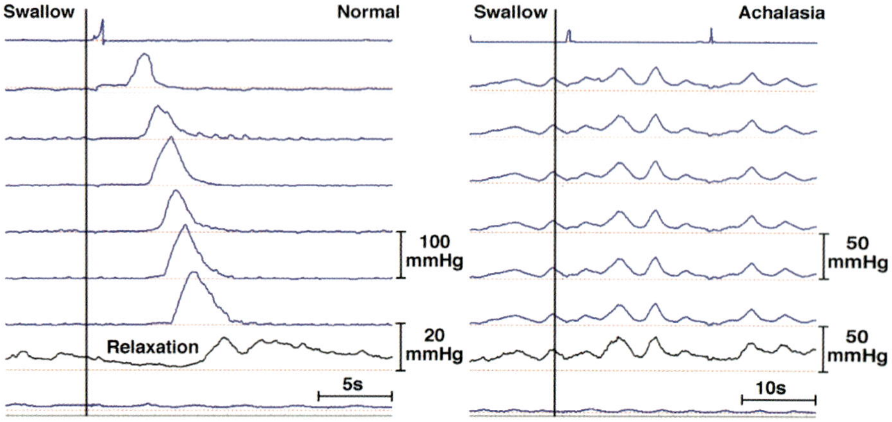

Figure 2. Example of manometry tracings from a normal subject (left) *and a patient with achalasia* (right). *Note the absent relaxation of the lower esophageal sphincter and the absence of peristaltic contractions in the patient with achalasia.*[2]

Manometry is the definitive diagnostic procedure. Findings that are revealed by the procedure include failed relaxation of the LES with swallowing and aperistalsis of the body of the esophagus (Figure 2). Pressure generated by the LES may be normal or increased. Finally, esophagogastroduodenoscopy (EGD) is used to rule out other etiologies such as Chagas' disease (pseudoachalasia secondary to Trypanosoma cruzi infection), eosinophilic esophagitis, and neoplasm, among other disorders.

Treatment

As the etiology of achalasia is still not fully understood, treatments to alter the neuromuscular changes seen in the esophagus at a cellular level are not available to date. Therapy, therefore, centers on the palliation of symptoms with the goal of decreasing LES tone. While this does not address the issue of aperistalsis, passive emptying of the esophagus is enabled, relieving dysphagia. Medical therapy most commonly employs calcium channel blockers and nitrates. Both treatments work through their ability to cause smooth muscle relaxation. However, systemic medical treatment provides only transient relaxation of the LES tone, requiring dosing prior to meals. Their use is limited by their side-effect profiles, including hypotension and headache. Medical therapy for achalasia has not been shown to be particularly successful in long-term management.[3,4]

Endoscopic modalities address the lowering of LES pressure via two approaches—botulinum toxin (Botox) injection and pneumatic dilation. Botulinum toxin is used to produce transient paralysis of the lower esophageal sphincter. The resting pressure of the LES can be lowered by at least 50%,[4] leading to symptomatic relief in approximately 66% of patients treated with this modality.[5] However, durability of Botox injection is lacking, with a recurrence of dysphagia noted in at least 50% of patients at 1 year, and in nearly all patients within 2 years.[6,7] Thus, it is a more effective treatment than oral medications, but requires repeat injections. Furthermore, the duration of the symptom-free interval may be unpredictable. In addition, these injections are noted to produce significant scarring in the submucosal plane, causing subsequent surgical approaches to the esophagus to be challenging. Many health-care professionals advocate reservation of this therapy for the severely infirm, elderly, or otherwise inoperable populations.

Pneumatic dilation of the LES is a mechanical tactic possible via an endoscopic approach. Notable improvements in symptoms are typically seen in 75–85% of patients treated with a single dilation.[8] However, only 40–60% will remain asymptomatic at 10 years following this single intervention.[9,10,11] Thus, serial dilations are advocated. Dilation for achalasia is complicated by a 2–4% risk of esophageal perforation with risk increasing with each subsequent dilation.[12] More aggressive dilation techniques with larger balloon or dilator sizes may result in better symptom relief, but are associated with an even higher risk of perforation. Esophageal perforation may be catastrophic, resulting in overwhelming sepsis, need for an operative intervention, or death. Despite the potential morbidity, pneumatic dilations remain a good treatment option for patients unfit to tolerate surgical intervention. In a randomized, prospective trial, balloon dilation was found to be 65% effective, compared to 95% for myotomy.[13]

Surgical approaches to the treatment of achalasia were pioneered by Ernst Heller, a German surgeon, who deduced that the LES could be modified by division of the outer longitudinal and inner circular muscular layers of the esophagus. He performed the first myotomy in 1913, which extended from the esophagus onto the cardia of the stomach.[14] His initial procedure involved an anterior as well as posterior myotomy. This was later modified to a single anterior myotomy. Heller noted that while one could extend the length of the myotomy, a longer myotomy is associated with a higher incidence of gastroesophageal reflux. The optimum length of the myotomy and extension onto the gastric cardia has been debated. Nonetheless, the modified Heller myotomy became and has remained the most effective and durable treatment for achalasia, with more than 90% of patients experiencing excellent relief of dysphagia over 5 years.[15] The addition of a partial fundoplication, or wrapping of the gastric fundus around the area of the LES, has been included to ameliorate reflux.

Heller's initial procedure was performed via an open abdominal approach. Later, transthoracic approaches were developed via a left thoracotomy incision. Either approach could be expected to provide relief of dysphagia in 90% of patients.[15] However, both techniques carried significant morbidity and could carry prohibitive operative risk to the elderly or comorbid patient despite the improved palliative outcome over medical management. Even suitable operative candidates were often dissuaded by the morbidity of a laparotomy or thoracotomy, leading to utilization of less effective treatments such as dilation and botulinum toxin injection.

Minimally Invasive Techniques

In the 1990s, advances in laparoscopic technology paved the way for the transition of the Heller myotomy to a minimally invasive procedure. Videoscopic modified

Heller myotomy was initially accessed through the thoracic cavity and allowed completion of an esophagomyotomy that provided success rates similar to that of the original open procedure.[16] Later, laparoscopic approaches accessed the abdomen via four or five small incisions, with, in some series, superior results to the thoracoscopic approach.[17] Additionally, an anti-reflux procedure could be performed more easily via a laparoscopic transabdominal approach.

Laparoscopic Modified Heller Myotomy: Technique

The general approach is transabdominal via four or five ports. Advances in available laparoscopic tools, such as the harmonic scalpel, make the dissection more efficient and accurate. Division of the muscular layers of the esophagus can be achieved by electrocautery or bluntly with a kittner. The proximal extent of the myotomy is easily reached by gentle downward traction of the esophagus, often facilitated by encircling the esophagus with a Penrose drain. Typically, the proximal myotomy should include 5–7 cm of the distal esophagus and should be continued onto the cardia where the more erratic orientation of gastric muscular fibers is readily evident. Failure of esophagomyotomy occurs if remnant fibers of either the circular or longitudinal layers remain. Conversely, carrying dissection beyond the muscular planes disrupts the mucosa, resulting in esophageal perforation. The surgeon must be meticulous with visualization and dissection. The added magnification of the laparoscope is beneficial during minimally invasive modified Heller myotomy.

Partial fundoplication can be achieved via the same port site access by mobilization of the fundus, via division of the proximal short gastric vessels. Debate as to the type of fundoplication continues, but it remains an accepted component of modified Heller myotomy. Several types of fundoplications exist, from full 360-degree wraps, such as the Nissen fundoplication, to varying degrees of partial fundoplication. Partial fundoplication may be oriented anterior to the esophagus or posterior, and the most common are the Dor (anterior) or Toupet (posterior) fundoplication (Figure 3). Nissen fundoplication is felt to be too restrictive; thus a Dor or Toupet is the most commonly used with laparoscopic modified Heller myotomy.

A prospective randomized control trial demonstrated that inclusion of a Dor fundoplication reduces postoperative reflux from 47.6% with myotomy alone to 9.1%.[18] A Dor fundoplication provides the benefit of the wrapped gastric fundus as a buttress over the exposed esophageal mucosa from the anterior myotomy. Critics of this approach argue that this may also act to re-approximate the edges of the myotomy, hampering its efficacy in relieving dysphagia. The Toupet fundoplication, in which the fundus passes posteriorly to the esophagus, avoids this potential issue. Proponents of the Toupet believe that tacking the wrapped gastric fundus to the edges of the myotomy help maintain the patency offered by the myotomy while still providing the anti-reflux benefit of the fundoplication.

Minimally invasive modified Heller myotomy has demonstrated significant decreases in morbidity, mortality, and length of stay.[19] Challenges with the minimally invasive approach include the perpendicular orientation of the instruments to

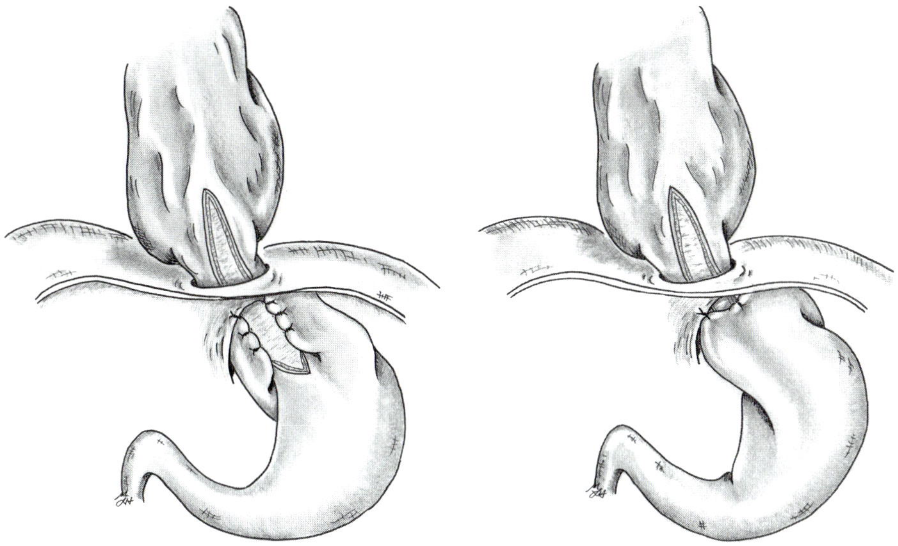

Figure 3. Toupet fundoplication, a posterior partial wrap (left). *Dor fundoplication, an anterior partial fundoplication* (right). *Either fundoplication is often used in conjunction with a modified Heller myotomy. Credit: LaWaun Hance, PA-C.*

the submucosal plane that cannot be violated. In addition, the length of the instruments passing through the ports in the abdominal wall and reaching toward the target anatomy cause a fulcrum effect that can make precise control of the tip of the instrument difficult. As with other types of laparoscopic operations, ergonomics for the surgeon are often awkward. Stable visualization is dependent upon the steady hand of an assistant holding the laparoscope. Surgical robotic assistance provides advantages by addressing many of these drawbacks.

Robotic-Assisted Modified Heller Myotomy: A Hybrid Technique

Since the 1990s, robotic techniques in surgery have been developed for a number of applications. Their utility in modified Heller myotomy is now well established. Robotic instruments have been developed with the same functionalities as many of the laparoscopic instruments. Their operation is unique in the wristlike mobility allowing a parallel orientation of the instruments to the tissue plane for completion of the myotomy (Figure 4). The built-in cancellation of tremor and adjustable scaling of movements enhance control and precision of the surgeon's movement.

Our approach to the modified Heller myotomy is to establish a pneumoperitoneum using a Veress needle technique to a pressure of 15 mmHg. A 12 mm port is then placed 6 finger-breadths below the level of the xiphoid process in the midline, which serves as the camera port. A 5 mm subxiphoid port is placed and removed to facilitate the insertion of a Nathanson liver retractor. Two left upper quadrant ports are placed (a 5 mm laparoscopic and an 8 mm robotic port), and two right upper

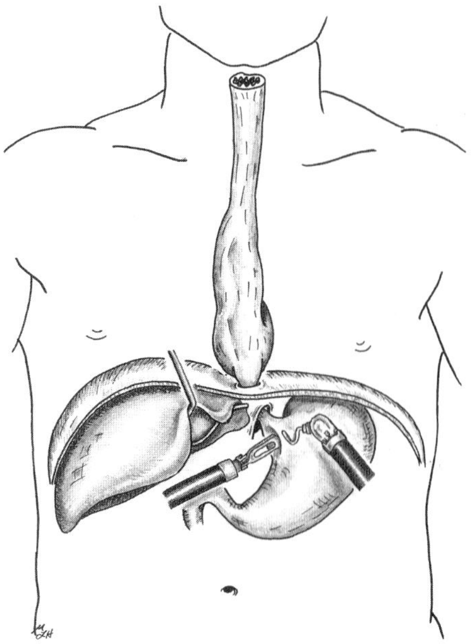

Figure 4. Schematic illustrating the anatomic location approached for a robotic-assisted modified Heller myotomy. Credit: LaWaun Hance, PA-C.

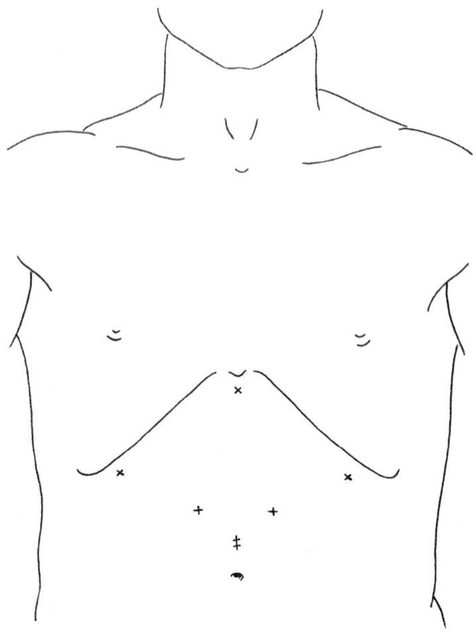

Figure 5. Port placement for robotic-assisted modified Heller myotomy and laparoscopic fundoplication. × = *robotic;* + = *laparoscopically;* ‡ = *camera port. Credit: LaWaun Hance, PA-C.*

quadrant mirror image ports are inserted as well. An additional 5 mm port can be placed in the left lower quadrant to facilitate retraction of a Penrose drain wrapped around the GE junction, if necessary (Figure 5).

The initial mobilization is performed laparoscopically. A harmonic scalpel is utilized to define the right and left diaphragmatic crura. The proximal short gastric vessels are ligated with the harmonic scalpel. A 0.25 inch Penrose drain is placed loosely around the esophagogastric junction and secured with an Endoloop® to facilitate retraction for completion of the myotomy. Under direct visualization, a 60 French bougie is placed. The surgical robotic platform is docked. A Cadiere forceps is placed into the left working arm and a hook cautery coagulation into the right working arm (set at 20 watts). Binocular three-dimensional vision is provided to the surgeon, allowing exceptional visualization of the esophageal muscular layers while performing the myotomy. A myotomy is created approximately 5–6 cm proximal to the esophagogastric junction and 1.5 cm distal to the junction onto the cardia of the stomach (Figure 6). The robotic platform is undocked.

Next, our preference is to perform a Toupet posterior 270-degree partial fundoplication with a laparoscope. This hybrid technique, utilizing a combined laparoscopic and robotic approach, has resulted in a balance of efficient operating times with superior accuracy and virtually no morbidity, even in higher-risk patients. Many centers perform a total robotic-assisted modified Heller myotomy with partial fundoplication with equally outstanding results.

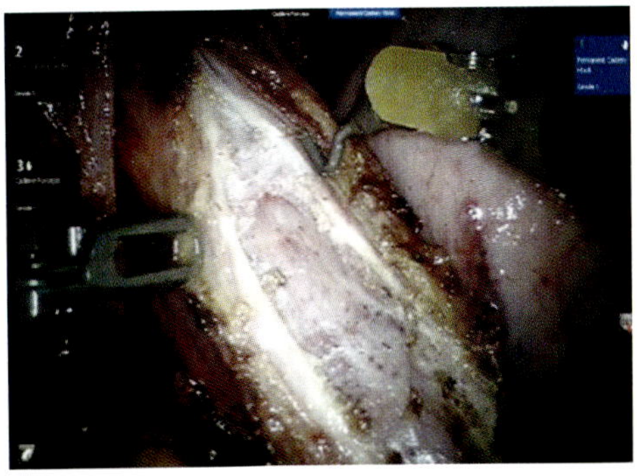

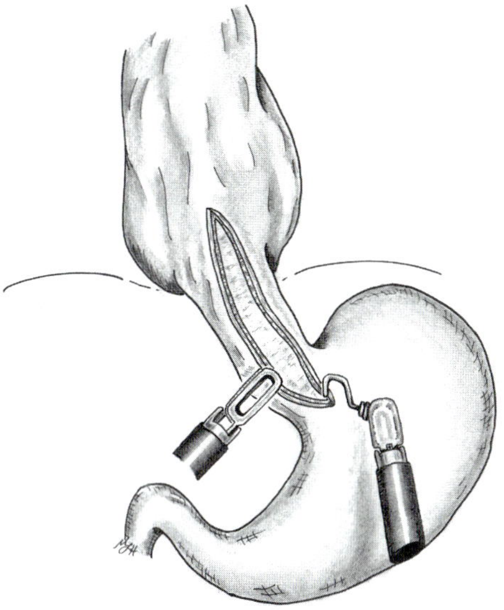

Figure 6. (left) *Modified Heller myotomy in progress, performed with surgical robotic assistance.* (right) *The myotomy must be extended from the esophagus, beyond the gastroesophageal junction, and onto the cardia of the stomach.*
Credit: LaWaun Hance, PA-C.

Robotic assistance in performing esophageal myotomy for achalasia is associated with a lower rate of esophageal perforation in multiple series.[20,21,22,23,24] Subjective reports obtained by patient surveys demonstrate at least equivalent, if not superior, improvement of overall health and well-being following robotic-assisted myotomy compared to laparoscopic myotomy.[25]

Criticisms of the use of robotic assistance include increased operating room time, cost, and device-associated technical problems. While the actual operating time for robotic-assisted cases is comparable to laparoscopic cases, additional time is needed to place sterile drapes on the arms of the robot and in docking the robot for use.[26] Draping can be performed prior to the patient's arrival in the operating suite, therefore reducing the duration of general anesthetic time for the patient. An analysis of 211 robotic-assisted procedures demonstrated that device-associated technical difficulties occurred in only 4% of cases, with only 2 requiring conversion to standard laparoscopy to complete the case.[27]

Complications of Modified Heller Myotomy

There are three main classes of complications associated with surgery for achalasia: esophageal perforation leading to leak, dysphagia secondary to incomplete myotomy or due to advanced disease not amenable to myotomy as primary therapy, and severe reflux as a consequence of myotomy. Esophageal perforation rates in open modified Heller myotomy range from 1% to 15%, and in experienced hands, esophageal perforation rates from laparoscopic modified Heller myotomy are equivalent.[22] Robotic-assisted modified Heller myotomy has demonstrated a clear benefit where the rate of esophageal perforation in multiple series approaches zero.[20,21,23,25] Regardless of the surgical approach, early detection of an esophageal perforation or leak remains *crucial* as delayed diagnosis is associated with significant morbidity and mortality.

While care must be exercised to avoid mucosal perforation, incomplete myotomy or surgical intervention on severely advanced disease ("burnt out esophagus") will fail to relieve dysphagia. Robotic assistance offers enhanced visualization with magnification and three-dimensional binocular optics aiding in the identification of remaining muscular fibers along the myotomy to minimize this complication. Failed minimally invasive myotomy may be palliated with attempted open myotomy. If there is convincing evidence of severely advanced disease, esophagectomy is the treatment of choice.

Patients with achalasia are at a 16-fold increased risk for squamous cell carcinoma of the esophagus.[28] Therefore, continued EGD surveillance is essential, but specific guidelines have not been agreed upon for interval or duration. Our practice has been to perform surveillance EGD 1 year after intervention with multiple random biopsies. If the biopsies are normal, then the EGD interval is lengthened to every 3 years. A change of symptoms will prompt earlier endoscopy.

Summary

Modified Heller myotomy in patients with acceptable operative risk is recommended as first line therapy for achalasia. This approach offers the most effective and durable treatment for this disease. While esophageal myotomy is possible following prior endoscopic dilations or botulinum toxin injections, scarring of the submucosal plane makes the procedure much more technically difficult. No statistical difference in perforation rate has been noted after previous endoscopic treatment, though a trend toward increased risk of perforation has been observed.[29] Minimally invasive modified Heller myotomy is well established in its safety and efficacy, making it the procedure of choice. Robotic-assisted modified Heller myotomy offers a particular advantage in this delicate and precise dissection, resulting in lower morbidity. Partial fundoplication is typically performed concomitantly to minimize postoperative reflux. Failed myotomy or severely advanced disease may require esophagectomy.

References

1. Iqbal A, Haider M, Desai K, et al. Technique and follow-up of minimally invasive Heller myotomy for achalasia. *Surg Endosc.* 2006 Mar;20(3):394–401.

2. Kessing BF, Bredenoord AJ, Smout AJPM. Erroneous diagnosis of gastroesophageal reflux disease in achalasia. *Clin Gastroenterol Hepatol.* 2011 Dec;9(12):1020–1024.

3. Eckardt AJ, Eckardt VF. Treatment and surveillance strategies in achalasia: an update. *Nat Rev Gastroenterol Hepatol.* 2011 Jun;8(6):311–9.

4. Hoogerwerf WA, Pasricha PJ. Pharamocologic therapy in treating achalasia. *Gastrointest Clin North Am.* 2001;11(2):311–324.

5. Pasricha PJ, Rai R, Ravich WJ, Hendrix TR, Kalloo AN. Botulinum toxin for achalasia: long-term outcome and predictors of response. *Gastroenterology.* 1996;110(5): 1410–1415.

6. Boeckxstaens, GEE. Achalasia. *Best Pract Res Clin Gastroenterol.* 2007;21(4): 595–608.

7. Allescher HD, Storr M, Seige M, et al. Treatment of achalasia: botulinum toxin injection vs. pneumatic balloon dilation. A prospective study with long-term follow-up. *Endoscopy.* 2001;33(12):1007–1017.

8. Kadakia SC, Wong RK. Pneumatic balloon dilation for esophageal achalasia. *Gastrointest Endosc Clin North Am.* 2001;11(2):325–346.

9. Chan KC, Wong SK, Lee DW, et al. Short-term and long-term results of endoscopic balloon dilation for achalasia: 12 years' experience. *Endoscopy.* 2004;36(8):690–694.

10. Karamanolis G, Sgouros S, Karatzias G, et al. Long-term outcome of pneumatic dilation in the treatment of achalasia. *Am J Gastroenterol.* 2005;100(2):270–274.

11. West RL, Hirsch DP, Bartelsman JF, et al. Long-term results of pneumatic dilation in achalasia followed for more than 5 years. *Am J Gastroenterol.* 2002;97(6):1346–1351.

12. Katzka DA, Castell DO. Review article: an analysis of the efficacy, perforation rates and methods used in pneumatic dilation for achalasia. *Aliment Pharmacol Ther.* 2011 Oct; 34(8):832–839.

13. Csendes A, Braghetto I, Burdiles P, Csendes P. Comparison of forceful dilatation and esophagomyotomy in patients with achalasia of the esophagus. *Hepatogastroenterology.* 1991;38(6):502–505.

14. Payne WS. Heller's contribution to the surgical treatment of achalasia of the esophagus. *Ann Thorac Surg.* 1989;48:876–881.

15. Ruurda JP, Gooszen HG, Broeders IA. Early experience in robot-assisted laparoscopic Heller myotomy. *Scand J Gastroenterol Suppl.* 2004;241:4–8.

16. Pellegrini C, Wetter LA, Patti M, et al. Thoracoscopic esophagomyotomy. Initial experience with a new approach for the treatment of achalasia. *Ann Surg.* 1992 Sept; 216(3): 291–6; discussion 296–299.

17. Ramacciato G, Mercantini P, Amodio PM, et al. The laparoscopic approach with antireflux surgery is superior to the thoracosopic approach for the treatment of esophageal achalasia. Experience of a single surgical unit. *Surg Endosc.* 2002 Oct;16(10):1431–1437.

18. Richards WO, Torquati A, Holzman MD, et al. Heller myotomy versus Heller myotomy with Dor fundoplication for achalasia: a prospective randomized double-blinded clinical trial. *Ann Surg.* 2004;240(3):405–412.

19. Leonard DS, Broe P. Oesophageal achalasia: an argument for primary surgical management. *Surgeon.* 2009 April;7(2):101–113.

20. Maeso S, Reza M, Mayol JA, et al. Efficacy of the da Vinci surgical system in abdominal surgery compared with that of laparoscopy: a systematic review. *Ann Surg.* 2010 Aug;252(2):254–62.

21. Melvin WS, Dundon JM, Talamini M, Horgan S. Computer-enhanced robotic telesurgery minimizes esophageal perforation during Heller myotomy. *Surgery.* 2005 Oct; 138(4):553–8; discussion 558–9.

22. Horgan S, Galvani C, Gorodner MV, Omelanczuck P, et al. Robotic-assisted Heller myotomy versus laparoscopic Heller myotomy for the treatment of esophageal achalasia: multicenter study. *J Gastrointest Surg.* 2005 Nov;9(8):1020–9; discussion 1029–30.

23. Galvani C, Gorodner MV, Moser F, Baptista P, Horgan S. Laparoscopic Heller myotomy for achalasia facilitated by robotic assistance. *Surg Endosc.* 2006 Jul;20(7):1105–12.

24. Shaligram A, Unnirevi J, Simorov A, Kothari VM, Oleynikov D. How does the robot affect outcomes? A retrospective review of open, laparoscopic, and robotic Heller myotomy for achalasia. *Surg Endosc.* 2012 Apr;26(4):1047–50.

25. Huffman LC, Pandalai PK, Boulton BJ, et al. Robotic Heller myotomy: a safe operation with higher postoperative quality-of-life indices. *Surgery.* 2007 Oct; 142(4):613–8; discussion 618–20.

26. Newlin ME, Mikami DJ, Melvin SW. Initial experience with the four-arm computer-enhanced telesurgery device in foregut surgery. *J Laparoendosc Adv Surg Tech A.* 2004 Jun; 14(3):121–4.

27. Talamini MA, Chapman S, Horgan S, Melvin WS; Academic Robotics Group. A prospective analysis of 211 robotic-assisted surgical procedures. *Surg Endosc.* 2003 Oct; 17(10):1521–4.

28. Sandler RS, Nyren O, Ekbom A, Eisen GM, Yuen J, Josefsson S. The risk of esophageal cancer in patients with achalasia. A population-based study. *JAMA.* 1995 Nov 1; 274(17):1359–62.

29. Bonavina L, Incarbone R, Antoniazzi L, Reitano M, Peracchia A. Previous endoscopic treatment does not affect complication rate and outcome of laparoscopic Heller myotomy and anterior fundoplication of oesophageal achalasia. *Ital J Gastroenterol Hepatol.* 1999 Dec; 31(9):827–830.

Chapter Eight

Robotic Partial Nephrectomy

Christodoulos G. Kaoutzanis, MD; Crystal M. Kavanagh, MD; Eduardo Kleer, MD

History and Techniques of Partial Nephrectomy

The modern era of renal surgery began in 1869 when Simon successfully performed the first planned nephrectomy to cure a urinary fistula.[1] In 1870, Simon also performed the first deliberate partial nephrectomy (PN) for hydronephrosis. Seventeen years later, Czerny was credited with being the first surgeon to perform PN for a renal tumor when he resected an angiosarcoma from the kidney of a young man.[2] Subsequent experimental studies established the feasibility of partial resection for localized kidney diseases by exploring numerous concerns, such as renal repair mechanisms, changes in renal and body function, as well as the amount of overall renal tissue required to support life following PN.

In the first half of the twentieth century, PN gradually replaced total nephrectomy for the treatment of localized benign diseases of the kidney, such as cysts, infarcts, and localized hydronephrosis. In 1950, Vermooten removed a 10 cm carcinoma from the left kidney of a woman with a normal right kidney and advocated that PN may be a reasonable option in the presence of a malignant growth involving the kidney.[3] However, total nephrectomy was still believed to be the optimal management of malignant renal neoplasms, given its lower complication rate and less technically demanding nature when compared to PN. Another major concern was the possibility of local tumor recurrence due to inadequate excision or multicentric tumors after partial resection. During that time, PN was used sparingly for tumors in a solitary kidney, bilateral renal tumors, and poor renal function.

Over the second half of the twentieth century, the enhanced understanding of the intrarenal vascular anatomy, the introduction of renal hypothermia, and the development of better surgical methods to reconstruct the kidney made PN a more attractive option. Furthermore, the shift in the beliefs of surgical oncology toward organ preservation in the treatment of certain malignancies and the ongoing improvement of the advanced radiological imaging techniques created a new class of small incidentally detected renal tumors that seemed appropriate for less radical surgical intervention.

In 1993, Licht and Novick introduced the phrase *nephron-sparing* in a report of 241 cases of PN with a normal contralateral kidney.[4] Although the median tumor size was 3.5 cm and the median follow-up was only 3 years, the survival was 95% with only 2 local recurrences. A few years later, Herr and Fergany et al. reported similar results for 10-year follow-up.[5,6] It was not until then that PN was widely accepted by most urologists as a suitable surgical option for localized renal tumors.

The first laparoscopic operation used to remove a major solid organ from a human being was done in 1991 by Clayman and his team when they removed the right kidney of an 85-year-old female for a 3 cm mass.[7,8] This led to a new era of minimally invasive kidney surgery. Dr. McDougall's laboratory work on laparoscopic PN was transformed into clinical reality in 1993 when Winfield and his colleagues performed the first transperitoneal laparoscopic PN for a lower-pole caliceal diverticulum containing a stone.[9,10] Since then, laparoscopic PN has demonstrated comparable long-term oncological control and functional outcomes to open PN, with the potential benefits of improved perioperative outcomes, convalescence, and better cosmesis.[11–14] However, widespread adoption of laparoscopic PN has been limited due to the lengthy learning curve and the technically challenging nature related to the difficult intracorporeal sutured reconstruction, leading to longer warm-ischemia times.[15]

In an effort to overcome the technical difficulties of laparoscopic nephron-sparing surgery, two novel approaches emerged—hand-assisted laparoscopic PN and robotic PN. Hand-assisted laparoscopic PN is less invasive than open surgery and technically less demanding than traditional laparoscopic surgery. It has been advocated to be an intermediate approach with numerous advantages, including better control of the renal pedicle, faster dissection and suturing, as well as more effective hemostasis. A shorter learning curve is evident given the use of the hand as a working instrument.

In 2004, Gettman et al. reported on a cohort of 13 patients who underwent renal tumor excision entirely robotically.[16] In more recent years, several investigators confirmed the safety and feasibility of robotic PN with oncologic results and perioperative outcomes comparable to open and laparoscopic PN.[17,18] This type of surgery was even shown to be effective for the treatment of larger renal tumors, over 4 cm in diameter.[19] By offering the surgeon a magnified, three-dimensional high-definition view, computer-aided elimination of tremor, and seven degrees of freedom at the distal ends of the instruments with superior maneuverability, robot assistance has the potential to reduce the technical challenges associated with critical portions of the procedure and thus to facilitate precise tumor excision and sutured renal reconstruction. Moreover, robotic PN has been reported to have a relatively shortened learning curve when compared to the traditional laparoscopic approach, offering the laparoscopically inexperienced surgeon a minimally invasive option for the treatment of small renal masses.[15]

Staging of Renal Tumors

An estimated 64,770 Americans will be diagnosed with renal cancer and 13,570 will die of the disease in the United States in 2012.[20] Renal cell carcinoma (RCC) is the most common kidney cancer and accounts for 3% of all adult malignancies and nearly 90% of all cases of primary renal malignancies.[21] Its incidence has increased steadily in the past few decades, a trend that has been observed across both sexes and all ethnic groups. The reason for this increased incidence is mainly due to the incidental finding of unsuspected renal cancers from abdominal imaging studies such as ultrasounds, CT scans, and MRIs. Most of these incidentally found renal cancers tend to be less than 4 cm, making most of them amenable to PN. Most renal cell cancers are aggressive tumors and, as a class, the most lethal of urologic neoplasms. An accurate cancer staging system is therefore of paramount importance. This can be used not only as a prognostic indicator but also to facilitate clinical decision-making and counseling, to simplify exchange of cancer data in clinical practice, and to elucidate targets for basic and clinical research.

The first formal staging system for RCC was developed by Flocks and Kadesky in 1958 and was based on anatomic characteristics and observed patterns of tumor spread.[22] The system was modified a few years later by Robson et al. with the addition of vascular involvement.[23] Robson's classification was useful, but it was soon found to be difficult to adapt to the increasing diagnostic and therapeutic capabilities due to a lack of variability.

In 1974, the International Union Against Cancer introduced the earliest version of the TNM system.[24] This was a more comprehensive classification system whose key elements were applicable to the description of the extent of any malignant tumor. This system distinguished between the local extension of the primary tumor (T-classification), the involvement of regional lymph nodes (N-classification), and the presence of distant or blood-borne metastases (M-classification). Over the last three decades, the TNM classification has become more widely accepted and evolved to keep pace with the demands of clinical practice. Several investigators have assessed the predictive ability of the system, which resulted in its continuous refinement.[25] The current TNM classification and staging system from 2009 is listed in Tables 1 and 2, respectively.[26]

Patient Positioning

The patient is initially placed in the supine position on the operating table. After induction of general anesthesia, the patient is placed in 30–60° lateral decubitus or flank position with the hips positioned on the break in the table and the affected side up (Figure 1). The table may be mildly flexed at the midpoint (15–20°) to increase the distance between the costal margin and iliac crest, thus maximizing the working space. The patient is secured to the table with heavy straps and cloth tape and all pressure points are padded. Positioning of the arms and legs is important. If the arm is brought across the body, a Mayo stand or arm braces can be used to support the arm that is secured at the level of the chin. Alternatively, the arm can be positioned with the upper arm along the side of the body to minimize collisions of the upper robotic arm with the elbow. The bottom leg is flexed while the top leg is kept straight. At this point, it is important to airplane the table as needed in order to increase the lateral decubitus angle to prevent the kidney from falling forward once the Gerota's fascia is incised. If flexion is not adequate prior to docking,

Table 1. TNM Classification

Classification	Description
Primary Tumor (T-classification)	
TX	Primary tumor cannot be assessed
T0	No evidence of primary tumor
T1	Tumor 7 cm or less in greatest dimension, limited to the kidney
T1a	Tumor 4 cm or less in greatest dimension, limited to the kidney
T1b	Tumor more than 4 cm but not more than 7 cm in greatest dimension, limited to the kidney
T2	Tumor more than 7 cm in greatest dimension, limited to the kidney
T2a	Tumor more than 7 cm but less than or equal to 10 cm in greatest dimension, limited to the kidney
T2b	Tumor more than 10 cm, limited to the kidney
T3	Tumor extends into major veins or perinephric tissues but not into the ipsilateral adrenal gland and not beyond Gerota's fascia
T3a	Tumor grossly extends into the renal vein or its segmental (muscle containing) branches, or tumor invades perirenal and/or renal sinus fat but not beyond Gerota's fascia
T3b	Tumor grossly extends into the vena cava below the diaphragm
T3c	Tumor grossly extends into the vena cava above the diaphragm or invades the wall of the vena cava
T4	Tumor invades beyond Gerota's fascia (including contiguous extension into the ipsilateral adrenal gland)
Regional Lymph Nodes (N-classification)	
NX	Regional lymph nodes cannot be assessed
N0	No regional lymph node metastasis
N1	Metastasis in regional lymph node(s)
Distant Metastasis (M-classification)	
M0	No distant metastasis
M1	Distant metastasis

Table 2. Staging System

Stage Grouping			
Stage I	T1	N0	M0
Stage II	T2	N0	M0
Stage III	T1 or T2	N1	M0
	T3	N0 or N1	M0
Stage IV	T4	Any N	M0
	Any T	Any N	M1

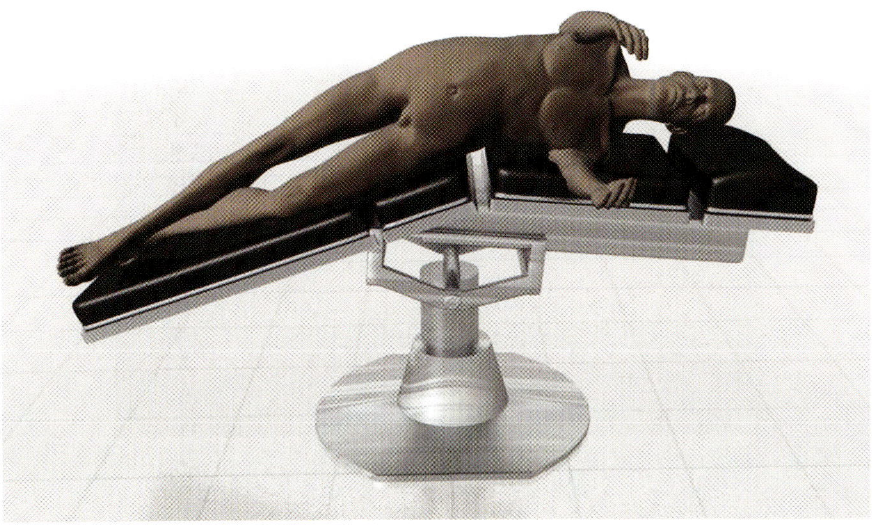

Figure 1. The patient is placed in flank position, with the hips positioned on the break in the table and the affected side up. Credit: © 2013 Intuitive Surgical, Inc.

undocking will be needed during the procedure to move back, which will cause unnecessary delay and increase operative time.

Trocar Placement

Although both transperitoneal and retroperitoneal approaches have been described, the majority of the reported experience is transperitoneal. Access to the peritoneal cavity is achieved using a Veress needle. Once pneumoperitoneum is established at a pressure of 15 mmHg, port placement ensues after marking the costal margin, iliac crest, and port sites. Trocar placement is based on the triangulation principle and varies according to surgeon's preference, patient's anatomy, and robot models.

In our practice, we use a modified lateral port placement. An incision is made off the patient's midline lateral to the border of the rectus muscle at the level of the renal hilum for the 12 mm camera port (Figure 2, blue port). Once the camera port has been placed, it is important to perform an initial assessment of the anatomy to decide if adjustment of the instrument ports' position is needed. An 8 mm robotic port is introduced at the lateral border of the ipsilateral rectus muscle, about 2–3 cm below the costal margin (Figure 2, yellow port). Another 8 mm robotic port is placed about 5 cm superior to the anterior superior iliac spine and 15 degrees inferior to the camera port (Figure 2, green port). It is advisable to place both robotic ports at a minimum distance of 8 cm from the camera port site in order to avoid arm collision. An 8 mm fourth arm instrument port can be placed 15 degrees inferior to the lower quadrant robotic arm while maintaining 8 cm of distance (Figure 2, red port). Occasionally, it is positioned medial and inferior to

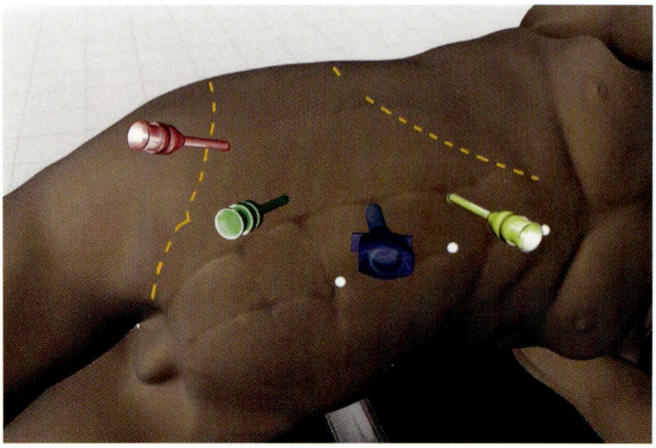

Figure 2. Port placement technique (right-sided procedure). Credit: © 2013 Intuitive Surgical, Inc.

the lower robotic port if the patient's habitus precludes a lateral placement. The instrument ports should be inserted under direct endoscopic view. Also, one should be aware that for obese patients, all ports may shift further laterally.

Two 12 mm assistant ports are placed in the midline (Figure 2). These two assistant ports are placed at a distance of 4 cm superior and inferior to the camera port. Occasionally, if liver retraction is required for right-sided renal tumors, an additional 5 mm port is placed 2–3 cm below the xiphoid along the midline.

The robot is then positioned over the patient's shoulder and centered at the camera arm with the camera oriented in line with the kidney (Figure 3). The robot is then docked to the patient.

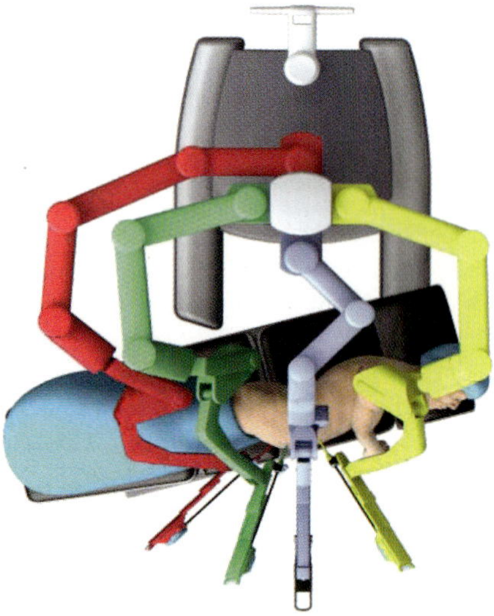

Figure 3. The patient cart is rolled in at an angle over the patient's shoulder to accommodate the natural position of the kidney. Credit: © 2013 Intuitive Surgical, Inc.

Surgical Technique Step-by-Step

The surgery is begun with a 30-degree up lens through the camera port using a modified lateral camera port placement (Figure 2). The right arm is fitted with a hot monopolar curved scissor. The left arm is fitted with a ProGrasp or Maryland. The fourth arm is fitted with a fenestrated bipolar grasper. The assistant uses a suction irrigator for one of the assistant ports and a wavy grasper for the other.

1. **Mobilizing the large colon medially.** This is begun by incising along the line of Toldt. The colon is mobilized medially in standard fashion medial

to the hilum of the kidney. The duodenum is kocherized for right-sided tumors.

2. **Accessing the hilum.** The next key step is to gain access to the hilum by finding the ureter. This is located just below the lower pole of the kidney as one exposes the psoas muscle. Once the ureter is identified, the fourth arm is used to pull the ureter straight up. This is a key maneuver that allows elevation of the kidney and the hilum to be placed on stretch, facilitating isolation of the renal artery and vein. One can readjust the fourth arm as one gets closer to the hilum to allow for more ureteral elevation and thus better stretch of the hilum. The fourth arm can also be used to pull up on the lower pole of the kidney, as well.

   As one approaches the hilum, it helps to be able to see the psoas muscle medially. Once the renal vein is identified, its surface is exposed by gently defatting it. One needs to dissect it circumferentially to allow for a bulldog clamp to be placed around it if needed later on in the procedure. The Pro-Grasp or Maryland is then gently placed underneath the edge of the renal vein and lifted superiorly. One then looks for a pulsation to identify the renal artery. It is best to isolate the renal artery medial to the insertion of the gonadal vein on the left side, since it tends to branch laterally to this point. It is usually not necessary to take the gonadal vein at this point, but this certainly can be done if necessary for easier access to the renal artery by the operating surgeon.

   On the right side, it is best to lift up on the renal vein just lateral to its insertion to the inferior vena cava. It is imperative that the operating surgeon be well-acquainted with the details of the hilar vascular anatomy prior to the start of the operation. Knowledge of the number of renal arteries supplying the kidney is also essential to the success of the operation. If it is difficult to find the renal artery(ies), one can use intraoperative robotic Doppler ultrasound probes to help find it (them); although from our experience, this is rarely necessary. Again one needs to be able to clean out an area large enough around the artery(ies) to allow for a laparoscopic or robotic bulldog clamp to be placed around it. The best way to clean out the fat and adventitia from the vessel is to get underneath the fat or adventitia with one of the open jaws of the curved scissors and to cauterize as one is pulling the tissue away from the vessel.

3. **Accessing the renal mass.** After the renal hilum has been prepared for future clamping, the ureteral traction can be released. The goal now is to find the mass and to prepare it for excision. The kidney may need to be mobilized, especially if the mass is polar or posteriorly located. The fourth arm can aid with this mobilization if needed. Of note is that once lateral kidney attachments are taken, the kidney will tend to flop down and will be more difficult to manipulate. If the mass is large enough, one can easily see it distorting the perinephric fat. However, most of the time, one needs to look for it.

   Begin by dissecting out the perinephric fat away from the kidney so that the renal capsule can be identified, being careful not to get subcapsular.

This is especially likely in patients with what is referred to as "sticky fat," which can actually make this part of the operation very challenging. Sticky fat is most common in obese men, although it can certainly be encountered with any patient undergoing this surgery. If one does get subcapsular, more bleeding can be expected for this portion of the operation. It is important to be able to get back to the appropriate plane of dissection. If the mass is difficult to find, the CT scan may need to be reviewed again to get a better appreciation of its potential anatomy. This has been facilitated with the incorporation of TilePro into the viewing console. Intraoperative ultrasound may be required as well to facilitate identification of the mass and its border.

Certainly the use of the da Vinci robot-controlled ultrasound probe, Aloka, can greatly help in this endeavor over traditional bedside ultrasound performed by the surgical assistant, especially for minimally exophytic or endophytic masses, as well as for small masses (Figure 4). The use of intraoperative photoluminescence, "Firefly Fluorescence," imaging can also help with identification of the renal mass. Once the mass is found, it is scored using cautery circumferentially with an ideal 2 cm margin (Figure 5). As this is being done, 12.5 g of mannitol is ordered to be given by the anesthesiologist to start a diuresis prior to renal arterial clamping. In those cases where one edge of the tumor abuts on the hilum, it may not be possible to score the parenchyma circumferentially. As one scores around the tumor, the fourth arm may need to be used to help fix the kidney in position, depending on the location of the tumor.

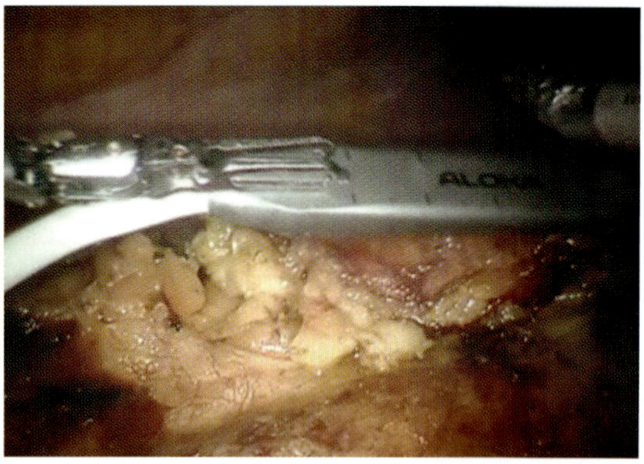

Figure 4. Robotically controlled ultrasound probe. Credit: © 2013 Intuitive Surgical, Inc.

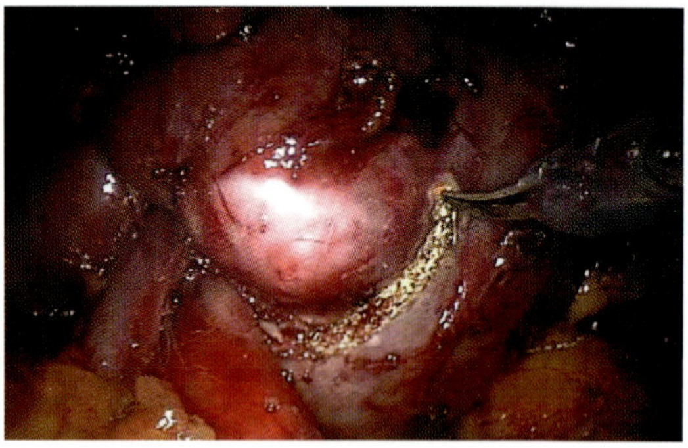

Figure 5. Scoring tumor using cautery. Credit: © 2013 Intuitive Surgical, Inc.

4. **Hilar clamping.** The fourth arm should again be used to pull up on the ureter or lower pole to facilitate access to the hilum and allow for identification of the dissected hilar vessel(s) to be clamped. We prefer the use of robotic bulldog clamps for clamping the hilar vessel(s) (Figure 6). For multiple hilar vessels, some surgeons advocate the use of a laparoscopic Satinsky clamp. We typically have not found it necessary to clamp the renal

vein. Some surgeons also advocate this process be used for hilar tumors. If the vein needs to be clamped, it is clamped last. Before clamping, it is confirmed that the mannitol has been administered. After clamping is accomplished, the circulating operating room nurse is asked to note the time at which this occurred. Clamp time should ideally be kept to 30 minutes or less. Also, operating room traffic should also be kept to a minimum to minimize distractions of the operating room team.

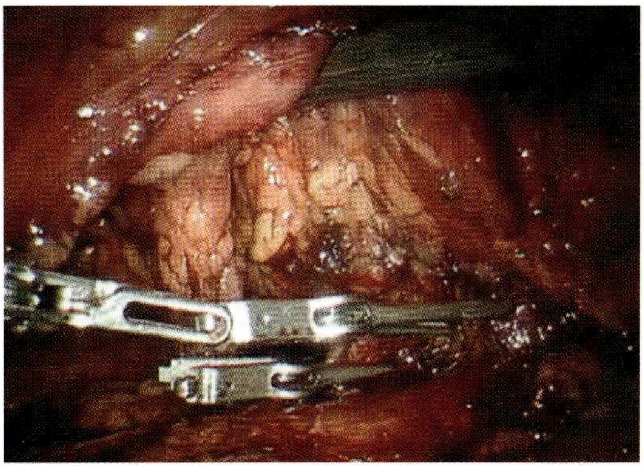

Figure 6. Clamping renal artery with robotically controlled bulldog clamp. Credit: © 2013 Intuitive Surgical, Inc.

5. **Tumor excision.** Again, the fourth arm is removed away from the ureter or lower pole and is used to help fix the kidney in position, if needed. The key to appropriate tumor excision is to create a circumferential trough around the tumor to allow one to get "under" the tumor and progress with its removal in the appropriate plane. One needs to be conscious of tumors that may abut the renal hilum to avoid cutting into the renal artery or vein.

   As one initially cuts into the renal parenchyma, some oozing that represents residual trapped blood in the kidney at the time of hilar clamping may be encountered. Excessive bleeding may indicate the presence of an accessory artery that has not been identified or poor compression of a clamped artery. The surgeon must act quickly to solve this issue prior to continuing tumor excision. Initially the curvature of the scissors should be pointing away from the tumor. However, as one gets under the tumor in the appropriate plane, it is easier to work with the curvature toward the tumor.

   Initially during tumor excision, it is particularly helpful to have the assistant's sucker tip retracting and sucking intermittently on the parenchymal edge away from the tumor, while the edge of the ProGrasp or Maryland should be retracting the specimen edge toward the tumor (Figure 7). This creates traction-countertraction for the surgeon, facilitating

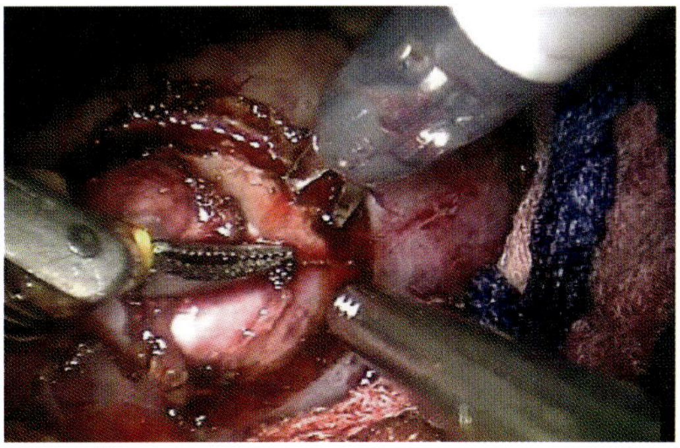

Figure 7. Use of assistant's sucker tip retracting and sucking intermittently on the parenchymal edge away from the tumor while the Maryland is retracting the specimen edge toward the tumor. This creates traction-countertraction for the surgeon, facilitating tumor excision. Credit: © 2013 Intuitive Surgical, Inc.

tumor excision. Based on preoperative study of the tumor depth, one needs to accurately gage where to begin to "get" under the tumor, based again on intraoperative ultrasound and Firefly fluorescence when applicable. If a tumor abuts the renal sinus, it is best to cut down into the sinus fat to be sure that one is all the way around the tumor. Because of the excellent robotic visualization, it is easy to visualize whether or not one may be beyond the edge of the tumor or too close for comfort. Appropriate adjustments can be made accordingly.

Of note is that once the surgeon has cut initially through the renal parenchyma, cautery is no longer utilized. After one gets under the tumor, provided that an appropriate trough has been created around the tumor, the rest of the dissection proceeds in a very straightforward manner. Often at this point, the traction from the ProGrasp or Maryland underneath the specimen edge may be all that is needed to excise the tumor from its bed. For deeper tumors, the fourth arm grasper, if it is not being used to fix the kidney in place, can be used for upward traction on the tumor specimen, helping to create further countertraction.

Once the tumor is excised, it is usually placed by the spleen on the left side or by the liver on the right side, in a position where it can easily be retrieved later. One may choose to send a specimen from the tumor base for frozen section at this point, particularly if there is any question as to the integrity of the specimen or as a routine part of the operation. This is based on surgeon preference. Before starting with suturing, the surgeon may choose to burn the cortical edge of the tumor bed with either electrocautery or the argon beam coagulator. However, we have found that this is typically not necessary and simply takes up warm-ischemia time (WIT).

6. **Management of the tumor bed.** The task at hand now is to close any collecting system openings and place hemostatic sutures before the hilum is unclamped. Before proceeding with the next step, one can switch to using two needle drivers for the right and left robotic arms or to switch out the scissors for a needle driver on the right robotic arm and keep the ProGrasp or Maryland to use as the other needle driver. We typically next like to run the tumor bed with a seven inch 2-0 V-lock suture, GS-21 needle. It has a large enough needle to allow for large bites, and, because it is braided, it maintains tension from bite to bite.

   From here to the end, all of the sutures, including this V-lock suture, are preloaded with a Lapra-Ty followed by a Hem-o-lok on its end. The first bite then goes from the parenchyma into the inside edge of the tumor bed. The suture is then pulled all the way through until the Lapra-Ty and Hem-o-lok clip prevent this end of the suture from traveling any further. One then runs the suture from one end of the tumor bed to the other (Figure 8). If collecting system and vascular defects are noted, they can all be incorporated with this suture. Intraoperative retrograde or antegrade indigo carmine or methylene blue are not typically used.

   The needle and suture then comes out the opposite end of where it entered into the tumor bed, and a Hem-o-lok clip is placed such that the

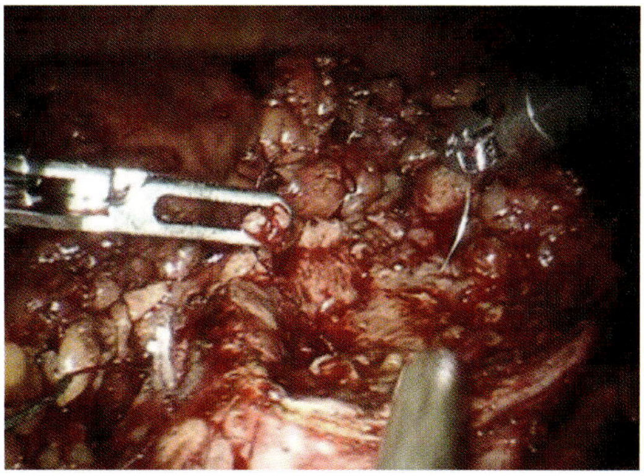

Figure 8. Running suture across the tumor bed for hemostasis from one end to the other. Credit: © 2013 Intuitive Surgical, Inc.

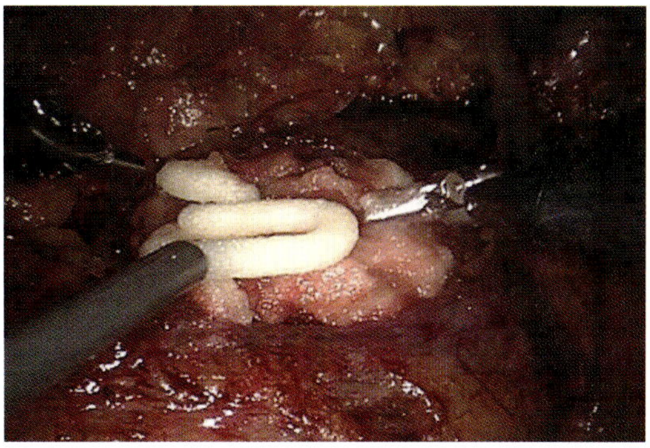

Figure 9. Applying Floseal to renal bed. Credit: © 2013 Intuitive Surgical, Inc.

suture is halfway between the ends of the clip by the bedside assistant. This allows the clip to be slid down onto the renal parenchyma by one arm of the robot while the other arm pulls up on the suture. The surgeon can come back and tighten this further after the remaining sutures are placed. These steps in the management of the Hem-o-lok clip placed by the assistant onto the suture are repeated for all subsequent hemostatic sutures placed to help bring the tumor bed edges together. After the V-lock running suture, all subsequent sutures are interrupted 0-Vicryl on a CT-1 needle, six inches long. These Vicryl sutures are placed approximately 1 cm apart extending from one tumor edge to the other. One can either tighten these sutures as one goes along or place some Surgicel +/– Floseal into the tumor base before tightening the sutures (Figure 9). In our experience, these hemostatic agents are rarely needed. Once all of the hemostatic sutures have been placed and tightened, attention is taken to unclamp the hilum.

7. **Hilar unclamping.** In order to again expose the renal hilum, the fourth arm is placed under the ureter or lower pole on traction, as previously described. If two needle drivers are in place for the right and left robotic arms, a ProGrasp needs to be switched out from the left needle driver in order to open up the jaws of the robotic bulldog clamp. Extreme care must be taken during hilar unclamping as the hilar vasculature can be inadvertently injured with the bulldog clamp. If the renal vein and artery have been clamped, the vein is unclamped first.

   After the entire hilum is unclamped, attention is turned to the reconstructed tumor bed to look for any active bleeding. The Hem-o-lok clips may be tightened further to help bring the parenchymal edges even closer together. If more bleeding than expected is noted, one can apply pressure, pushing down on a piece of Surgicel or thrombin-soaked Gelfoam with either one of the robotic arms or the sucker tip on top of the area of suspected bleeding. One may also try and inject more Floseal in between the edges of the reconstructed parenchyma. Additional hemostatic 0-Vicryl sutures may be placed. The pneumoperitoneum can be increased from 15 to 20 mmHg. As a last resort, if bleeding continues to be excessive, the hilum may need to be reclamped and the tumor bed re-exposed and inspected. This, however, would be very unusual. Finally, before proceeding to the next portion of the operation, one can slide down Lapra-Ties on top of the Hem-o-loks to stabilize them in place. This, however, is optional.

8. **Suture removal, drain placement, tumor extraction, and termination of the procedure.** The next step is to ensure that all of the needles are cut from each suture and removed one by one, verifying a correct final needle count. The specimen is then bagged using the Endo Catch bag through one of the 12 mm assistant ports. A 10 French flat Jackson-Pratt drain is then placed through one of the 12 mm assistant ports and grasped with a Maryland grasper by the bedside assistant through the fourth arm port after the fourth arm has been undocked. The drain is pulled so the holes of the drain are in the vicinity of the reconstructed parenchyma. The next step is to close the 12 mm port sites using the Carter-Thomason laparoscopic closing device, except for the port site where the Endo Catch bag will be extracted. All port sites are observed by the robotic camera as they are pulled out. Finally, the 12 mm port site where the Endo Catch bag is extracted is elongated enough at the skin and fascial level to allow for removal of the specimen inside it. The fascia is then closed with a 0-Vicryl suture on a UR-6 needle. All skin sites are closed using subcuticular 4-0 monocryl suture.

Outcomes of Robotic Partial Nephrectomy

Surgical resection remains the gold standard for treatment of localized RCC. Over the last two decades, the excellent oncologic outcomes following PN and the higher incidence of chronic kidney disease with radical nephrectomy, even with good preoperative contralateral kidney function, led away from radical nephrectomy and toward nephron-sparing surgery for small renal masses.[27] Although open PN used to be the gold standard treatment, this is now open to debate with the rapid and progressive improvements in minimally invasive technology and expanding laparoscopic surgical expertise.

Open PN often requires a muscle-cutting flank incision and occasional removal of a lower rib, which can lead to chronic morbidity such as pain, paresthesia, and hernia formation.[28–30] Laparoscopic PN remains prohibitively technically challenging for a significant portion of urologists, requiring acquisition of advanced skills and a steep learning curve. The two-dimensional visualization and poor ergonomics due to the use of rigid instrumentation make tumor excision and intracorporeal suture reconstruction under minimal ischemia time challenging. When compared to open PN, laparoscopic PN was shown to have comparable intermediate oncologic and functional outcomes with shorter convalescence, but longer ischemia times and increased risk of postoperative hemorrhage and major urologic complications.[12,15,31]

The realization of the benefits of a robotic approach to PN in combination with some of the disadvantages of open and traditional laparoscopic techniques has led to an increase in the use of the robot for small renal masses. Robotic instruments can bridge the gap between open and laparoscopic PN, providing the surgeon the benefit of open technique and the value of a minimally invasive approach. The magnified three-dimensional vision, tremor filtration, and articulating instruments facilitate precise tumor resection and sutured renal reconstruction with reduced operative times, blood loss, as well as WITs.[19,32,33] Moreover, most series published to date showed oncologic control similar to open and laparoscopic PN. Although it has not been extensively studied, robotic PN has been reported to have a reduced learning curve when compared to laparoscopic PN, for both the inexperienced laparoscopic surgeons and surgeons with substantial prior robotic experience.[32,34,35] It is important to mention the cost differential between robotic PN and laparoscopic or open PN. Certainly, the robotic procedure is more expensive to both implement and perform; however, its wider use and availability appear to make this technology more cost effective.

Intraoperative Outcomes

The mean operative time for robotic PN varies between 82.7 and 279 minutes, and the estimated blood loss (EBL) varies between 92 and 360 cc.[36–40] There appears to be wide variability across published studies, which may be attributed to the fact that data are reported at different points on institutional learning curves. One of the largest single-institution series to date reported mean operative times and EBL of 206 minutes and 127 cc, respectively, which compare favorably with historic open and laparoscopic PN series.[12,33] In another large single-institution study by Wang and Bhayani, a comparison between laparoscopic and robotic PN revealed a statistically significant reduction in operative time for robotic PN (140 vs. 156 minutes, $P = 0.04$), while there was no difference in EBL between the two groups.[41]

On the other hand, Benway and colleagues compared laparoscopic and robotic PN in a large multi-institutional series and reported no significant difference in operative times (189 vs. 174 minutes) between the two groups, but reduced EBL (155 vs. 196 cc; $P = 0.03$) in the robotic PN group.[15] It is apparent that comparative data are inconsistent so far and have failed to demonstrate definite superiority of robotic techniques with regard to operative times and EBL. However, careful interpretation of these results is important given the fact that in most of these series, surgeons were experienced in the open and laparoscopic technique but were at the beginning of their learning curve for robotic techniques when the study was performed. This may have influenced the study outcomes.

WIT is the term created to describe the length of time the renal vessels are clamped without cooling during minimally invasive PN. Recently, WIT has been the subject of debate because it not only gives an indication of the efficiency of the surgeon to perform renorrhaphy, but also allows prediction of the short- and long-term renal function outcomes.[42,43] Although the “safe” period of warm ischemia during minimally invasive PN remains controversial, it has been suggested that WIT under 30 minutes provides satisfactory postoperative renal function. When comparing laparoscopic and robotic PN, several studies have shown a significantly shorter WIT in patients undergoing robotic PN.[15,41,44] This was even demonstrated with complex renal tumors.[15] This may be a result of the technically demanding nature of the laparoscopic technique as opposed to the easier renal reconstruction with the robotic approach.

Postoperative Outcomes

Length of hospital stay, a surrogate for return to function, is an important consideration that can affect a patient’s decision about which treatment option to choose. As expected, minimally invasive PN has been associated with shorter hospital stays when compared to open PN. Indeed, length of hospital stay after robotic PN has been comparable to laparoscopic PN and has ranged from a mean of 2.0–4.8 days in contemporary series.[45] Some series have reported even significantly shorter postoperative hospital stay with robotic PN when compared to laparoscopic PN.[34,41]

The overall complication rate is also crucial when evaluating the safety of new surgical procedures. The reported complication rate in large series of robotic PN varies from 8.2 to 25%.[18,19,33,41,46,47] These results compare favorably to the postoperative complication rate in both open PN (13.7%) and laparoscopic PN (18.6%).[12] A multi-institutional analysis by Benway et al. revealed similar rates of postoperative complications for robotic and laparoscopic PN (8.6% vs. 10.2%).[15] A few of the most commonly described complications in the recently published series were urinary leaks, hematomas, and cardiopulmonary problems.

Oncological outcomes of robotic PN are perhaps the most important determinants of the effectiveness and future of this procedure. The early oncologic efficacy of robotic PN is promising and appears to be equivalent to open and laparoscopic PN. Given the short follow-up periods of the current robotic series, which makes assessment of local recurrence and metastatic spread difficult, the rate of positive surgical margins has been utilized as a primary oncologic outcome. The initial large, single-institution robotic PN series demonstrated positive surgical margin rates ranging from 1.5% to 5.7%.[19,34,41,46] A multi-institutional study by Benway et al. also showed a low positive margin rate of 3.8%.[15] These results compare favorably with historical rates for open PN (1.3%) and laparoscopic PN (2.9%) in experienced hands.[12] Interestingly, Lane and Gill showed equivalent 5-year and 7-year cancer-specific survival rates for both open and laparoscopic PN in patients with renal tumors less than 7 cm.[48] It is very likely that the long-term oncologic efficacy of robotic PN will be comparable to the other two techniques; however, until long-term data are available for the robotic approach, urologists should be cautious when discussing the different surgical approaches with their patients.

References

1. Simon G. *Chirurgie der Nieren.* Stuttgart: Ferdinand Enke; 1871.

2. Czerny V. Reported by Herczel E: *Über Nierenextir-pation.* Beitr Z Klin Chir 1890;6:485.

3. Vermooten V. Indications for conservative surgery in certain renal tumors: a study based on the growth pattern of the cell carcinoma. *J Urol.* 1950;64:200–8.

4. Licht MR, Novick AC. Nephron sparing surgery for renal cell carcinoma. *J Urol.* 1993;149:1–7.

5. Herr HW. Partial nephrectomy for unilateral renal carcinoma and a normal contralateral kidney: 10-year followup. *J Urol.* 1999;161:33-4; discussion 4–5.

6. Fergany AF, Hafez KS, Novick AC. Long-term results of nephron sparing surgery for localized renal cell carcinoma: 10-year followup. *J Urol.* 2000;163:442–5.

7. Clayman RV, Kavoussi LR, Soper NJ, et al. Laparoscopic nephrectomy: initial case report. *J Urol.* 1991;146:278–82.

8. Clayman RV, Kavoussi LR, Soper NJ, et al. Laparoscopic nephrectomy. *N Engl J Med.* 1991;324:1370–1.

9. McDougall EM, Clayman RV, Chandhoke PS, et al. Laparoscopic partial nephrectomy in the pig model. *J Urol.* 1993;149:1633–6.

10. Winfield HN, Donovan JF, Godet AS, Clayman RV. Laparoscopic partial nephrectomy: initial case report for benign disease. *J Endourol.* 1993;7:521–6.

11. Allaf ME, Bhayani SB, Rogers C, et al. Laparoscopic partial nephrectomy: evaluation of long-term oncological outcome. *J Urol.* 2004;172:871–3.

12. Gill IS, Kavoussi LR, Lane BR, et al. Comparison of 1,800 laparoscopic and open partial nephrectomies for single renal tumors. *J Urol.* 2007;178:41–6.

13. Lane BR, Gill IS. 5-Year outcomes of laparoscopic partial nephrectomy. *J Urol.* 2007;177:70–4; discussion 4.

14. Porpiglia F, Volpe A, Billia M, Scarpa RM. Laparoscopic versus open partial nephrectomy: analysis of the current literature. *Eur Urol.* 2008;53:732–42; discussion 42–3.

15. Benway BM, Bhayani SB, Rogers CG, et al. Robot assisted partial nephrectomy versus laparoscopic partial nephrectomy for renal tumors: a multi-institutional analysis of perioperative outcomes. *J Urol.* 2009;182:866–72.

16. Gettman MT, Blute ML, Chow GK, Neururer R, Bartsch G, Peschel R. Robotic-assisted laparoscopic partial nephrectomy: technique and initial clinical experience with da Vinci robotic system. *Urology.* 2004;64:914–8.

17. Rogers CG, Metwalli A, Blatt AM, et al. Robotic partial nephrectomy for renal hilar tumors: a multi-institutional analysis. *J Urol.* 2008;180:2353–6; discussion 6.

18. Benway BM, Bhayani SB, Rogers CG, et al. Robot-assisted partial nephrectomy: an international experience. *Eur Urol.* 2010;57:815–20.

19. Patel MN, Krane LS, Bhandari A, et al. Robotic partial nephrectomy for renal tumors larger than 4 cm. *Eur Urol.* 2010;57:310–6.

20. Siegel R, Naishadham D, Jemal A. Cancer statistics, 2012. *CA Cancer J Clin.* 2012; 62:10–29.

21. Karumanchi SA, Merchan J, Sukhatme VP. Renal cancer: molecular mechanisms and newer therapeutic options. *Curr Opin Nephrol Hypertens.* 2002;11:37–42.

22. Flocks RH, Kadesky MC. Malignant neoplasms of the kidney; an analysis of 353 patients followed five years or more. *J Urol.* 1958;79:196–201.

23. Robson CJ, Churchill BM, Anderson W. The results of radical nephrectomy for renal cell carcinoma. *J Urol.* 1969;101:297–301.

24. Harmer M. *TNM Classification of Malignant Tumors,* 2nd ed. Geneva: International Union Against Cancer; 1974.

25. Moch H, Artibani W, Delahunt B, et al. Reassessing the current UICC/AJCC TNM staging for renal cell carcinoma. *Eur Urol.* 2009;56:636–43.

26. Edge SB, Byrd DR, Compton CC, et al. Eds. *AJCC Cancer Staging Manual.* 7th ed. New York: Springer-Verlag; 2009.

27. Kim SP, Thompson RH, Boorjian SA, et al. Comparative effectiveness for survival and renal function of partial and radical nephrectomy for localized renal tumors: a systematic review and meta-analysis. *J Urol.* 2012;188:51–7.

28. Brandina R, Aron M. Laparoscopic partial nephrectomy: advances since 2005. *Curr Opin Urol.* 2010;20:111–8.

29. Yoshimura K, Ohara H, Ichioka K, et al. Body image alteration after flank incision: relationship between the results of objective evaluation using computerized tomography and patient perception. *J Urol.* 2003;169:182–5.

30. Chatterjee S, Nam R, Fleshner N, Klotz L. Permanent flank bulge is a consequence of flank incision for radical nephrectomy in one half of patients. *Urol Oncol.* 2004;22:36–9.

31. Campbell SC, Novick AC, Belldegrun A, et al. Guideline for management of the clinical T1 renal mass. *J Urol.* 2009;182:1271–9.

32. Mottrie A, De Naeyer G, Schatteman P, Carpentier P, Sangalli M, Ficarra V. Impact of the learning curve on perioperative outcomes in patients who underwent robotic partial nephrectomy for parenchymal renal tumours. *Eur Urol.* 2010;58:127–32.

33. Scoll BJ, Uzzo RG, Chen DY, et al. Robot-assisted partial nephrectomy: a large single-institutional experience. *Urology.* 2010;75:1328–34.

34. Deane LA, Lee HJ, Box GN, et al. Robotic versus standard laparoscopic partial/wedge nephrectomy: a comparison of intraoperative and perioperative results from a single institution. *J Endourol.* 2008;22:947–52.

35. Ellison JS, Montgomery JS, Wolf JS Jr, Hafez KS, Miller DC, Weizer AZ. A matched comparison of perioperative outcomes of a single laparoscopic surgeon versus a multisurgeon robot-assisted cohort for partial nephrectomy. *J Urol.* 2012;188:45–50.

36. Boris R, Proano M, Linehan WM, Pinto PA, Bratslavsky G. Initial experience with robot assisted partial nephrectomy for multiple renal masses. *J Urol.* 2009;182:1280–6.

37. Caruso RP, Phillips CK, Kau E, Taneja SS, Stifelman MD. Robot assisted laparoscopic partial nephrectomy: initial experience. *J Urol.* 2006;176:36–9.

38. Ho H, Schwentner C, Neururer R, Steiner H, Bartsch G, Peschel R. Robotic-assisted laparoscopic partial nephrectomy: surgical technique and clinical outcomes at 1 year. *BJU Int.* 2009;103:663–8.

39. Aron M, Koenig P, Kaouk JH, Nguyen MM, Desai MM, Gill IS. Robotic and laparoscopic partial nephrectomy: a matched-pair comparison from a high-volume centre. *BJU Int.* 2008;102:86–92.

40. Kaul S, Laungani R, Sarle R, et al. da Vinci-assisted robotic partial nephrectomy: technique and results at a mean of 15 months of follow-up. *Eur Urol.* 2007;51:186–91; discussion 91–2.

41. Wang AJ, Bhayani SB. Robotic partial nephrectomy versus laparoscopic partial nephrectomy for renal cell carcinoma: single-surgeon analysis of >100 consecutive procedures. *Urology.* 2009;73:306–10.

42. Thompson RH, Lane BR, Lohse CM, et al. Every minute counts when the renal hilum is clamped during partial nephrectomy. *Eur Urol.* 2010;58:340–5.

43. Becker F, Van Poppel H, Hakenberg OW, et al. Assessing the impact of ischaemia time during partial nephrectomy. *Eur Urol.* 2009;56:625–34.

44. Thompson RH, Lane BR, Lohse CM, et al. Comparison of warm ischemia versus no ischemia during partial nephrectomy on a solitary kidney. *Eur Urol.* 2010;58:331–6.

45. Gautam G, Benway BM, Bhayani SB, Zorn KC. Robot-assisted partial nephrectomy: current perspectives and future prospects. *Urology.* 2009;74:735–40.

46. Gupta GN, Boris R, Chung P, Marston Linehan W, Pinto PA, Bratslavsky G. Robot-assisted laparoscopic partial nephrectomy for tumors greater than 4 cm and high nephrometry score: Feasibility, renal functional, and oncological outcomes with minimum 1 year follow-up. *Urol Oncol.* 2011: Epub.

47. White MA, Haber GP, Autorino R, et al. Outcomes of robotic partial nephrectomy for renal masses with nephrometry score of ≥7. *Urology.* 2011;77:809–13.

48. Lane BR, Gill IS. 7-year oncological outcomes after laparoscopic and open partial nephrectomy. *J Urol.* 2010;183:473–9.

Chapter Nine

Robotic Prostatectomy

Crystal M. Kavanagh, MD; Christodoulos G. Kaoutzanis, MD; Eduardo Kleer, MD

Epidemiology

Prostate cancer is the most frequently diagnosed non-skin cancer in the United States, with roughly 240,890 new cases diagnosed in 2011. Projected lifetime risk for this diagnosis is currently estimated at 1 in 6 for American men. The risk of prostate cancer death is 1 in 33.[1,2] These figures, however, assumed that screening protocols as initiated in the 1990s would remain unchanged.[1] The US Preventative Services Task Force published revised recommendations in 2012 endorsing the cessation of non-targeted screening, citing an imbalance between risk and benefit.[3] Among the reasons for this shift was the observation that one-third of all prostate-specific antigen (PSA) levels are obtained in men greater than age 70, a significant number of whom are facing competing mortality. The lack of individualization of care often means that patients are directed toward curative treatment when their risk of death from prostate cancer is secondary.[3,4,5,6] Proponents of continued screening by way of PSA and digital rectal exam (DRE) cite strong evidence of a reduction in the rates of advanced disease.[7,8]

Despite the ongoing debate surrounding screening for the disease, radical prostatectomy has been established as the treatment with the best evidence for reducing cancer-specific mortality in men.[9] As such, it remains the standard of care for patients with localized prostate cancer and a life expectancy that exceeds 10 years.[10,11] For those patients with more advanced disease, the addition of adjunct therapies, including chemotherapy, radiation, and hormonal therapies, has improved overall all-stage five-year survival rates to 99.6%.[2] A review recently published in the *New England Journal of Medicine* randomized 731 men with localized prostate cancer to radical prostatectomy versus observation over an 8-year period. The authors concluded no advantage for the cohort randomized to surgical intervention. While this is a single study, the results are significant in terms of how newly diagnosed men are counseled.[6]

Prostate Cancer Staging

The first formal clinical staging system for prostate cancer was introduced by Whitmore in 1956, and later refined by Jewett in 1975. Despite amendments, however, this system lacked the refinement to accurately describe the extent of local disease or sites of metastasis.[12] As such, the contemporary modality in the staging of prostate cancer is based upon the tumor-node-metastases (TNM) classification system. This system has undergone multiple revisions in conjunction with the American Joint Committee on Cancer (AJCC), the most recent of which occurred in 2010 (Table 1). The updated guidelines incorporate a more risk-based approach that utilizes the Gleason grading system and current PSA value in the staging system, bringing it more in line with risk-adapted approaches[13] (Table 2). Additionally, microscopic bladder neck invasion as a form of extracapsular extension was incorporated into T3 disease rather than T4, given the more favorable outcomes of this subgroup of men. Controversy remains in the current model as it relates to nonpalable lesions identified by transrectal ultrasound (TRUS), which are categorized as T2. Because TRUS findings do not predict tumor extent in PSA-detected non-palpable lesions,[6,14,15] these malignancies are often classified as T1c in clinical practice, irrespective of TRUS findings.

Therefore, the following items are noted:

1. A tumor found in one or both sites by needle biopsy, but not palpable or reliably visible by imaging, is classified T1c.
2. Invasion into the prostatic apex or into (but not beyond) the prostatic capsule is classified as T2.
3. There is no pathologic T1 classification.
4. Positive surgical margins should be indicated by an R1 descriptor (residual macroscopic disease).
5. When more than one site of metastasis is present, the most advanced category is used. PM1c is most advanced.

History of Radical Prostatectomy

Hugh Hampton Young is credited with performing the first open prostatectomy for carcinoma in 1905. In 1947, Millin described the first radical retropubic prostatectomy (RRP).[12,16,17] These approaches were complicated by a high incidence of erectile dysfunction, impotence, hemorrhage, and incontinence. In the late 1970s and early 1980s, however, further delineation of surgical anatomy, specifically defining the dorsal venous complex, the striated sphincter, and the neurovascular bundle, led to marked reduction in postoperative morbidity.[10,12,16] As such, while innovations in approaches have emerged, the tenets of the anatomic, nerve-sparing radical prostatectomy have remained largely unchanged over the past three decades.

In their series of nine patients, Schuessler et al. were the first to describe laparoscopic radical prostatectomy (LRP).[18] While cure rates were determined to be comparable to open surgery, operative duration and technical difficulty deterred its adoption for mass use. Advances in both technology and technique, led by two large French centers,[19] culminated in the development of a systematic and reproducible approach that translated into broader use of LRP, primarily in large academic

Table 1. TNM Classification for Prostatic Adenocarcinoma

Classification	Description
Primary Tumor	
TX	Primary tumor cannot be assessed.
T0	No evidence of primary tumor.
T1	Clinically unapparent tumor neither palpable nor visible by imaging.
T1a	Tumor incidental histologic finding in ≤5% of tissue resected.
T1b	Tumor incidental histologic finding in >5% of tissue resected.
T1c	Tumor identified by needle biopsy (e.g., because of elevated PSA).
T2	Tumor confined within prostate.[1]
T2a	Tumor involves = one-half of one lobe.
T2b	Tumor involves >one-half of one lobe but not both lobes.
T2c	Tumor involves both lobes.
T3	Tumor extends through the prostate capsule.[2]
T3a	Extracapsular extension (unilateral or bilateral).
T3b	Tumor invades seminal vesicle(s).
T4	Tumor is fixed or invades adjacent structures other than seminal vesicles such as external sphincter, rectum, bladder, levator muscles, and/or pelvic wall.
Pathologic (pT)[3]	
pT2	Organ Confined
pT2a	Unilateral, one-half of one side or less
pT2b	Unilateral, involving more than one-half but not both sides
pT2c	Bilateral disease
pT3	Extraprostatic disease
pT3a	Extraprostatic extension or microscopic invasion of the bladder neck[4]
pT3b	Seminal vesicle invasion
pT4	Invasion of rectum, levator muscles and/or pelvic wall
Regional Lymph Nodes (N)	
Clinical	
NX	Regional nodes not assessed
N0	No regional lymph node metastasis
N1	Metastasis in regional lymph node(s)
Pathologic	
pNX	Regional nodes not sampled
pN0	No positive regional nodes
pN1	Metastasis in regional node(s)
Distant Metastasis[5]	
M0	No distant metastasis
M1	Distant metastasis
M1a	Non-regional lymph nodes
M1b	Bone(s)
M1c	Other site(s) with or without bone disease

Table 2. Prostate Cancer Staging

Stage	T	N	M	PSA*	Gleason
I	T1a-c	N0	M0	PSA < 10	Gleason =6
	T2a	N0	M0	PSA < 10	Gleason =6
	T1-T2a	N0	M0	PSA X	Gleason X
IIA	T1a-c	N0	M0	PSA < 20	Gleason 7
	T1a-c	N0	M0	PSA =10 but < 20	Gleason =6
	T2a	N0	M0	PSA < 20	Gleason = 7
	T2b	N0	M0	PSA < 20	Gleason =7
	T2b	N0	M0	PSA X	Gleason X
IIB	T2c	N0	M0	Any PSA	Any Gleason
	T1-2	N0	M0	PSA =20	Any Gleason
	T1-2	N0	M0	Any PSA	Gleason =8
III	T3a-b	N0	M0	Any PSA	Any Gleason
IV	T4	N0	M0	Any PSA	Any Gleason
	Any T	N1	M0	Any PSA	Any Gleason
	Any T	Any N	M1	Any PSA	Any Gleason

* If PSA or Gleason is not available, grouping should be determined by T stage and/or either PSA or Gleason, as available.

centers. However, successful completion of LRP had a challenging learning curve. To discern complex anatomical landmarks utilizing only visual cues displayed on a television monitor in two dimensions is especially challenging. Additionally, suturing of the vesicourethral anastomosis with rigid instruments that prevent articulated wrist motion impedes proficiency.[12]

The development of robotic-assisted devices, such as the da Vinci robotic surgical system and its application in prostatectomy, has provided the benefit of a minimally invasive approach while addressing the technical limitations of conventional laparoscopy. Robotic-assisted laparoscopic prostatectomy (RALP) was first performed in the United States by Binder and Kramer in 2000, and since that time a rapid growth in RALP has been noted, driven both by patient demand and surgeon preference. Its use continues to expand such that in 2007 roughly 85% of radical prostatectomies were completed using this approach; less than 1% of all radical prostatectomies were performed via purely laparoscopic means.[9] Debate surrounding the merit of RALP versus conventional open approaches is ongoing, primarily concerning cost and the learning curve of the surgeon and operative team. Despite the controversy, RALP has led to a revolutionary shift in the management of prostate disease, and its use is expected to continue to expand.

Patient Selection

The indications to proceed with RALP match those for conventional open surgery. The highest cure rates from surgery alone are observed among those patients who have a clinical diagnosis of T1 or T2 cancer with no evidence of metastatic disease, PSA levels <10, and a Gleason score <8. Patients who present with clinical stage T3 cancers, a Gleason score >8, and PSA >10 are still potential surgical candidates, provided that metastatic preoperative evaluation is negative. These patients must also be advised of the possible need for adjunct therapies based on pathological findings. In general, patients less than age 70 should be selected; however, age-based determinations rely heavily on functional status.

As with any operative intervention, an uncorrectable bleeding diathesis or the presence of severe cardiopulmonary disease that would preclude tolerance of general anesthesia are absolute contraindications to RALP. Patients who are morbidly obese pose limitations from a technical standpoint related to working space and trocar length. Additionally, Trendelenburg positioning can incite respiratory compromise in this group. While not a contraindication, patients with a history of treatment failure following radiation or ablation therapies or those who have undergone neo-adjuvant hormonal therapy often have loss of planar definition. Obliteration and fibrosis, specifically between the anterior rectum and posterior prostate, can lead to increased risk of rectal perforation.[20,21]

In those patients with a history of complex lower abdominal or pelvic surgery, technical challenges present owing to distortion of normal anatomy in combination with adhesion formation. Patients who have a history of laparoscopic extraperitoneal mesh herniorrhaphy may benefit from a transperitoneal approach, which avoids dense adhesions in the retropubic space.[12,16,22,23]

Patient Positioning

On induction of endotracheal anesthesia, the patient is placed supine and into steep Trendelenburg (>20 degrees). Arms are tucked and all bony prominences padded. The patient's legs are spread apart and placed into stirrups in low lithotomy position in order to allow for access to the rectum and perineum. A safety strap is placed across the patient's chest. Orogastric and urethral catheters are placed.

Trocar Placement

The most common approach to RALP is via the transperitoneal anterior approach, which allows for immediate access to the space of Retzius and anterior dissection of the prostate gland, seminal vesicle, and vasa. In this method, pneumoperitoneum is established using either an open Hassan or Veress needle approach just above the umbilicus, and a trocar is inserted.

The maximum working length of the da Vinci instruments is 25 cm. As such, ports should be placed on an arc at a distance of roughly 15 cm from the pubic bone. The stereo endoscope is placed in a 12 mm cannula port 1–2 cm above the umbilicus. In patients who are tall or obese, infraumbilical camera placement may be preferable. The right instrument arm port is an 8 mm cannula that is placed 8 cm to the right of the camera port, intersecting a line one finger-breadth below the umbilicus. The left instrument port is also an 8 mm cannula placed 8 cm to the left of the midline, mirroring the right arm port. If using a third instrument arm port, this would be placed on an 8 mm cannula at the patient's left side approximately 8 cm (or one hand-breadth) away from the left instrument arm port, slightly more proximal. The assistant port is a 12 mm cannula placed on the patient's right side at distance 8 cm away from the right arm instrument port and slightly more proximal (Figure 1).

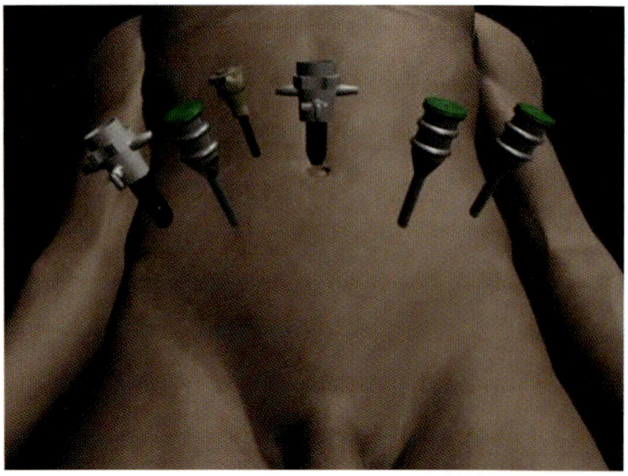

Figure 1. Trocar placement in standard four-arm da Vinci prostatectomy. Credit: © 2013 Intuitive Surgical, Inc.

In the extraperitoneal approach, a 1.5 cm incision is made at the level of the umbilicus. Dissection is carried down through the anterior rectus sheath and a space is developed over the posterior rectus sheath. A trocar-mounted balloon dilator is placed into this space and advanced down to the pubis. A 0-degree, 10 mm endoscope is inserted through the trocar and 500 mL of air is inflated, thus developing the space of Retzius. The remainder of the trocars are inserted as previously described. This approach may be of benefit in patients with extensive abdominal surgical history or in the morbidly obese.

Working in the pre-peritoneal space inherently reduces the risk of bowel injury. Furthermore, should a leak from the vesicourethral anastomosis occur, urine would be excluded from the peritoneal cavity. The extraperitoneal approach, however, is associated with longer operative times and is more technically challenging given the limited working space compared to transperitoneal access.

In the following section, this chapter will describe the transperitoneal approach.

Transperitoneal RALP: Surgical Technique Step-by-Step

The surgery is initiated with a 0 degree lens. The right arm is fitted with hot monopolar curved scissors and the left arm with a bipolar Maryland grasper. The fourth arm is fitted with a ProGrasp. The assistant uses a suction irrigator through the 5 mm port and a wavy grasper through the 12 mm assistant port.

1. **Establishment of the retropubic space.** The anterior peritoneal attachments to the posterior rectal fascia just lateral to the right and left of the medial umbilical ligaments are incised as high up as one can reach. This is best achieved by applying heat to one blade of the scissors while they are open. This maneuver results in the appearance of a "wispy" or "cotton-candy" looking connective tissue (Figure 2). One can then continue this incision inferior-laterally down toward the vas deferens, which establishes

the lateral border of the incision. That "wispy" looking tissue is then moved anteriorly and inferiorly using blunt dissection until the pubic bone is encountered. After this is accomplished bilaterally, the operator transects horizontally high up across the median and medial umbilical ligaments. The previously established plane of dissection comes into view. One can then follow this plane containing the "wispy" tissue anteriorly straight down to the pubic bone, safely dropping the bladder out of harm's way.

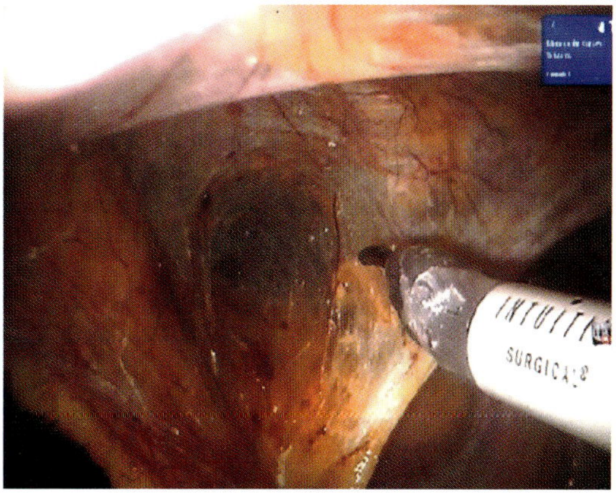

Figure 2. "Wispy" or "cotton-candy" appearance of tissue as one dissects into the retropubic space.

The operator then bluntly separates the remaining attachments between the bladder and pelvic sidewall laterally, until reaching the vas deferens on either side. The next step is to "defat" the area over the surface above the prostate, as distally as the puboprostatic ligaments, laterally above the endopelvic fascia, and proximally to the bladder neck as possible. Cephalad traction on the bladder with the ProGrasp facilitates this portion of the surgery. The next step is to incise the endopelvic fascia from the base of the prostate all the way up to the puboprostatic ligament. Lateral levator muscular attachments are bluntly separated from the lateral prostate. The puboprostatic ligaments are incised at the level of the pubis.

2. **Ligation of the deep dorsal vein complex (DVC) and anterior urethropexy.** The da Vinci needle drivers are switched into the right and left robot arms. The DVC is suture-ligated using a 0-Vicryl suture on a CT-1 needle (Figure 3). One can use either one throw with a slipknot to tie it down securely or a figure of eight throw. It is important to check that the indwelling Foley catheter slides easily and is not caught by the stitch before tying it down. Some surgeons prefer to take the DVC using an endovascular stapler instead of suture. The next stitch is the anterior urethropexy stitch. This is done with a 0-Vicryl suture on a CT-2 needle with a Lapra-Ty on the end. The first throw of the suture is to the back of the pubic symphysis going from left to right. The suture is pulled up

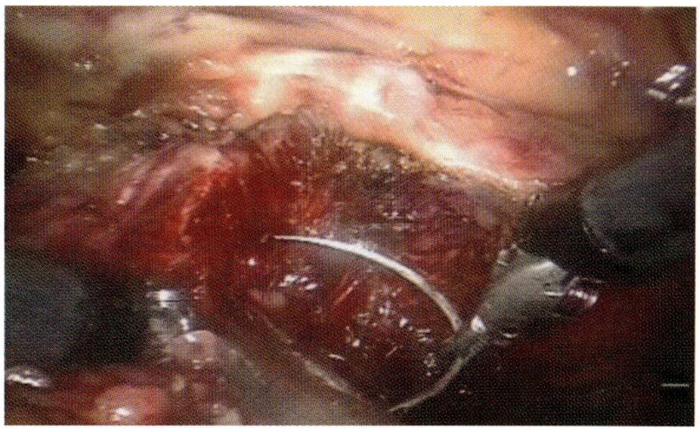

Figure 3. Driving of the CT-1 needle during suture ligation of the dorsal venous complex. Credit: © 2013 Intuitive Surgical, Inc.

until the Lapra-Ty is flush against the pubis. The needle is then passed right to left through the same plane as the first DVC stitch. Finally, the suture is again passed into the back of the pubis, left to right. As this stitch is pulled upward, it also pulls up the DVC and anterior urethra. A Lapra-Ty is placed to the suture next to the back of the pubis by the assistant to maintain its tension. Again, it is advised to check that the indwelling Foley catheter slides easily again. The purpose of this stitch is to help with hemostatic control of the DVC and to help with continence by minimizing postoperative urethral hypermobility.

3. **Bladder neck transection.** The hot monopolar curved scissors and bipolar Maryland graspers are switched back into the right and left robotic arms, respectively. A lens 30 degrees down helps to better delineate the prostatovesical junction and to look down into the bladder neck once it is entered. The fourth arm ProGrasp continues with cephalad tension on the bladder. The bladder neck incision starts through the prostatovesical junction using cautery at the 12 o'clock position, where one can appreciate anterior bladder fibers attaching to the prostate. The left arm places traction just proximal to where the right arm is incising. As one does this, the bladder springs back proximally. At this point, one can also score the fat lateral to the prostatovesical junction. This fat dissection lateral to the bladder neck helps to establish a landmark that can be followed after the bladder neck is transected (Figure 4).

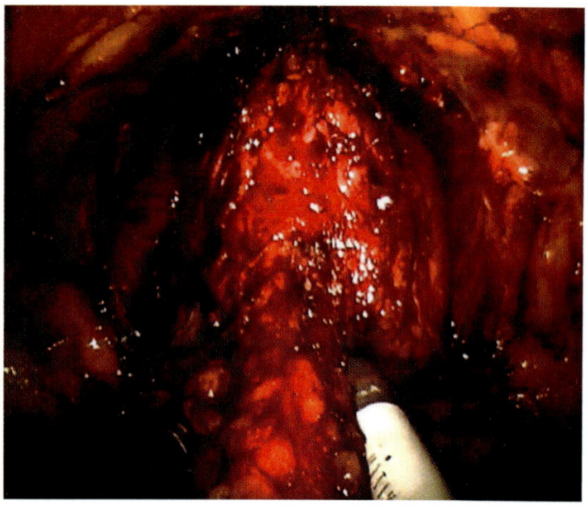

Figure 4. Bladder neck is isolated prior to incising it anteriorly.

Once the anterior bladder neck is incised, the tip of the Foley catheter is grasped using the fourth arm ProGrasp and is pulled up high in the pelvis anteriorly behind the pubis. The distal end of the Foley is then placed on stretch by the bedside assistant. This elevates the posterior bladder neck, which facilitates its visualization. At this point, one looks for the presence of a median lobe. If no median lobe is present, the operator incises the posterior bladder neck at the 6 o'clock position and carries the dissection through, following the contour of the bladder neck laterally to help establish a plane between the bladder neck and prostate. This lateral posterior bladder neck dissection helps to preserve a more muscular bladder neck.

As one continues with the dissection posteriorly, it is important to maintain it straight down at 90 degrees. Angling the dissection toward the bladder neck will result in thinning of the bladder neck or even buttonholing the trigone. Angling the dissection anteriorly can result in inadvertent entrance into the prostate. Identification of the previously scored fat, lateral to the vesical neck, also facilitates this dissection. If a median lobe is present after entering the posterior bladder neck, one needs to follow this lobe circumferentially and score its junction to the bladder (Figure 5).

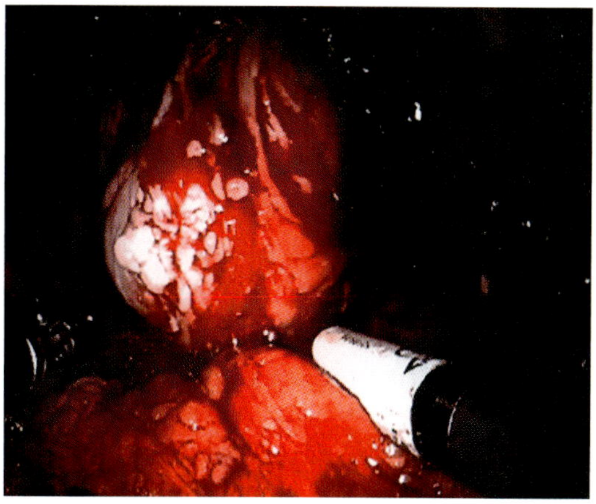
Figure 5. A large median lobe is appreciated.

This is easier done if the median lobe can be lifted anteriorly by the fourth arm. It is at this junction that the bladder is incised to full thickness. Once the bladder is incised full thickness, the dissection then continues posteriorly, which allows one to gain more space between the bladder and prostate by taking down the upper portion of the lateral pedicles. Eventually, the anterior layer of Denonvilliers' fascia, which covers the vasa deferentia and seminal vesicles, is reached.

4. **Dissection of vasa deferentia and seminal vesicles.** The anterior Denonvilliers' fascia is incised longitudinally exposing the underlying vasa deferentia. It is important not to skeletonize and transect the vas early in this dissection. The vas essentially helps to pull up the tip of the seminal vesicle. The vas is first pulled up anteriorly with the fourth arm. The operator should stay medial to the vas, allowing identification of the medial wall of the seminal vesicle. The fourth arm is repositioned and is used to pull this up. One can then trace the seminal vesicle medially down to its tip (Figure 6). The fourth arm is again used to pull up the tip of the seminal vesicle. It is at this point that the vas is transected. The vasal artery is encountered posterior to the vas at this portion of the procedure. The blood supply to the tip of the seminal vesicle is clearly seen. The blood supply is then taken with clips rather than cautery if a nerve-sparing prostatectomy is being performed. The rest of the lateral seminal vesicle is then traced to the base of the prostate. An additional artery supplying the seminal vesicle is often found during this portion of the procedure. The identical procedure is performed on the contralateral side.

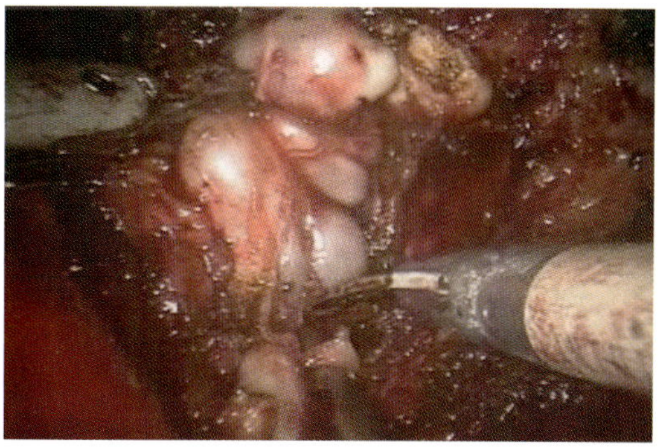
Figure 6. Dissection of the seminal vesicles.
Credit: © 2013 Intuitive Surgical, Inc.

5. **Separation of prostate away from rectum.** The fourth arm is used to pull the vas and seminal vesicle straight up on one side and the assistant does the same on the contralateral side using a wavy grasper. This upward traction facilitates entrance to the posterior layer of Denonvilliers' fascia. The initial establishment of this plane is achieved through a combination of sharp and blunt dissection. If one is in the right plane, this dissection progresses smoothly and quickly on top of a pearly white looking fascia anterior to the rectum. One can facilitate the dissection distally if the assistant pushes down on the anterior rectal surface with the sucker tip. The dissection can generally be advanced distally, all the way up to the apex of the prostate.
6. **Nerve sparing.** The fourth arm is used to pull the base of the prostate contralaterally to the side of the nerve sparing. Any residual levator fibers attached laterally to the prostate are mobilized away. One then finds a superficial fascial plane in the posterolateral prostate just above the location of the bundles that can be incised sharply, the lateral prostatic fascia. This is done at the mid prostate level. This is a very superficial layer. Dissection then continues straight posteriorly to try to completely separate the bundle away from the prostatic capsule. There is often some bleeding encountered during this maneuver. This is managed by the assistant's sucker being placed in this plane, allowing for adequate visualization. It is critical that one does not dissect too medially, since inadvertent entrance into the prostatic capsule will occur. Once the bundle is completely freed from the side of the prostate and a dissection plane has been established between the bundle and prostate, it can gently be developed using a combination of sharp and blunt dissection proximally and distally as far as the tissues will allow (Figures 7a–d).

   The more proximally the plane at the base of the prostate can be developed, the less likely one will injure the bundle during separation of the base of the prostate away from its vascular pedicle. At this point, the assistant pulls the seminal vesicle anteriorly and medially while the fourth arm pulls up on the ipsilateral aspect of the bladder base. This allows for the delineation of the prostatic vascular pedicle, which is divided. Cautery is avoided.

   As one dissects from the base of the prostate toward the apex, away from the neurovascular bundle, some residual attachments that typically separate with blunt dissection are encountered. This allows for complete separation of the neurovascular bundle away from the side of the prostate. As the apex is approached, the neurovascular bundle can become more difficult to separate away from the side of the prostate. Caution must be taken not to injure the bundle or inadvertently enter the prostate at this point. As the dissection progresses, the assistant can pull the prostate contralaterally more distally to allow for better traction. If this apical portion of the bundle is difficult to dissect out, it may help to dissect out the contralateral neurovascular bundle to better help mobilize the prostate.
7. **Incision through the dorsal vein complex (DVC) and urethra.** The 0-degree or 30-degree lens may be used for this step. The fourth arm is now placed midline in the base of the prostate, pulling it cephalad. It is impor-

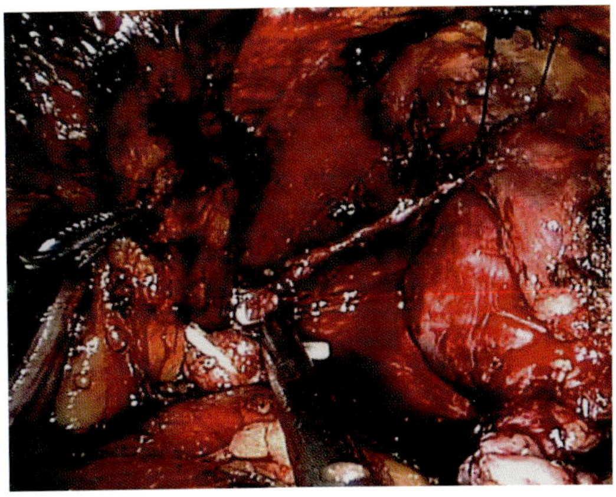

Figure 7a. The neurovascular bundle having been separated from the left side of the prostate.

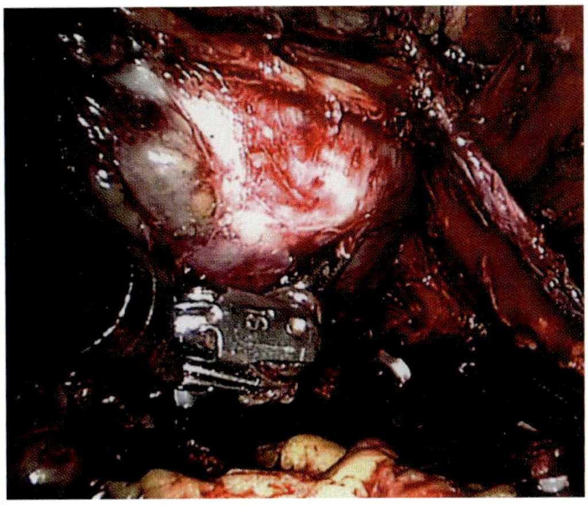

Figure 7b. The neurovascular bundle having been separated from the right side of the prostate.

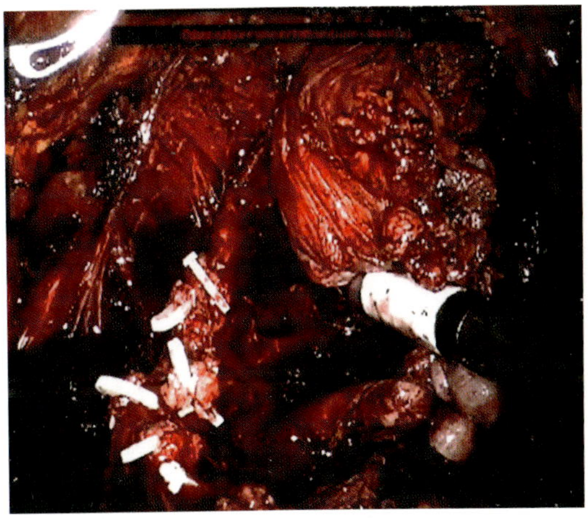

Figure 7c. The neurovascular bundle having been separated from the left side of the prostate.

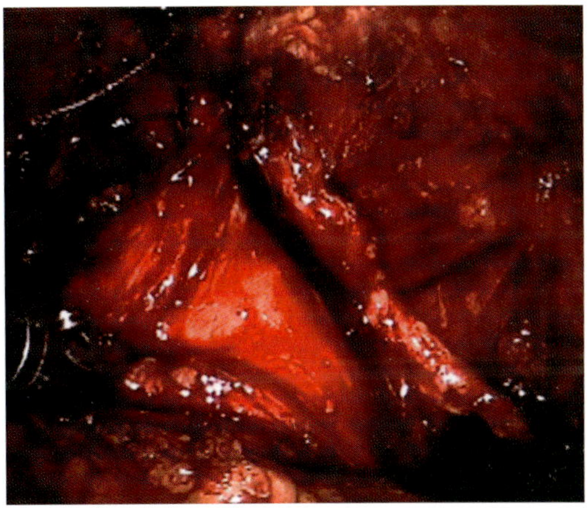

Figure 7d. The neurovascular bundle having been separated from the right side of the prostate.

tant to ensure that the Foley catheter is all the way in through the prostate. Using cautery, a plane is initiated between the DVC and urethra. Adjusting the fourth arm traction as this plane is developing facilitates this step of the procedure. After one is past the DVC, one continues the plane of dissection sharply. Once the urethra is isolated (Figures 8a–d), its anterior wall is incised sharply just distal to the apical prostatic notch (Figures 9a–b).

The left arm with the Maryland is placed underneath the posterior urethral wall with gentle upward traction. The Foley is then pulled back so just the tip is visible through the urethral lumen (Figure 10).

The posterior urethral wall is then incised at the level of the verumontanum to maximize sphincteric length. As the separation of the remaining

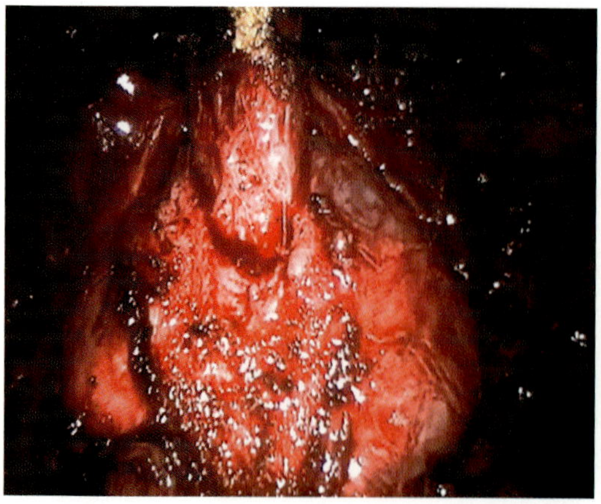

Figure 8a. Membranous urethra exposed prior to incision.

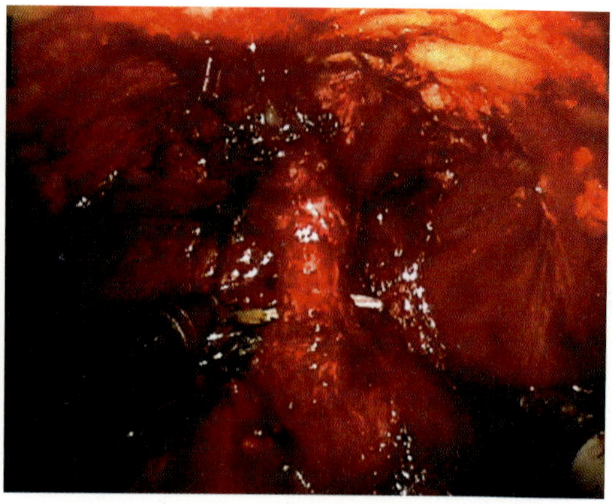

Figure 8b. Membranous urethra isolated prior to incision with Maryland underneath it.

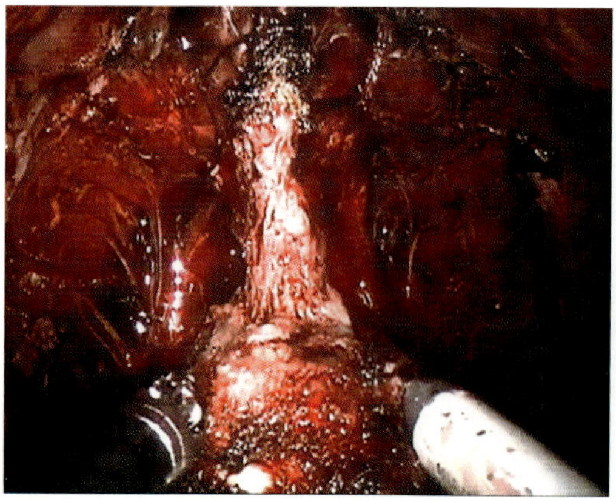

Figure 8c. Long membranous urethra isolated prior to its incision.

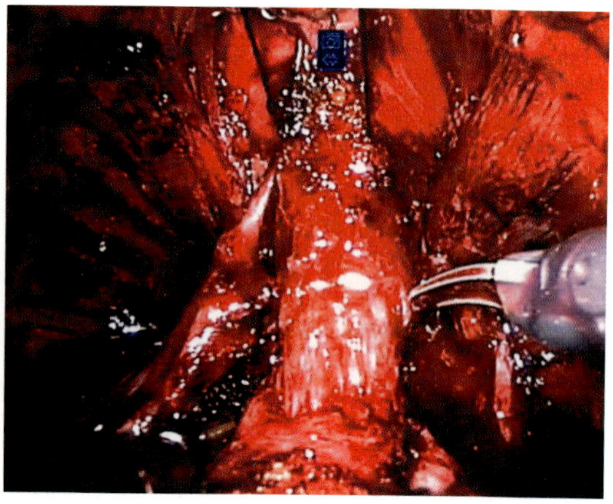

Figures 8d. Long membranous urethra prior to incision.

attachments of the prostatic apex to the pelvic floor is completed, it is important to look for a posterior lip of prostate that extends distally to again avoid cutting into it and leaving a positive margin. It is also important to be aware of the location of the neurovascular bundles, if they have been preserved, to avoid their inadvertent injury during this part. Finally, the operator needs to be certain that the rectum is fully separated below from the prostatic apex before cutting through this posterior connection. Once the prostate is completely freed, it is then placed into an Endo Catch bag for subsequent retrieval. If a full bilateral nerve-sparing prostatectomy has been performed, one should be able to appreciate a "railroad track" appearance to the bundles with the urethral stump in between them (Figures 11a–d).

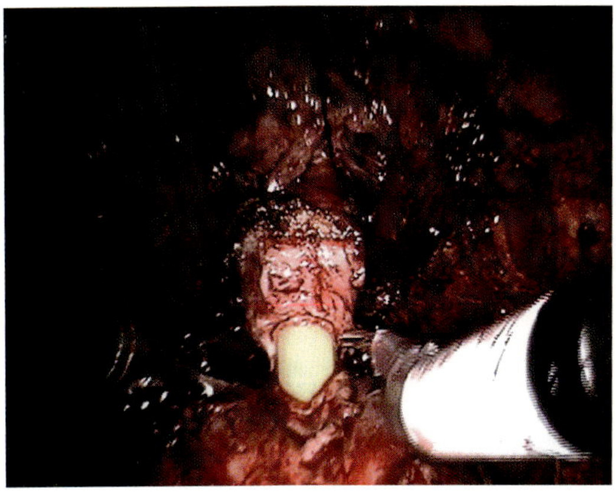

Figure 9a. Anterior urethral wall incised distal to apical prostatic notch.

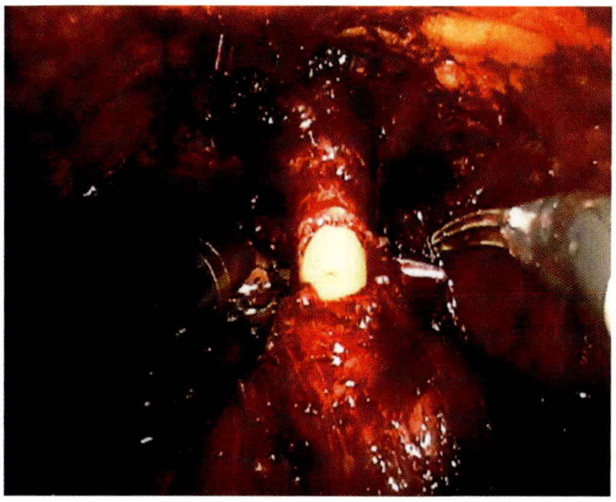

Figure 9b. Anterior urethral wall incised distal to apical prostatic notch.

8. **Vesicourethral anastomosis.** The 0-degree or 30-degree lens may be used for this step. One may use a double armed barbed suture such as a 2-0 Quill on an HR-17 needle, which is specifically made for this anastomosis. Alternatively, two 3-0 monocryl sutures are prepared on RB-1 needles, each 7 inches in length, one dyed and the other undyed, tied to each other, creating a double armed suture. Given that the suture will not pull back, the advantage of the barbed suture is it consists in keeping continuous tension on the suture while performing the anastomosis. On the other hand, a potential disadvantage is that one cannot pull out a stitch once placed.

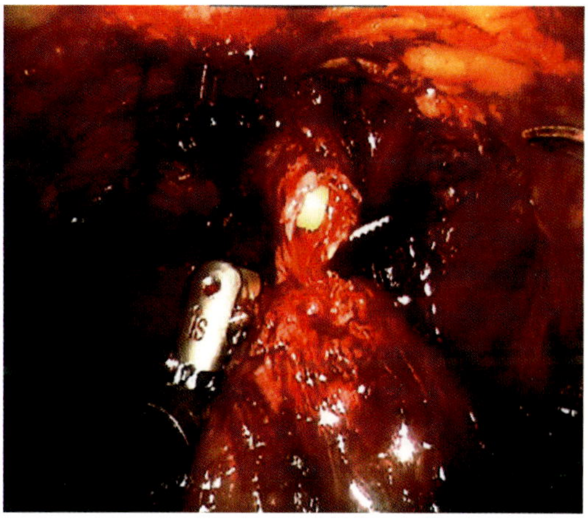

Figure 10. The Foley catheter is pulled back so that its tip is visible through the urethral lumen.

If using the 2-0 Quill suture, the anastomosis should be started by going out to in, through the bladder mucosa at the six o'clock position with the two needles next to each other and pulling up on both symmetrically. The urethral bite is then continued inside out at the corresponding site. A Foley catheter is pulled in and out of the urethral stump during the anastomosis to help identify the urethral mucosa. One then continues clockwise and counterclockwise symmetrically up both sides of the anastomosis. After an additional 4 bites on each side of the anastomosis (two on the urethral end and two on the bladder mucosal end), the bladder is brought all the way down to the posterior suture line by pulling the ends of the suture coming

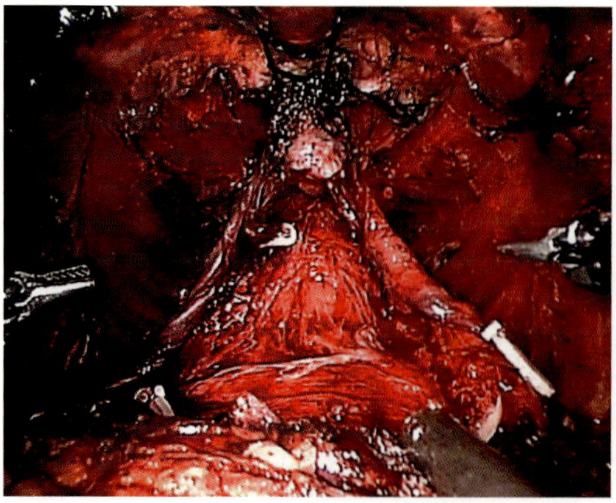

Figure 11a. Bilateral preservation of neurovascular bundles.

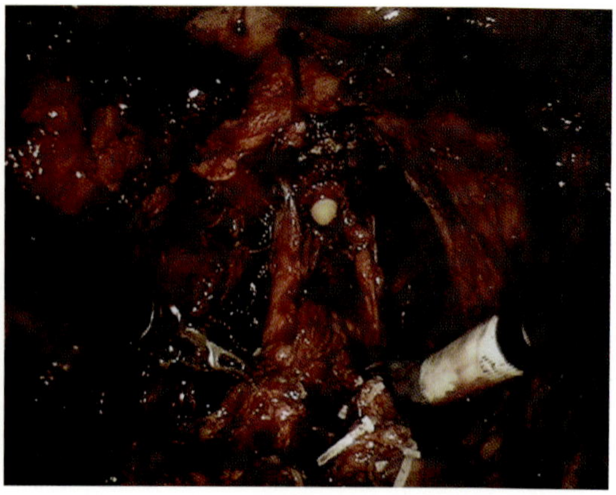

Figure 11b. Bilateral preservation of neurovascular bundles.

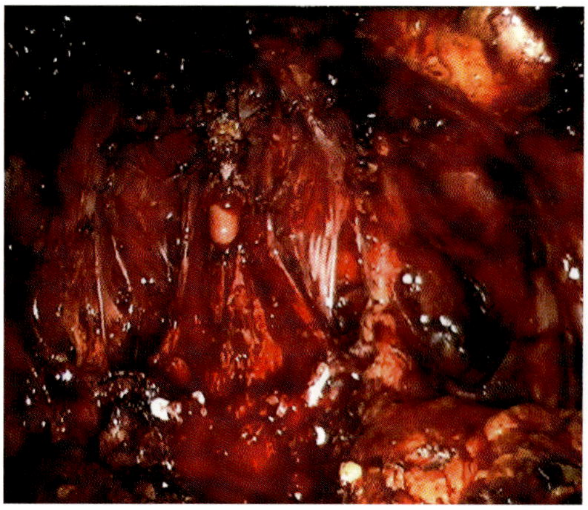

Figure 11c. Bilateral preservation of neurovascular bundles.

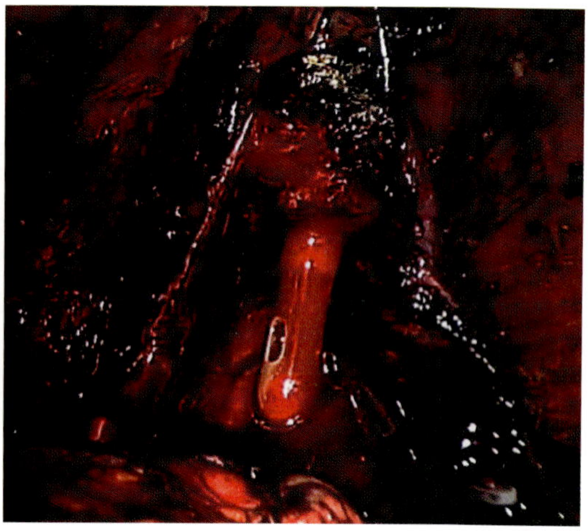

Figures 11d. Appearance of bilateral remaining neurovascular bundles following prostatectomy with the urethral stump in between them.

out on each side of the urethra gently straight up. This maneuver allows the posterior bladder wall to "parachute" straight down on to the posterior urethral wall (Figure 12).

The operator should avoid pulling the sutures in a cephalad direction as this could result in tearing of the suture through the tissues. It is important to obtain mucosa-to-mucosa bites. As one comes around the anastomosis, one of the arms of the suture is transitioned in its direction of insertion into the urethra. Thus, after going inside out, the suture is brought outside in and then inside out on the bladder neck as one progresses through the anastomosis. This will allow the operator to tie the two arms of the suture

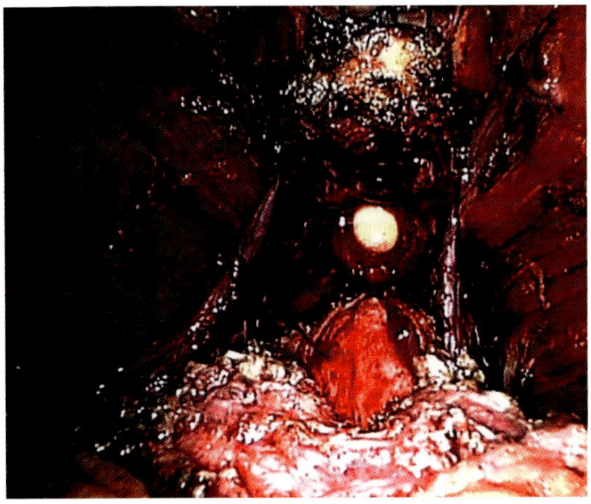

Figure 12. Posterior bladder wall has come down to the posterior urethral wall early in the anastomosis. The spared nerves are visible bilaterally.

across the anastomosis rather than over the urethral stump. A fresh 18 French Foley catheter is placed at the end of the anastomosis and irrigated to confirm a watertight anastomosis. If two sutures of 3-0 monocryl tied to each other are used, the anastomosis can be completed as described above. Tension must be kept continuously on the suture, however, to prevent potential gaps in the anastomosis. The anastomosis can also be constructed with the monocryl suture by starting outside in with the dyed end of the suture at the 4 o'clock or 5 o'clock position at the bladder neck and then inside out at the corresponding site at the urethral stump.

After three throws into the bladder and two into the urethra in a clockwise direction, one can start to bring the posterior lip of the anastomosis together by gently pulling the suture straight up. Once the 11 o'clock position through the urethral stump is approached, the fourth arm ProGrasp can be used to maintain tension on this end of the suture while the undyed end is run in a counterclockwise direction. The two ends are then tied to each other, and the anastomosis is completed the same way as described for the barbed suture.

9. **Lymph node dissection.** This portion of the surgery can be done at the beginning of the surgery if positive lymph node involvement on frozen section is suspected. This may affect the course of the operation. One may also decide to do it toward the end of the surgery per surgeon preference. This section of the surgery is carried out just like in the open technique. For a standard modified pelvic lymphadenectomy, the lymph node packet between the external iliac vein anteriorly, the obturator nerve inferiorly, the lymph node of Cloquet distally, and the angle between the external iliac vein and obturator nerve proximally is removed. The nodes are removed by the assistant out of the 12 mm port.

   A more extensive lymphadenectomy, with the lateral margin of the dissection being the genitofemoral nerve and the proximal margin being the bifurcation of the iliac vessels, is performed for patients who present with a high PSA, high Gleason grade, or clinically locally advanced disease. Of note is that if more than the expected oozing is encountered from the lymphadenectomy bed, and if no particular bleeding point is identified, one can place a hemostatic agent into the bed, such as Surgicel, to achieve hemostasis.

10. **Drain placement, prostate extraction, and termination of the procedure.** A size 10 French Jackson-Pratt flat drain is advanced into the surgical bed through the assistant 12 mm port. The distal end of the drain is then brought out using the fourth arm port with a Maryland grasper manipulated by the bedside assistant after the robot has been undocked from this port. The drain is advanced such that the ends of the flat portion of the drain are located close to the obturator spaces and the body of the drain is across the bladder. Care is taken to avoid placing the drain too close to the anastomosis so that it does not create a leak by placing suction over it. After this is accomplished, the robot is undocked.

    The robot camera is repositioned through the lateral 12 mm assistant port. The string attached to the Endo Catch bag is brought out of the supraumbilical 12 mm midline port with a grasper and secured with a hemostat. All ports are then removed under direct visualization to look for any bleeding. The patient is taken out of the Trendelenburg position. The Jackson-Pratt drain is anchored to the skin using 2-0 nonabsorbable sutures. The midline supraumbilical incision is elongated at the skin and fascia just enough to allow removal of the Endo Catch bag with the prostate inside it. The fascia is then closed with a running 0-Vicryl suture using a UR-6 needle. Local anesthesia is infiltrated into all incision sites and the skin is closed with subcuticular 4-0 monocryl on a PS-2 needle. An age appropriate parenteral dose (assuming normal renal function) of ketorolac is administered during skin closure.

Postoperative Care

Parenteral narcotics are typically given for the first 24 hours postoperatively then transitioned to an oral regimen. A urethral catheter is maintained for a variable period based on surgeon preference and degree of bladder neck reconstruction. For most patients, one to two weeks of catheterization is sufficient for the anastomosis to heal. A cystogram is not required routinely prior to catheter removal, but may be valid should the catheter need to be removed prematurely or if there are any concerns about the integrity of the anastomosis.

Outcomes of Robotic Prostatectomy

Perioperative Outcomes

Intraoperative Blood Loss. The antegrade approach utilized in RALP allows for earlier control of the prostatic pedicle and late division of the dorsal venous complex, thus reducing ongoing bleeding risk. Additionally, pneumoperitoneum has a tamponade effect on bleeding from venous sinuses, which are the cause of the majority of blood loss during radical prostatectomy. Most studies have proven a decreased transfusion requirement in patients undergoing minimally invasive approaches compared to RRP.[12,24] Blood transfusions are extremely rare for RALP.

Length of Hospital Stay. In general, owing mainly to programs focusing on early discharge, even for patients undergoing RRP, no significant difference in hospital length of stay has been noted. Delays in discharge are typically secondary to ileus and, less frequently, pain. Even for RRP, however, patient reported pain is similar in intensity as reported following minimally invasive approaches. Most patients are discharged home following RALP the day after surgery.

Functional Outcomes

Erectile dysfunction (ED) and urinary incontinence are the complications that assert the biggest impact on quality of life post-RALP.[25] The data comparing open vs. minimally invasive approaches reflect significant divergence on the question of which approach can predict the best functional outcomes.

Urinary Incontinence. Urinary incontinence post radical prostatectomy typically manifests as stress incontinence. While the vast proportion of patients can be expected to regain urinary control (some may take up to a full year), for surgical centers performing frequent RALP, 5–10% of patients can be expected to have persistent stress incontinence to some degree. Challenges in applying a strict definition of incontinence have led to significant variance in the observed rates in several large series.[24,26] Several anatomic based technical modifications in RALP have been made with the aim of reducing rates of incontinence with an arguably marginal effect on outcomes.[27] Recent interest has been placed on preserving the anatomic relationships of the puboprostatic complex in its entirety, such that both posterior and anterior support of the vesicourethral complex is provided with good early results.[24,28] In general, advanced patient age is the most significant predictor of failure to achieve continence at six weeks.[5]

Erectile Dysfunction. As a consequence of screening and early detection of localized cancers, an increasing number of prostatectomies are being performed in younger men for whom postoperative ED is particularly concerning. In some series, the rates of ED exceed 80% for all radical prostatectomies without consideration of technique.[12] It is well established, however, that in order to maintain postoperative potency, meticulous interfascial dissection and preservation of the cavernous nerves within the neurovascular bundle are essential.[10,12] Avoiding electrocautery during dissection and preventing excess traction on the cavernosal nerves are also known to reduce the rate of ED.[10]

The frequency of post-RALP ED varies greatly among published reviews. A recent meta-analysis examining ED revealed 12-month potency rates of 54–90%.[29] More significantly, however, this review was the first to demonstrate with statistical significance a clear advantage in 12- and 24-month potency rate for those patients who underwent RALP compared to RRP (odds ratio [OR]: 2.84; 95% confidence interval [CI]: 1.46–5.43; $p = 0.002$).[29] Proponents of a minimally invasive approach suggest the finer degree of precision afforded by robotic instrumentation, in combination with enhanced visualization of anatomic detail and decreased bleeding in the surgical field, may account for this finding. As is the case for urinary incontinence, however, the lack of a standardized definition for potency and no consensus regarding the optimal instrument for assessing recovery of erectile function after prostatectomy make comparison among different series extremely difficult. Additionally, the use of adjunctive therapies, including phospho-diesterase-5 inhibitors or vasoactive injections, can substantially influence results.

Although extended pelvic lymph node dissection can be associated with damage to the pelvic plexus and therefore associated with ED, a recent review suggests no impact on functional outcomes.[29] Patient factors predictive of ED include advanced age, preexisting vasculopathy, and a preoperative history of ED.[30,31] Where wide excision of nerve bundles is necessary, nerve advancement and grafting have been described. However, the efficacy of these techniques remains unproven.[32]

Oncologic Outcomes

Surgical Margins. Given that a predominant proportion of prostatic adenocarcinomas occur in the peripheral zone, encroaching on the capsular margin, variations in surgical technique can influence oncologic outcomes. While attempting to preserve continence or potency, dissection too close to the apex or posterolateral aspect of the prostate can negatively impact margin status.[33]

In general, the rates of positive surgical margins observed after RALP, RRP, and LLP have been found to be mostly similar.[12,34] However, inadequate training and rapid adoption of RALP have been noted to lead to higher margin positive rates and subsequent progression to salvage therapy within 6 months of operation.[4,10,23]

The comparison of margin positivity between centers is further complicated by the method and detail of pathologic analysis. The World Health Organization International Consultation Consensus Committee estimated that whole mount histological sectioning might miss positive margins in 12% of cases compared to conventional sectioning in which thinner slices are used.[12]

Biochemical Recurrence. Oncologic control is thought to be better defined by the absence of biochemical recurrence (BCR) than by margin status. In general, the presence of extracapsular extension, seminal vesicle invasion, and adjuvant radiotherapy are significantly associated with BCR. The longest follow-up data to date were published by Suardi et al., who reported 3-, 5-, and 7-year BCR-free survival rates of 94%, 86%, and 81%, respectively. These rates were 97%, 93%, and 85% for pT2 disease; 94%, 84%, and 84% for pT3a; and 69%, 43%, and 43% for pT3b tumors.[35] After adjusting for clinical and pathological features, recent retrospective comparison of RALP and RRP suggests no difference in the rate of BCR.[36]

Complications

Vascular or Enteral Injury. Vascular or bowel perforations generally occur on trocar placement, and the majority can be repaired laparoscopically. Rectal injuries, although uncommon, require prompt intraoperative recognition. If suspected but not readily identified, insufflation of air into the rectum after placing fluid in the pelvis and observing for air bubbles is diagnostic. Multilayered repair with omental interposition, if there is a prior history of radiation, is recommended.

Anastomotic Failure. Anastomotic leak can lead to dissemination of urine through the abdominal cavity if a transperitoneal approach is performed. Typically, urinary anastomotic leaks seal with conservative management. This characteristically consists of removing suction from the drain and slowly withdrawing the drain over time. Despite intraoperative drain placement, fluid collections can form, necessitating percutaneous drainage. Complete anastomotic disruption requires surgical revision. Anastomotic stricture and subsequent contraction of the bladder neck occurs to a much lesser extent in RALP compared to RRP. Achieving a watertight anastomosis with appropriate approximation of the mucosa is thought to be key in preventing bladder neck contraction.[14,37]

Embolic Complications. RALP is associated with a low rate of thromboembolic phenomena (0.5%) given Trendelenburg positioning intraoperatively and postoperative early patient mobilization strategies. The use of preoperative anticoagulation is only advocated for patients with known risk factors including obesity, venous stasis, and hypercoagulability.[38] Complications related to pelvic lymph node dissection are rare.[12]

Summary

RALP has become a standard modality in the treatment of localized prostatic carcinoma. The technique, once mastered, is performed in a length of time that approaches that for standard RRP and provides ergonomic advantages, compared to pure laparoscopic technique.

Oncologic and functional outcomes for RALP have been shown to approximate RRP, despite challenges in comparing available data and taking into account operator learning curve. While equipment expense is a concern that precludes the introduction of RALP in some centers, its use continues to expand among community-based and tertiary centers. Driven both by patient and surgeon preference, RALP is the dominant surgical treatment modality in the management of prostatic carcinoma. Further improvements in technological capability will only serve to promote its use and are predicted to further improve patient outcomes. Ongoing reviews of long-term follow-up data are needed to improve risk stratification and selection of the most appropriate surgical modality based on patient specific factors.

References

1. Brawley OW. Prostate cancer epidemiology in the United States. *World J Urology.* 2012;30:195–200.

2. National Cancer Institute. *SEER Stat Fact Sheets: Prostate.* Bethesda, MD: National Cancer Institute; 2010.

3. Carlsoon S, Vickers AJ, Roobol M. Prostate cancer screening: Facts, statistics and interpretation in response to the US Preventive Services Task Force Review. *J Clin Oncol.* 2012;30:1–3.

4. Altekruse SF, Krapacho M, Neyman N, Aminou R, et al. *Seer Cancer Statistics Review*. 1975–2007; 2010: National Cancer Institute, Bethesda.

5. Loeb S, Carter HB. Early detection, diagnosis and staging of prostate cancer. In: Wein AJ, Kavoussi LR, Novick AC, Partin, AW, Peters CA, eds. *Campbell-Walsh Urology.* 10th ed. Vol 3. Philadelphia, PA: Saunders; 2012:2763–70.

6. Wilt TJ, Brawer MK, Jones KM, et al. Radical prostatectomy versus observation for localized prostate cancer. *N Engl J Med.* 2012;367:203–13.

7. Smith JA Jr, Scardino PT, Resnick MI, et al. Transrectal ultrasound versus digital rectal examination for the staging of carcinoma of the prostate: results of a prospective, multi-institutional trial. *J Urol.* 1997;157:902–6.

8. Van der Cruijsen-Koeter IW, Vis AN, Roobol MJ, Wildhagen MF, et al. Comparison of screen detected and clinically diagnosed prostate cancer in the European randomized study of screening for prostate cancer, section Rotterdam. *J Urol.* 2005;174:121–5.

9. Barry MJ, Gallagher PM, Skinner JS, Fowler FJ. Adverse effects of robotic-assisted laparoscopic versus open retropubic radical prostatectomy among a nationwide random sample of Medicare-age men. *J Clin Oncol.* 2012;30:513–518.

10. Ficarra V, Novara G, Artibani W, Gestari A, et al. Retropubic, laparoscopic, and robot-assisted radical prostatectomy: a systematic review and cumulative analysis of comparative studies. *Eur Urol.* 2009;55:1037–1063.

11. Walsh PC. Radical prostatectomy for localized prostate cancer provides a durable cancer control with excellent quality of life: a structured debate. *J Urol.* 2000;163:1802–7.

12. Su LM, Smith JA. Laparoscopic and robotic assisted radical prostatectomy and pelvic lymphadenectomy. In: Wein AJ, Kavoussi LR, Novick AC, Partin, AW, Peters CA, eds. *Campbell-Walsh Urology.* 10th ed. Vol 4. Philadelphia, PA: Saunders; 2012:2830–49.

13. American Cancer Society. *Cancer Facts & Figures 2010.* Atlanta, GA: American Cancer Society; 2010.

14. Sroughi M, Paranhos K, Leite KM, et al. The influence of bladder neck mucosal eversion and early urinary extravasation on patient outcome after radical retropubic prostatectomy: a prospective controlled trial. *BJU Int.* 2005;96:757–760.

15. Washington SL, Bonham M, Whitson JM, Cowan JF, Carroll PR. Transurethral ultrasonography-guided biopsy does not reliably identify dominant cancer location in men with low-risk prostate cancer. *BJU Int.* 2012;110:50–5.

16. Millin T. Retropubic prostatectomy: a new extravesical technique report on 20 cases. *Lancet.* 1945;2:693–6.

17. Qiang Fu, Moul JW, Sun L. Contemporary radical prostatectomy. *Prostate Cancer.* 2011;1–13.

18. Schuessler WW, Schulam PG, Clayman RV, Kavoussi LR. Laparoscopic radical prostatectomy: initial short-term experience. *Urology.* 1997;50:854–7.

19. Abbou CC, Salomon L, Hoznek A, et al. Laparoscopic radical prostatectomy: preliminary results. *Urology.* 2000;55:630–5.

20. Boris RS, Bhandar A, Krane LS, et al. Salvage robotic-assisted radical prostatectomy: initial results and early report of outcomes. *BJU Int.* 2009;103:952–6.

21. Kaouk JH, Hafron J, Goel R, et al. Robotic salvage retropubic prostatectomy after radiation/brachytherapy. *BJU Int.* 2008;102:93–6.

22. Rajesh LG, Sanjeev J, Muhletaler F, Ketan BK, et al. Impacts of previous inguinal hernia repair on transperitoneal robotic prostectomy. *Can J Urol.* 2007;14:3635–9.

23. Rassweiler J, Schulze M, Teber D, et al. Laparoscopic radical prostatectomy: functional and oncologic outcomes. *Curr Opin Urol.* 2004;14:75–82.

24. Tewari AK, Bigeolow K, Rao S, et al. Anastomotic restoration technique of continence mechanism and preservation of puboprostatic collar: a novel modification to achieve early urinary continence in men undergoing robotic prostatectomy. *Urology.* 2007; 69:726–31.

25. Sanda MG, Dunn RL, Michalski J, et al. Quality of life and satisfaction with outcome among prostate-cancer survivors. *N Engl J Med.* 2008;358:1250–1261.

26. Reynolds WS, Shikanov SA, Katz MH, Zagaja GP, Shalhav AL, Zorn KC. Analysis of continence rates following robot-assisted radical prostatectomy: strict leak-free and pad-free continence. *Urology.* 2007;75(2):431–6.

27. Lee DJ, Cheetham P, Badani KK. Predictors of early urinary continence after robotic prostatectomy. *Can J Urol.* 2010;17:5200–5.

28. Hurtes X, Roupret M, Vaessen C, et al. Anterior suspension combined with posterior reconstruction during robot-assisted laparoscopic prostatectomy improves early return of urinary continence: a prospective randomized multicenter trial. *BJU Int.* 2012; Epub ahead of print.

29. Ficarra V, Novara G, Ahlering TE, et al. Systematic review and meta-analysis of studies reporting potency rates after robot-assisted radical prostatectomy. *Eur Urol.* 2012; 62:418–30.

30. Gandaglia G, Suradi N, Gallina A, et al. Extended pelvic lymph node dissection does not affect erectile function recovery in patients treated with bilateral nerve-sparing radical prostatectomy. *J Sex Med.* 2012; Epub ahead of print.

31. Teloken PE, Nelson CJ, Karellas M, et al. Defining the impact of vascular risk factors on erectile function recovery after radical prostatectomy. *BJU Int.* 2012; Epub ahead of print.

32. Zorn KC, Bernstein AJ, Gofrit ON, et al. Long-term functional and oncologic outcomes of patients undergoing sural nerve interposition grafting during robot-assisted laparoscopic radical prostatectomy. *J Endourol.* 2008;22:1005–12.

33. Touijer K, Kuroiwa K, Saranchuk JW, et al. Quality improvement in laparoscopic radical prostatectomy for pT2 prostate cancer: impact of video documentation review on positive surgical margin. *J Urol.* 2005;173:765–8.

34. Lance RS, Freidrichs PA, Kane C, et al. A comparison of radical retropubic with perineal prostatectomy for localized prostate cancer within the Uniformed Services Urology Research Group. *BJU Int.* 2001;87:61–65.

35. Suardi N, Ficarra V, Willemsen P, et al. Long-term biochemical recurrence rates after robot-assisted radical prostatectomy: analysis of a single-center series of patients with a minimum follow-up of 5 years. *Urology.* 2012;79:133–8.

36. Schroeck FR, Sun L, Freedland SJ, et al. Comparison of prostate-specific antigen recurrence free-survival in a contemporary cohort of patients undergoing either radical retropubic or robot-assisted laparoscopic radical prostatectomy. *BJU Int.* 2008;102:28–32.

37. Msezane LP, Reynolds WS, Gofrit ON, et al. Bladder neck contracture after robot-assisted laparoscopic radical prostatectomy: evaluation of incidence and risk factors and impact on urinary function. *J Endourology.* 2008;22:97–104.

38. Secin FP, Jiborn T, Bjartell AS, et al. Multi-institutional study of symptomatic deep venous thrombosis and pulmonary embolism in prostate cancer patients undergoing laparoscopic or robot-assisted laparoscopic radical prostatectomy. *J Urol.* 2005;173:552–4.

Chapter Ten

General and Pediatric Surgery

Seema Kapur, MD; Stefan W. Leichtle, MD; Daniel S. Rhee, MD

Overview

Compared to the sea of change that the advent of laparoscopic cholecystectomy brought to the field of general surgery, the adoption of robotic technology has been a rather sedate process. From their pioneering applications in neurosurgery and urology, the use of surgical robotic systems is currently most prevalent in the surgical specialties of cardiac and colorectal surgery, urology, and otolaryngology.[1-4] However, at the first "transatlantic cholecystectomy" in 2001, an operative robot demonstrated its impressive performance in general surgery to a broader audience.[5] Prior to that, surgical robots had already been used for gastric banding, Nissen fundoplication, and cholecystectomy.[6,7]

In the 1980s, the era of minimally invasive general surgery began, with reports of the first laparoscopic cholecystectomies and appendectomies.[8,9] Allowing for smaller incisions, decreased blood loss, fewer wound infections, shorter hospital stays, and reduced recovery times, laparoscopic techniques have all but replaced open surgery for many elective operations. With their superior imaging capabilities, improved ergonomics, and increased dexterity, surgical robotic systems are particularly useful in those general surgical operations where visibility and maneuverability are limited. However, adoption of robotics has been slower than expected when compared to laparoscopic techniques. Reasons may include higher costs, poor haptics, and the current lack of certain instruments such as a stapling device. Additionally, operations in general surgery frequently require access to more than one quadrant, which could result in excessive redocking maneuvers. Despite the above limitations, imaginative surgeons have been developing robotic adaptations that expand the repertoire of the minimally invasive general surgeon.

In the following paragraphs, some common applications of robotics in general surgery are highlighted. While not an exhaustive review of the entire spectrum of robotic applications in the field, the focus of this section is to review the indications and delineate some of the unique considerations when applying robotic techniques to specific clinical scenarios.

Robotic Cholecystectomy

Robot-assisted cholecystectomy was first reported in 1997.[10] With large case numbers and a fairly standardized operative approach, this operation frequently represents the first exposure of interested general surgeons to surgical robotic systems.[11] Several studies compared laparoscopic and robotic techniques and demonstrated the feasibility and safety of the latter. However, none of the studies could identify any significant advantages of using the robot.[12] Operative times, particularly instrument set-up times and costs, are generally higher for robotic cholecystectomy than for conventional laparoscopy. Not surprisingly, the use of a surgical robotic system for elective, uncomplicated cholecystectomies appears to be an overutilization of resources. However, these cases provide an opportunity for surgical teams to gain experience with robotic surgical systems and to establish effective team techniques in the operating room for more complex procedures.

Operative Steps. At our institution, we use the da Vinci Surgical Robot System to perform elective cholecystectomies. A standard port placement is utilized, with subxiphoid and medial subcostal incisions for the robotic arms. The robot is docked over the right shoulder, and a 5 mm lateral subcostal port is manned by the assistant. Alternatively, a surgeon operating alone can use the third arm for retracting the fundus of the gallbladder, thus obviating the need for an assistant (Figure 1). The perioperative nurse would then perform instrument changes and delivery maneuvers. Dissection and transection of the cystic artery are performed with the harmonic scalpel, while medium or large Hem-o-lok® clips secure the duct. An Endoloop® can be used when performing the cholecystectomy via a top down approach. We prefer to use a bag introduced via the optical port for specimen retrieval. This is then left in situ until the end of the case.

A well-established disadvantage of the laparoscopic technique is the higher rate of common bile duct (CBD) injury compared to open cholecystectomy. Though an extremely rare complication (approximately 0.1% in open and 0.5% in laparoscopic cases), CBD injury can result in severe morbidity and is most likely to occur

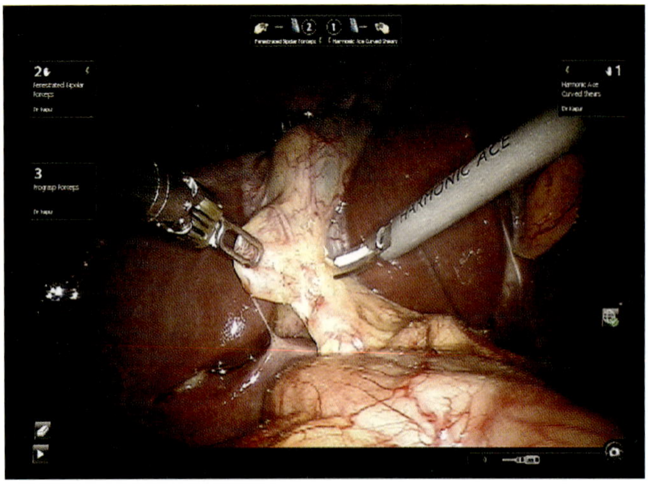

Figure 1. Retraction of the gallbladder is greatly facilitated by the third robotic arm.

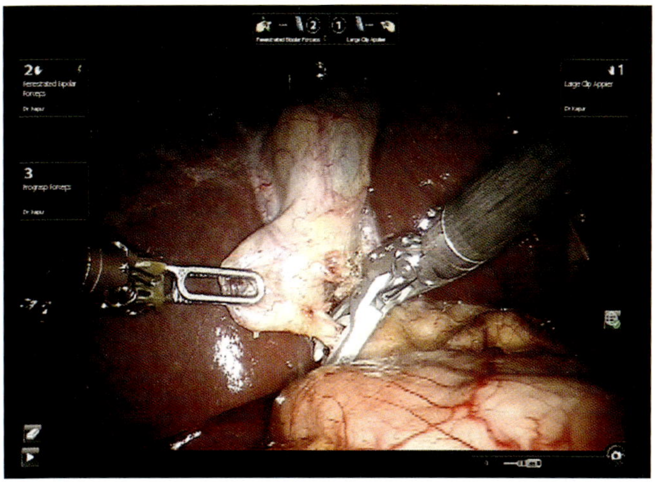

Figure 2. Wristed instruments and three-dimensional view allow for more precise dissection and clipping.

secondary to inadequate visualization of the anatomy, e.g., in the setting of a non-elective operation for acute inflammation. As such, it could be hypothesized that a robotic approach with its high-resolution, three-dimensional viewing field would result in fewer common CBD injuries and/or conversions to open surgery in the acute setting (Figure 2). However, very few facilities have the capability to keep a surgical robotic system and team available for emergent cases, and none of the studies comparing robotic versus traditional cholecystectomy have adequately studied this potential advantage.

Single Incision Laparoscopic Surgery (SILS). Another setting with potential advantages for the robotic system versus conventional laparoscopy is SILS. Currently most SILS platforms are limited by triangulation difficulties and left-right distortion, which tends to unnecessarily increase the complexity of what would be a straight forward procedure. However, the prospect of a single, small incision has been the impetus for continued research in this area. The advent of an approved SILS setup for the da Vinci System has renewed the enthusiasm for minimally invasive operations through a single incision, with the hope of avoiding the associated technical difficulties. The robotic arms are crossed to provide triangulation. Changing the settings of the robot arms via the surgical console allows for a normal left-right configuration. Indeed, first reports of SILS cholecystectomies using the da Vinci System have demonstrated that they can be performed safely, and as fast as conventional SILS operations.[13,14]

In summary, robotic cholecystectomy does not appear to offer significant advantages over conventional laparoscopy in the elective setting. However, in SILS, and potentially in the acute setting, or when expecting difficult anatomical problems, robot assistance might offer unique advantages. Moreover, it represents an excellent introduction to the field of robotic surgery for the general surgeon.

Antireflux Surgery and Hiatus Hernia Repair

Gastroesophageal reflux disease (GERD) is very common in developed countries, with increasing rates worldwide. In the United States, the incidence of reflux esophagitis documented on esophagogastroduodenoscopy is approximately 20%, and a majority of patients are managed medically with antisecretory medication.[15] Classic symptoms include pyrosis and regurgitation. However, many patients also suffer from dysphagia, chest pain, globus sensation, pulmonary symptoms, and hoarseness. The etiology of GERD is multifactorial and includes one or more of the following: a lax gastroesophageal valve or hypotensive lower esophageal sphincter; a hiatal hernia; esophageal dysmotility; obesity; and poor gastric emptying. In addition to causing the above-mentioned symptoms, long-standing reflux can lead to esophagitis, ulcerations, strictures, and esophageal shortening. Of even greater concern is the development of intestinal metaplasia (Barrett's esophagus), with progression to dysplasia, and eventually esophageal adenocarcinoma.

Initial treatment has traditionally focused on lifestyle modifications and antisecretory medication. Weight loss and modification of eating habits can have a profound impact on symptomatic GERD. Lifelong antisecretory medications, especially proton-pump inhibitors (PPI), work very well to control symptoms and reduce the esophageal mucosal damage from gastric acid. However, in cases of cervical reflux, regurgitation as the primary symptom, or when a hiatus hernia is present, nonsurgical treatment is often insufficient. Surgical correction of GERD focuses on restoring an adequate intra-abdominal esophagus, tightening the gastroesophageal valve, and repairing a hiatus hernia if present. Although there is plenty of controversy regarding the best method of correction and the important components of the operation, the above treatment plan represents a general consensus.

Indications for Surgical Treatment. Indications for surgical treatment include GERD refractory to medical management, esophagitis, squamocolumnar metaplasia, pulmonary symptoms, and regurgitation. Preoperative work-up in a patient with classic symptoms and good response to PPIs should include a dynamic esophagogram and upper endoscopy. In patients with unusual symptoms, or in the presence of dysphagia, additional diagnostic testing is indicated, such as pH measurements, manometry and, rarely, gastric emptying studies and computed tomography. Additionally, patients should be assessed for their ability to tolerate general anesthesia (GETA) and a pneumoperitoneum. A thorough preoperative work-up is essential to produce consistent results, reduce the risk of postoperative dysphagia, and choose the optimal repair method.

Laparoscopic fundoplication has an established role in the surgical treatment of GERD. Compared to the open approach, it offers advantages with regard to perioperative morbidity, hospital stay, and return to work.[16] Concerns about the durability of the laparoscopic repair have not been borne out by long-term data.[17]

Operative Steps. With the patient in a supine position, GETA is administered, a Foley catheter placed, and the left arm tucked to the patient's side. The operative table has to be positioned in such a way that the anesthesiologist can access the patient between the right arm and head. Standard laparoscopic equipment does not have to be opened routinely, and initial access for the camera port in the epigastrium (2 to 3 cm to the left of the midline) is accomplished via open technique. This step is necessary to ensure that the robotic camera has a direct line of sight to the hiatus. Unlike conventional laparoscopy, the robotic camera is less flexible; i.e., a change of view from 30 degrees up to 30 degrees down would require an instrument change. Eight millimeter left and right subcostal ports are placed to achieve triangulation with the camera port over the patient's left shoulder. A 10 mm assistant port is placed in the left lateral subcostal area, while taking care to place it inferiorly enough as to avoid collisions between the assistant and robotic arms.

An additional 5 mm assistant port is sometimes necessary for retraction in patients with large paraesophageal hernias or obscuring intra-abdominal obesity. A 5 mm subxiphoid incision is used for the Nathanson retractor to elevate the left lobe of the liver. Alternatively, the third arm coming from the right lateral subcostal area can be used to retract the liver (Figure 3).

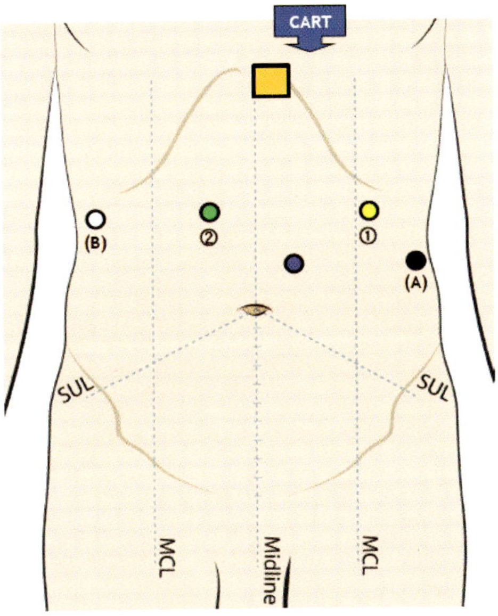

Figure 3. Port placement for robotic Nissen fundoplication. Credit: modified from Intuitive Surgical, Inc.

Using a harmonic scalpel, full mobilization of the gastroesophageal junction is performed, and the short gastrics are taken. Additional mobilization of the esophagus into the mediastinum is performed to achieve 2 to 3 cm of intra-abdominal esophagus, while taking care to protect both vagus nerves. If there is a larger hernia with a grade III or IV paraesophageal component, it is essential to dissect the hernia sac out of the mediastinum completely. The superior degrees of freedom and three-dimensional visualization of the robot are a distinct advantage during this portion of the procedure to avoid injury to the esophagus and mediastinal structures. Mobilization can be extended cephalad as far as the inferior pulmonary veins to obtain the required intra-abdominal length. The hiatus is approximated with Ethibond® sutures until a partially open grasper "snaps" through the opening to signify an orifice appropriate to prevent herniation or dysphagia. Mesh is not routinely applied, though if the defect is large, the primary approximation can be reinforced with a biologic prosthesis such as Surgisis®.

Subsequently, a 56 to 60 Fr bougie is placed, and a wrap is constructed by bringing the posterior fundus through the retroesophageal space. When performing a Nissen, it is approximated to the anterior fundus over the right anterior aspect of the esophagus. Partial anterior or posterior wraps are performed if there are preexisting esophageal dysmotility and dysphagia, or if any degree of postoperative dysphagia is unacceptable to the patient. Best clinical results with fundoplication are achieved in those patients who have been adequately counseled regarding postoperative expectations. We confirm the appropriateness of the repair via intraoperative endoscopy demonstrating a Hill grade I gastroesophageal valve. Postoperatively, the patient is discharged on a liquid diet, which is slowly advanced as tolerated. Early postoperative outcome is measured clinically via interview and objectively via esophagogram.

The Nissen fundoplication was one of the first general surgical operations performed with the robot. As a moderately complex procedure in one quadrant, it is well suited for the robot and is one of the few general surgical applications for which class I evidence is available. Several small randomized trials comparing the robot-assisted versus laparoscopic technique demonstrated the equivalence of both approaches with regard to postoperative complications and hospital stays, but also noted significantly longer total operative times (difference: 24.05 minutes, 95% CI, 5.19, 42.92; P = .01) and higher costs associated with the robotic system.[18] Interestingly, in one study performed by an experienced robotic surgery team, shorter operative times (88 vs. 102 min, P = .03) could be achieved using the robot,[19] with superior maneuverability and dexterity presumed as responsible factors.

With equivalence already documented regarding outcomes, safety, and feasibility, the only objections to more widespread adoption of the robotic system are cost factors and longer operative times. It has been shown that docking and console times follow a predictable inverse relationship to the number of cases performed and the experience of the team.[20] Although the initial capital costs cannot be avoided, operating costs and cost per case can be better managed with a consistent, well-planned case cart and a well-trained team.

Achalasia and Heller Myotomy

Achalasia is a primary esophageal motility disorder affecting 1 in 100,000 individuals in North America. Loss of the postganglionic inhibitory neurons in the plexus of Auerbach, via an unknown mechanism, causes unopposed lower esophageal sphincter (LES) constriction with hypertension. The primary symptoms are progressive liquid to solid dysphagia and poor esophageal emptying with prestenotic dilation and stasis leading to regurgitation, aspiration, and chest pain. Diagnosis is made via the classic "bird's beak" tapering of contrast at the gastroesophageal junction (GEJ) on a barium swallow. Other required preoperative work-ups include upper endoscopy to rule out malignancy and manometry to demonstrate increased pressures and the absence of relaxation of the LES on swallowing. Documentation of aperistalsis is also used. A CT scan helps to delineate the anatomical relationships.

Treatment in the past has focused on symptom control with GEJ dilation and Botox injection to relax the sphincter. With disease progression, operative myotomy was eventually offered. Since the advent of a minimally invasive option, and with studies demonstrating superior long-term results with operative treatment, Heller myotomy is now the treatment of choice in an acceptable risk patient. Dilation remains a viable option for patients not willing or able to undergo operative intervention or in cases of recurrence.

Robotic Heller Myotomy. The most morbid complication during Heller myotomy is injury to the esophagus and stomach during myotomy. This concern was the impetus for developing a robotic approach to this procedure, which was pioneered by Horgan et al. and reported in 2005.[21] The advantages of the surgical robotic system with regard to instrument dexterity and improved visibility are especially suited to the control and precision required during the dissection and transection of the variably oriented sling fibers on the stomach.

The operating room and table setup is similar to that for the anti-reflux surgery described above. After the robot is docked, dissection is begun at the right crus with the Harmonic Scalpel® and Cadiere grasper. Blunt dissection in a bloodless plane is used as much as possible to avoid any injuries. The phreno-esophageal ligament and peritoneal attachments over the anterior esophagus are dissected, while taking care to protect the anterior vagus nerve. The anterior fat pad over the GEJ is removed, the vagus nerve is encircled with a vessel loop, and retracted to the right. Anterior mobilization is continued over the left crus, and subsequently the short gastrics are taken. The posterior attachments are left intact.

Over a bougie, the myotomy is begun at the GEJ and first extended cephalad onto the esophagus for 6 to 8 cm. During this step, care must be taken to divide both longitudinal and circular muscle layers and to distract the two edges. This can be done with a hook cautery or scissors with cautery. Bleeding is controlled with the application of pressure. Using hook cautery, the myotomy is then extended inferiorly in a hockey stick fashion over the stomach for a distance of 2 to 3 cm. Once the myotomy is completed successfully, an anterior Dor wrap is constructed. The apex of the fundus is folded over the anterior esophagus, and two rows of 3-0 silk sutures are used to affix the left and right side of the fundus to the right and left edges of the myotomy, respectively. The superior most stitches incorporate the crura, and additional anterior sutures are placed between the diaphragm and the fundus as needed.

Application of robotic technology in the surgical treatment of achalasia has seen the most dramatic outcomes. Studies documenting results superior to conventional laparoscopy with zero leak rates are creating a new standard of care for this disease.[22]

Hepatobiliary and Pancreas

Minimally invasive hepatobiliary and pancreatic surgery offers some of the most complex and technically challenging operations. Nevertheless, there is accumulating data on complex liver and pancreatic resections done laparoscopically that speak to their safety and feasibility.[23,24] Unfortunately, the laparoscopic skill set and experience required for these procedures have limited universal adoption outside the realm of large research institutions. However, the learning curve for robotic surgery is shorter than for traditional laparoscopy. Many of the technical advantages of robotic systems, such as wristed movements, less ergonomic fatigue, and improved tremor control increase the utility and benefit, particularly for more complex operations. The currently available literature suggests that in a situation adequately planned and prepared for, adoption of robotic techniques in hepatobiliary and pancreatic surgery offers the benefits of shorter recovery and decreased blood loss. As compared to open surgery in similar contexts, robotic surgery presents decreased morbidity and mortality.[25] Early data suggest lower leak rates for reconstructions, especially after the initial learning curve has been achieved.[26]

The use of robotic techniques for complex hepatobiliary and pancreatic surgery is still in its infancy, as evidenced by the very limited number of authors and institutions supplying the available literature. It remains to be seen whether the interest in minimally invasive surgery in this discipline will trend toward increasing adoption of the da Vinci system with its purported advantages.

Endocrine

Thyroid Surgery. Robot-assisted operative techniques have also been introduced to the field of endocrine surgery, most notably for thyroid and adrenal disease. While the traditional open technique for thyroid operations using a Kocher neck incision is a safe operation with good outcomes, concerns about cosmesis have led to the development of alternative procedures that completely avoid a skin incision in the sensitive area of the anterior neck. Several studies have demonstrated the feasibility of video-assisted thyroidectomy,[27,28] but have also demonstrated the difficulties of working in a small space with limited, two-dimensional visualization and reliance on an assistant who holds a camera. To overcome these limitations, gasless robotic transaxillary thyroidectomy using the da Vinci Robot System has been pioneered recently.[29] This technique was found to be feasible[30] and potentially superior to endoscopic approaches.[31] Moreover, with increasing experience, operative times could be reduced to slightly over 100 minutes, which is comparable to a nonrobotic, conventional endoscopic approach, but still longer than for open operations.[30,32–34] Comparisons of robotic and open techniques demonstrate the effectiveness and oncologic safety of the minimally invasive approach.[34] While one study suggested improved patient comfort in the immediate postoperative period and superior cosmesis,[33] another study demonstrated the potential for complications such as brachial plexus injuries with a transaxillary approach.[32]

In summary, robot-assisted thyroidectomy appears to be a reasonable and possibly superior alternative to conventional endoscopic thyroidectomy, but clear advantages to such a well-established, safe, and efficient technique as open thyroidectomy are lacking.

Adrenal Surgery. Surgical resection of the adrenal gland was first performed almost a century ago, and the laparoscopic approach introduced in the early 1990s has now become the preferred technique.[35,36] The advantages generally associated with minimally invasive operations such as decreased postoperative pain, shorter recovery time, and decreased incidence of surgical site infections also apply to adrenalectomy, as do the well-known limitations of conventional laparoscopy including limited visibility and instrument dexterity.

Based on the positive experiences in other surgical specialties and promising results in animal models,[37] the technique of robot-assisted adrenalectomy was introduced a decade ago.[37,38] Analogous to the use of robotic surgical systems for other operations, operative times were initially substantially higher than for conventional laparoscopy, but decreased rapidly with increasing experience.[35,39]

Consistently reported advantages of using the robotic surgical system were precise movements, increased range of motion, improved visualization, and superior surgeon comfort.[36] Robotic adrenalectomies were found to be safe, and conversion rates were demonstrated to be low (less than 10%) in several studies.[35,36]

Direct comparisons between laparoscopic and robot-assisted adrenalectomy demonstrated that robotic operations may result in less blood loss and may be superior to conventional laparoscopy in technically difficult situations, such as operating on obese patients or large tumors.[40,41] Cost comparisons yielded highly variable results, ranging from no cost differences[42] to more than twice the cost[39] for robotic operations. In general, increasing frequency of robotic operations and longer time-intervals studied decreased the costliness of the robotic approach.[39]

Bariatric Surgery

Since the National Institute of Health approved vertical-banded gastroplasty and Roux-en-Y gastric bypass (RYGB) as suitable treatments for the obesity epidemic in 1991, the number of such procedures performed has steadily increased.[43] In recent years, in excess of 190,000 procedures were performed annually for morbid obesity in the United States. Although the laparoscopic approach is the preferred and most common approach for bariatric surgery, the complication rate remains significant at 5% due to the complexity of the RYGB and the high skill set required of the operating surgeon. Other challenges include the fatigue related to increased torque at the abdominal wall in morbidly obese patients.

In 1998, Cadiere et al. first used the robot to perform gastric banding,[7] and since then an increasing number of surgeons have adapted the robot to obesity surgery. Although gastric banding and the RYGB are the most commonly performed obesity procedures, any benefit the robot offers to gastric banding—a relatively simple procedure—is strictly related to improved ergonomics. In the case of the RYGB, the most significant findings have been the ease with which hand-sewn anastomoses can be created with the robot and the associated lower morbidity and gastrointestinal leak rates using robotic techniques.[44]

Interestingly, this lower morbidity comes with the added benefit of a shorter learning curve, i.e., well short of the 100 cases required to obtain comfort in the laparoscopic technique.[45,46] And finally, the improved ergonomics using robotics in this setting, including reduced fatigue, future loss of productivity, and minimizing abdominal wall torque and related tremor, fatigue, and errors, cannot be overemphasized.[47,48]

Pediatric Surgery

The use and adoption of robotic surgery in children has been limited compared to adults, due to challenges of adapting to the sizes of small infants and children.

However, more research is being published on the safety, feasibility, and effectiveness of pediatric robotic surgery.

The first reported pediatric robot-assisted surgery was a Nissen fundoplication in a 10-year-old girl in 2001.[49] Since that time, robot-assisted fundoplications have been compared to laparoscopic and open procedures. Robot-assisted fundoplications were found to have equivalent hospital stays, analgesic requirements, time to feeding, relief of preoperative symptoms, safety profiles, and postoperative complications compared to laparoscopic fundoplications.[50,51] The existing literature supports robotic surgery as safe, feasible, and effective in children. Additionally, robotic surgery gives the surgeon better dexterity to dissect tissues, place sutures, and tie knots.

The wide variation in children's sizes creates special technical concerns, including limited working space, a thinner abdominal wall, and the need for smaller instruments. Special attention is required to maintain anesthesia access to the patient while the robot is docked and also trocar positioning to allow adequate working space while avoiding collisions between the arms and the table. In addition, the robot is calibrated to have the trocars placed at a certain depth from the abdominal wall. This can further limit the intra-corporeal working space, since the robotic instruments will not open unless fully beyond the trocar.[52]

Evaluations of cost implications are limited in robot-assisted surgery in children. However, early comparisons between robotic, laparoscopic, and open fundoplications found that the mean cost for robotic surgery was lower than for open surgery, but higher than for conventional laparoscopic surgery. Robotic surgery had the highest intraoperative costs, which can be attributed to the cost of equipment and increased operating room time. However, hospital length of stay was decreased in robotic operations compared to open procedures, offsetting and even decreasing the overall cost of each fundoplication compared to open operations.[53]

The spectrum of operations in which robotic surgery is used in pediatric surgery continues to expand. Current uses include urologic surgery, cardiac surgery, hepatobiliary including Kasai procedures and choledochal cyst resections,[54,55] duodenal atresia,[56] repair of congenital diaphragmatic hernias,[57–59] splenectomies, pulmonary resections,[58] mediastinal masses,[60] esophageal diseases,[61,62] and anorectal malformations.[63]

Robotic surgery in the pediatric population requires special attention to the wide variety of size differences in patients. However, there is increasing evidence of the efficacy, safety, and cost-effectiveness of robot-assisted surgery in children. This, in combination with surgeon reports of improved performance of complex operations, will likely lead to wider utilization in the future.

Outlook

Compared to the surgical specialties, the current use of robotic systems in general surgery is rather limited. This may be explained by the lack of distinct, substantial advantages of robotic systems in many general surgical procedures.

The achievement of significant, measurable advantages that can compensate for the increased cost and time seen with robotic systems might change this situation. These advantages are less likely to be seen in basic operations such as cholecystectomy, but might be achieved in more complex cases such as hepatobiliary, pancreas, or stomach operations.

References

1. Davies BL, Hibberd RD, Ng WS, Timoney AG, Wickham JE. The development of a surgeon robot for prostatectomies. *Proc Inst Mech Eng H.* 1991;205:35–8.
2. Kwoh YS, Hou J, Jonckheere EA, Hayati S. A robot with improved absolute positioning accuracy for CT guided stereotactic brain surgery. *IEEE Trans Biomed Eng.* 1988; 35:153–60.
3. Reichenspurner H, Damiano RJ, Mack M, et al. Use of the voice-controlled and computer-assisted surgical system ZEUS for endoscopic coronary artery bypass grafting. *J Thorac Cardiovasc Surg.* 1999;118:11–6.
4. Weber PA, Merola S, Wasielewski A, Ballantyne GH. Telerobotic-assisted laparoscopic right and sigmoid colectomies for benign disease. *Dis Colon Rectum.* 2002;45:1689–94; discussion 95–6.
5. Marescaux J, Leroy J, Gagner M, et al. Transatlantic robot-assisted telesurgery. *Nature.* 2001;413:379–80.
6. Cadiere GB, Himpens J, Vertruyen M, et al. Evaluation of telesurgical (robotic) NISSEN fundoplication. *Surg Endosc.* 2001;15:918–23.
7. Cadiere GB, Himpens J, Vertruyen M, Favretti F. The world's first obesity surgery performed by a surgeon at a distance. *Obes Surg.* 1999;9:206–9.
8. Semm K. Endoscopic appendectomy. *Endoscopy.* 1983;15:59–64.
9. Muhe E. [Laparoscopic cholecystectomy]. *Zeitschrift fur Gastroenterologie Verhandlungsband.* 1991;26:204–6.
10. Himpens J, Leman G, Cadiere GB. Telesurgical laparoscopic cholecystectomy. *Surg Endosc.* 1998;12:1091.
11. Jayaraman S, Davies W, Schlachta CM. Getting started with robotics in general surgery with cholecystectomy: the Canadian experience. *Can J Surg.* 2009;52:374–8.
12. Gurusamy KS, Samraj K, Fusai G, Davidson BR. Robot assistant for laparoscopic cholecystectomy. *Cochrane Database Syst Rev.* 2009; CD006578.
13. Kroh M, El-Hayek K, Rosenblatt S, et al. First human surgery with a novel single-port robotic system: cholecystectomy using the da Vinci Single-Site platform. *Surg Endosc.* 2011;25:3566–73.
14. Wren SM, Curet MJ. Single-port robotic cholecystectomy: results from a first human use clinical study of the new da Vinci single-site surgical platform. *Arch Surg.* 2011; 146:1122–7.
15. Spechler SJ. Epidemiology and natural history of gastro-esophageal reflux disease. *Digestion.* 1992;51 Suppl 1:24–9.
16. Catarci M, Gentileschi P, Papi C, et al. Evidence-based appraisal of antireflux fundoplication. *Ann Surg.* 2004;239:325–37.
17. Draaisma WA, Rijnhart-de Jong HG, Broeders IA, Smout AJ, Furnee EJ, Gooszen HG. Five-year subjective and objective results of laparoscopic and conventional Nissen fundoplication: a randomized trial. *Ann Surg.* 2006;244:34–41.

18. Mi J, Kang Y, Chen X, Wang B, Wang Z. Whether robot-assisted laparoscopic fundoplication is better for gastroesophageal reflux disease in adults: a systematic review and meta-analysis. *Surg Endosc.* 2010;24:1803–14.

19. Muller-Stich BP, Reiter MA, Wente MN, et al. Robot-assisted versus conventional laparoscopic fundoplication: short-term outcome of a pilot randomized controlled trial. *Surg Endosc.* 2007;21:1800–5.

20. Giulianotti PC, Coratti A, Angelini M, et al. Robotics in general surgery: personal experience in a large community hospital. *Arch Surg.* 2003;138:777–84.

21. Horgan S, Galvani C, Gorodner MV, et al. Robotic-assisted Heller myotomy versus laparoscopic Heller myotomy for the treatment of esophageal achalasia: multicenter study. *J Gastrointest Surg.* 2005;9:1020–9; discussion 9–30.

22. Melvin WS, Dundon JM, Talamini M, Horgan S. Computer-enhanced robotic telesurgery minimizes esophageal perforation during Heller myotomy. *Surgery.* 2005; 138:553–8;discussion 8–9.

23. Dagher I, Di Giuro G, Dubrez J, Lainas P, Smadja C, Franco D. Laparoscopic versus open right hepatectomy: a comparative study. *Am J Surg.* 2009;198:173–7.

24. Kendrick ML, Cusati D. Total laparoscopic pancreaticoduodenectomy: feasibility and outcome in an early experience. *Arch Surg.* 2010;145:19–23.

25. Giulianotti PC, Coratti A, Sbrana F, et al. Robotic liver surgery: results for 70 resections. *Surgery.* 2011;149:29–39.

26. Giulianotti PC, Sbrana F, Bianco FM, et al. Robot-assisted laparoscopic pancreatic surgery: single-surgeon experience. *Surg Endosc.* 2010;24:1646–57.

27. Lombardi CP, Raffaelli M, Princi P, De Crea C, Bellantone R. Video-assisted thyroidectomy: report of a 7-year experience in Rome. *Langenbecks Arch Surg.* 2006; 391:174–7.

28. Bellantone R, Lombardi CP, Raffaelli M, Boscherini M, De Crea C, Traini E. Video-assisted thyroidectomy. *J Am Coll Surg.* 2002;194:610–4.

29. Kang SW, Lee SC, Lee SH, et al. Robotic thyroid surgery using a gasless, transaxillary approach and the da Vinci S system: the operative outcomes of 338 consecutive patients. *Surgery.* 2009;146:1048–55.

30. Kandil EH, Noureldine SI, Yao L, Slakey DP. Robotic transaxillary thyroidectomy: an examination of the first one hundred cases. *J Am Coll Surg.* 2012;214:558–64; discussion 64–6.

31. Lee S, Ryu HR, Park JH, et al. Excellence in robotic thyroid surgery: a comparative study of robot-assisted versus conventional endoscopic thyroidectomy in papillary thyroid microcarcinoma patients. *Ann Surg.* 2011;253:1060–6.

32. Landry CS, Grubbs EG, Warneke CL, et al. Robot-assisted transaxillary thyroid surgery in the United States: is it comparable to open thyroid lobectomy? *Ann Surg Oncol.* 2012;19:1269–74.

33. Lee J, Nah KY, Kim RM, Ahn YH, Soh EY, Chung WY. Differences in postoperative outcomes, function, and cosmesis: open versus robotic thyroidectomy. *Surg Endosc.* 2010;24:3186–94.

34. Lee S, Ryu HR, Park JH, et al. Early surgical outcomes comparison between robotic and conventional open thyroid surgery for papillary thyroid microcarcinoma. *Surgery.* 2012;151:724–30.

35. Brunaud L, Germain A, Zarnegar R, Cuny T, Ayav A, Bresler L. Robot-assisted adrenalectomy. *Surg Laparosc Endosc Percutan Tech.* 2011;21:248–54.

36. Rosoff JS, Otto BJ, Del Pizzo JJ. The emerging role of robotics in adrenal surgery. *Curr Urol Rep.* 2010;11:38–43.

37. Gill IS, Sung GT, Hsu TH, Meraney AM. Robotic remote laparoscopic nephrectomy and adrenalectomy: the initial experience. *J Urol.* 2000;164:2082–5.

38. Horgan S, Vanuno D. Robots in laparoscopic surgery. *J Laparoendosc Adv Surg Tech A.* 2001;11:415–9.

39. Brunaud L, Ayav A, Zarnegar R, et al. Prospective evaluation of 100 robotic-assisted unilateral adrenalectomies. *Surgery.* 2008;144:995–1001; discussion 1001.

40. Brunaud L, Bresler L, Ayav A, et al. Robotic-assisted adrenalectomy: what advantages compared to lateral transperitoneal laparoscopic adrenalectomy? *Am J Surg.* 2008; 195:433–8.

41. Agcaoglu O, Aliyev S, Karabulut K, Mitchell J, Siperstein A, Berber E. Robotic versus laparoscopic resection of large adrenal tumors. *Ann Surg Oncol.* 2012;19:2288–94.

42. Winter JM, Talamini MA, Stanfield CL, et al. Thirty robotic adrenalectomies: a single institution's experience. *Surg Endosc.* 2006;20:119–24.

43. NIH conference. Gastrointestinal surgery for severe obesity. Consensus Development Conference Panel. *Ann Intern Med.* 1991;115:956–61.

44. Snyder BE, Wilson T, Leong BY, Klein C, Wilson EB. Robotic-assisted Roux-en-Y gastric bypass: minimizing morbidity and mortality. *Obes Surg.* 2010;20:265–70.

45. Schauer P, Ikramuddin S, Hamad G, Gourash W. The learning curve for laparoscopic Roux-en-Y gastric bypass in 100 cases. Surg Endosc. 2003;17:212–5.

46. Mohr CJ, Nadzam GS, Curet MJ. Totally robotic Roux-en-Y gastric bypass. *Arch Surg.* 2005;140:779–86.

47. Talamini MA, Chapman S, Horgan S, Melvin WS. A prospective analysis of 211 robotic-assisted surgical procedures. *Surg Endosc.* 2003;17:1521–4.

48. Jacobsen G, Berger R, Horgan S. The role of robotic surgery in morbid obesity. *J Laparoendosc Adv Surg Tech A.* 2003;13:279–83.

49. Meininger DD, Byhahn C, Heller K, Gutt CN, Westphal K. Totally endoscopic Nissen fundoplication with a robotic system in a child. *Surg Endosc.* 2001;15:1360.

50. Margaron FC, Oiticica C, Lanning DA. Robotic-assisted laparoscopic Nissen fundoplication with gastrostomy preservation in neurologically impaired children. *J Laparoendosc Adv Surg Tech A.* 2010;20:489-92.

51. Albassam AA, Mallick MS, Gado A, Shoukry M. Nissen fundoplication, robotic-assisted versus laparoscopic procedure: a comparative study in children. *Eur J Pediatr Surg.* 2009;19:316–9.

52. Meehan JJ. Robotic surgery in small children: is there room for this? *J Laparoendosc Adv Surg Tech A.* 2009;19:707–12.

53. Anderberg M, Kockum CC, Arnbjornsson E. Paediatric robotic surgery in clinical practice: a cost analysis. *Eur J Pediatr Surg.* 2009;19:311–5.

54. Meehan JJ, Elliott S, Sandler A. The robotic approach to complex hepatobiliary anomalies in children: preliminary report. *J Pediatr Surg.* 2007;42:2110–4.

55. Chang EY, Hong YJ, Chang HK, Oh JT, Han SJ. Lessons and tips from the experience of pediatric robotic choledochal cyst resection. *J Laparoendosc Adv Surg Tech A.* 2012; 22:609–14.

56. Meehan JJ. Robotic repair of congenital duodenal atresia: a case report. *J Pediatr Surg.* 2007;42:E31–3.

57. Anderberg M, Kockum CC, Arnbjornsson E. Morgagni hernia repair in a small child using da Vinci robotic instruments—a case report. *Eur J Pediatr Surg.* 2009;19:110–2.

58. Meehan JJ, Phearman L, Sandler A. Robotic pulmonary resections in children: series report and introduction of a new robotic instrument. *J Laparoendosc Adv Surg Tech A.* 2008;18:293–5.

59. Meehan JJ, Sandler A. Robotic repair of a Bochdalek congenital diaphragmatic hernia in a small neonate: robotic advantages and limitations. *J Pediatr Surg.* 2007;42: 1757–60.

60. Meehan JJ, Sandler AD. Robotic resection of mediastinal masses in children. *J Laparoendosc Adv Surg Tech A.* 2008;18:114–9.

61. DeUgarte DA, Teitelbaum D, Hirschl RB, Geiger JD. Robotic extirpation of complex massive esophageal leiomyoma. *J Laparoendosc Adv Surg Tech A.* 2008;18:286–9.

62. Obasi PC, Hebra A, Varela JC. Excision of esophageal duplication cysts with robotic-assisted thoracoscopic surgery. *JSLS.* 2011;15:244–7.

63. Albassam A, Gado A, Mallick MS, Alnaami M, Al-Shenawy W. Robotic-assisted anorectal pull-through for anorectal malformations. *J Pediatr Surg.* 2011;46:1794–7.

Chapter Eleven

The Colon and Rectum

Stefan W. Leichtle, MD; Amanda Y. Yang, MD; Robert K. Cleary, MD

History and Introduction

Descriptions of colon and anorectal disease date back to the beginning of human civilization. Ancient Greek and Byzantine texts detailed instructions for the surgical treatment of hemorrhoids, fissures, and fistulas.[1] More complex procedures were not described until the eighteenth century, when the first successful colostomies were created for congenital diseases, acute obstructions, and cancer. More advanced surgical treatment options for the wide array of colon and rectal illnesses did not evolve until the twentieth century.

Innovations in minimally invasive surgery ultimately led to the first laparoscopic appendectomy in 1983,[2] the first laparoscopic cholecystectomy in 1985,[3,4] and the first reported series of laparoscopic colectomies in 1991.[5] Minimally invasive colon and rectal surgery poses several challenges: an operation in multiple abdominal quadrants; an organ that is not entirely fixed to surrounding structures; and the presence of the small bowel, which may obscure the view. Not surprisingly, the learning curve to acquire minimally invasive skills is steep, particularly for procedures in the pelvis. While colon and rectal surgeons were initially hesitant to adopt laparoscopic techniques widely, recent studies suggest that a third to half of colon and rectal operations across the United States are now conducted using minimally invasive techniques.[6,7]

Several large randomized controlled trials and meta-analyses comparing laparoscopic and open techniques demonstrated that minimally invasive laparoscopic surgery does not compromise oncologic outcomes and confers the advantages of shorter incisions, less tissue damage, decreased postoperative pain, quicker return of bowel function, shorter hospital stays, better cosmesis, quicker recovery time, and faster return to normal activities.[8–22] However, laparoscopic surgery for colon and rectal disease is limited by two-dimensional imaging, restricted instrument dexterity with only four degrees of freedom, and limited working space around the patient for the operating surgeon, camera assistant, and perioperative nurse. Furthermore, the laparoscopic technique does not allow for fixed retraction and requires an experienced assistant.[23] Because the laparoscopic camera is not on a stable platform and is not generally held by the operating surgeon, lens soiling may be a persistent limitation of visualization, thereby contributing to surgeon frustration and possibly premature conversion to open techniques.

Robot-Assisted Colon and Rectal Surgery

Largely as a result of the successful application in urology, colon and rectal surgeons began to investigate the role of robot-assisted surgery for operations on the colon and rectum. In 2002, Weber et al. reported the first robotic colon and rectal procedure.[23] Since that time, the number of colon and rectal surgeons performing robot-assisted operations has been steadily increasing, as has the volume of literature describing these experiences.[24] The availability of robotic systems in hospitals across the country is increasing, and several surgical residency programs have already incorporated robotic training into their educational curriculum. Therefore, it is expected that robot-assisted colon and rectal operations will be offered to patients by an increasing number of board-certified colon and rectal surgeons in upcoming years. Furthermore, skilled laparoscopic surgeons may find the transition to robotic surgery far less difficult than the transition from open to laparoscopic surgery.

The advantages of colon and rectal operations using robotic assistance include three-dimensional imaging, fine motion scaling, the availability of a third arm for fixed retraction, and superior dexterity with articulated instruments allowing for seven degrees of freedom. An additional benefit is the stable robotic camera platform that is more resistant to lens soiling and controlled by the surgeon rather than an assistant. These robotic advantages are particularly pertinent for rectal neoplasms and other diseases in the pelvis, where laparoscopic retraction and visualization are very challenging, and where robotic-assisted surgery affords better visualization and more precise movements.[25,26]

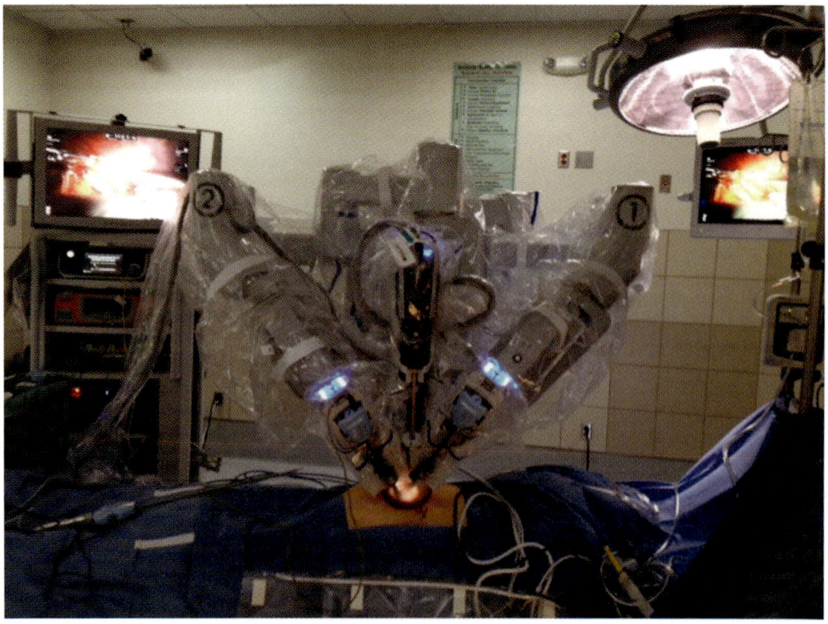

Figure 1. Colon and rectal surgery with the da Vinci Robotic System.

Several nuances of robotic colon and rectal surgery require attention when transitioning from the laparoscopic to the robotic approach.

The Three-Dimensional Image. This allows the operating surgeon to feel very close to the target anatomy, as if one was actually inside the patient's abdomen. It is important to keep all instruments in view to avoid tissue damage by an instrument outside the visual field. Additionally, the lack of direct haptic feedback in conjunction with the strength of the robotic instruments requires careful and precise handling. The feeling for the strength of the grasp can be improved when the tip of the instrument is fully visualized. In addition, it sometimes helps to pull the camera back for broader visualization so as not to "lose the forest for the trees."

Clutching. This essential technique enables the surgeon to "uncouple" the robotic arms from their controls and allows for comfortable repositioning of the surgeon's upper extremities, while maintaining the position of the operating instruments. The surgeon can therefore have the operating hands and arms in a comfortable position throughout the course of the operation, thereby minimizing fatigue and discomfort. Along with the ergonomically comfortable position of the surgeon's head and neck in the console viewport, this significantly decreases surgeon fatigue throughout lengthy colorectal operations and may result in fewer neck and back ailments.[27]

The Technical Details. Though most of us are not engineers, it is important for the surgeon to understand the basics of the robotic system and to be able to troubleshoot common problems and errors involving the operating instruments. System failures are rare, but it is helpful to have a knowledgeable vendor or circulating nurse to assist if these should occur.

Trocar Placement. Colon and rectal operations often span multiple quadrants. Therefore, strategic trocar placement to limit external and internal collisions between robotic arms is essential in robot-assisted operations, even more so than in laparoscopic operations. Experienced laparoscopic surgeons often have to make only minor adjustments to their usual trocar placement when transitioning to robotic surgery. With regard to trocar placement, novice robotic surgeons typically emulate those surgeons who have trained them, often with minor changes to accommodate their individual preferences.

Training Future Robotic Surgeons

As the technology of robotic surgery systems continues to evolve, the training and education of residents, fellows, and staff in robotic techniques is subject to change. Training options include the utilization of computer simulators, inanimate models, animal and cadaver lab workshops, as well as case observations. Attending staff should be proctored for their first three to five cases. This number will vary from institution to institution depending on privileging criteria and department regulations. Residents need to be trained in both established and emerging minimally invasive techniques. Training in the use of computer simulators and dual consoles can help prepare residents for work with the da Vinci Robotic System. Some institutions have already incorporated robotic training into their residency training programs.[28]

The da Vinci Skills Simulator is a software package that provides the operating surgeon with an opportunity to learn and practice robotic skills on a real operating robotic console. For novice learners, modules for hand-eye-foot coordination, camera movements, clutching, retraction, dissection, suturing, and the use of energy devices are available. More advanced trainees can practice complex operating maneuvers in a realistic fashion. The software also contains metrics that allow graded assessments and feedback, as well as the ability to track progress. The simulator is a method of training residents and staff and may be considered a prerequisite for preparing them to sit at the dual console during a live operation. The dual console technique involves the utilization of two consoles during a real-time operation. An experienced surgeon at one console is able to monitor and control the movements of the novice robotic surgeon at the second console.

Animal and cadaver laboratory training utilizing live porcine and cadaver models is available for robotic training. These training sessions are sponsored by industry. Candidates for training in these labs are determined on an individual basis.

Outcomes of Robotic Colon and Rectal Surgery

Several case series and nonrandomized comparative studies have now been published, demonstrating the safety and feasibility of robot-assisted colon and rectal surgery.[23,28–31] Complication rates for robotic surgery range from 5.4% to 43.2% and are comparable to conventional and hand-assisted laparoscopic surgery.[23,24,31] Some authors report even lower complication rates for robotic versus conventional laparoscopic operations.[30]

Operating Time. Longer operating times have been identified as a potential disadvantage of robot-assisted surgery when compared to conventional laparoscopic surgery. In a randomized study comparing robotic and laparoscopic total mesorectal excisions (TME) for rectal cancer, Baik et al. found that the operating time for the robotic approach was only 13 minutes longer.[32] Patel et al. compared robot-assisted to conventional and hand-assisted laparoscopy and found no difference in operating times for pelvic operations requiring a low anastomosis.[31] In a review of robotic surgery for rectal cancer, Leong and Kim found that two of five studies comparing robotic and laparoscopic rectal surgery revealed shorter operating times for robot-assisted surgery, though the difference was not statistically significant.[33] Operating times in the literature are difficult to interpret, because many "robotic operations" are in fact hybrid laparoscopic-robotic approaches, and operating time by any approach may be surgeon-dependent.

Length of Hospital Stay (LOS). The LOS after robotic operations is comparable to the LOS after conventional laparoscopic operations, with some studies demonstrating a shorter length of stay following robotic surgery.[30,31] These findings are consistent with the experience at our institution, where a preliminary analysis suggested shorter LOS for segmental colectomies (unpublished data).

Conversion to Open Surgery. This may be necessary for multiple reasons, most commonly due to adhesions from previous operations and morbid obesity. Morbid obesity represents a particular challenge for pelvic operations, where the consequences, including a narrow male pelvis and a heavy mesorectum, often compound the degree of difficulty and may make conversion necessary. Among the five comparative studies reviewed by Leong and Kim, the conversion rate for laparoscopic surgery was 6.2%. There were no conversions in the robotic groups.[33] Conversion rates reported for operations for rectal cancer vary from 0 to 4.9% for robotic and 12 to 20% for laparoscopic surgery.[23] Luca et al. suggested that a long, stressful operation may be more likely to be converted, and that the superior image quality and comfort of the robotic console may be important factors in explaining the decreased risk for conversion during robotic surgery.[34]

Oncologic Outcomes and Lymph Node Harvest. These important factors do not appear to be compromised when employing robotic surgery for colon and rectal cancer.[24,25,30,31,35–37] In a short-term analysis of open, laparoscopic, and robotic resection with curative intent for rectal cancer, Park et al. demonstrated that patients who had undergone laparoscopic or robotic resection had significantly faster recoveries than their open surgery counterparts. At the same time, distal and circumferential margins, lymph node yields, and complication rates were equivalent.[38]

Initial reports from case series for pelvic operations for rectal cancer were favorable for the robotic approach. Compared to laparoscopic LAR, robotic-assisted surgery resulted in better pathologic mesorectal grading, with more intact mesorectums in the pathologic specimens.[32,39,40] In addition, the robot-assisted surgery afforded a lower conversion rate (0% versus 10.5%) and a shorter mean LOS of 4.7 days versus 5.5 days. Baek et al. also published early outcomes data with a median follow up of 20.2 months that appeared favorable for robotic surgery, reporting a median lymph node harvest of 14.5, a local recurrence rate of 3.1%, and a conversion rate to open surgery of 9.4%.[41] In this study, circumferential and distal margins were uninvolved with tumor. Similar advantages for robotic surgery in the pelvis have been reported in subsequent case series.[42]

There are two randomized studies in progress addressing outcomes in this patient population. The first is the Robotic versus Laparoscopic Resection for Rectal Cancer (ROLARR) study, a randomized prospective trial comparing outcomes in patients undergoing robotic versus laparoscopic total mesorectal excision.[43] The second study is the ACOSOG Z6051 study, an international, multicenter trial comparing open and laparoscopic surgery for cancer of the rectum, which now includes robotic surgery in the laparoscopic arm. End points in these trials include short- and long-term oncologic outcomes, quality of the mesorectal excision, local recurrence, disease-free survival, quality of life metrics, sexual function, and cost analysis. These randomized trials should provide definitive data that answer the questions raised and commented on in the small case series and other comparative studies done to date.

Ergonomics. A point of interest that may gain momentum for future study is the notion that ergonomics of robotic surgery may compare favorably to laparoscopic and open surgery with regard to surgeon comfort, neck and back ailments, physical stress, and, ultimately, to performance.[44,45]

Economics. The da Vinci surgical robot is an example of a technological advance that has not yet proven its cost-effectiveness. With a unit cost of between one million to over $2 million, the da Vinci surgical robot is undeniably expensive.[46] It was first introduced into the United States in 1995, but was not available for general purchase until 1998. And yet, its worldwide use has increased substantially, from 80,000 procedures in 2007 to 205,000 procedures in 2011.[46]

The question remains whether or not robotic surgery provides benefits for both patients and the health-care system that outweigh the costs of the technology it represents, particularly when compared to existing, older technology. The da Vinci robot has been adopted by multiple specialties, including general surgery, thoracic/cardiac surgery, urology, gynecologic surgery, vascular surgery, and otorhinolaryngology. It is perhaps salient to ask whether da Vinci surgery has introduced benefits to the colorectal surgery population, a population that, prior to the introduction of robotic surgery, was beginning to reap the benefits of laparoscopic surgery.

In several studies, elective laparoscopic colorectal surgery has been shown to be more cost-effective than traditional open colorectal procedures. In a study by Klarenbeek et al., patients undergoing elective laparoscopic sigmoid resection for diverticular disease showed a 15.4% reduction in major complication rates when compared to the open elective sigmoid resection group.[47] In addition, patients undergoing laparoscopic surgery had less pain, shorter hospitalizations, and improved quality of life.[47]

Similarly, in a study by Senagore et al., patients undergoing elective laparoscopic sigmoid resection had a significantly lower cost per case when compared to their open procedure cohort ($3,458 ±437 vs. $4,321 ±501, $P < .05$), with a significantly shorter length of stay (3.1 ±0.2 vs. 6.8 ±0.4 days), fewer pulmonary complications (1.6 vs. 5.6%), and fewer wound infections (0 vs. 7%).[48] Both studies found that, although operative costs can be higher for laparoscopic operations, these costs were made up for by savings in laboratory studies, pharmacy costs, and overall hospitalization costs.

While patient outcomes have not been shown to be significantly different, literature to date has shown that robotic colectomy is more costly than its laparoscopic counterpart. Bertani et al. concluded that the da Vinci's depreciation costs were the main contributor to its overall greater expense: robotic colectomy was estimated to cost €2,059 more than a similar laparoscopic procedure, assuming that depreciation occurred at a rate of 15 robotic procedures performed each week.[49] Turchetti et al. performed a meta-analysis of 11 American and European studies comparing the economic analysis of the da Vinci robot to laparoscopic surgery. Research found that higher operative costs associated with the da Vinci robot were due to its high purchase price and maintenance costs and, to a lesser extent, to the longer operative times.[46]

In a preliminary cost analysis at our institution, we analyzed 101 colon resections done in fiscal year 2011, including 44 open, 47 robotic, and 10 laparoscopic procedures. An analysis of direct costs (those costs that are directly related to patient care) and indirect costs (costs which are incurred regardless of patient volume) suggested that open procedures were significantly more expensive than either laparoscopic or robotic procedures. In a direct comparison, direct and indirect costs were less for robotic than for laparoscopic surgery, without reaching statistical significance.

These findings at our institution might be explained by the high robotic volume across multiple disciplines, thereby making robotic surgery a financially feasible option despite the high purchase and maintenance costs. Therefore, achieving a certain economy of scale may be necessary to support a da Vinci robotic program. Depending on surgical discipline, the critical number for financial success is likely between 500 and 600 cases per year. The potential for shorter postoperative LOS and patients interested in robotic surgery are additional factors that can contribute to financial success. Though the data from fiscal year 2011 are hampered by a limited number of laparoscopic procedures and limited financial categorization data, the analysis to date suggests that robotic colorectal surgery is not more costly than the laparoscopic counterpart at our institution.

Operative Considerations

The robotic operations described in this chapter include segmental right and sigmoid colectomy, low anterior resection (LAR), and abdominoperineal resection (APR). In addition to benign diseases such as diverticulitis, these procedures are commonly performed for colon and rectal cancer.

As the fourth most common malignancy in the United States, colorectal cancer represents the second leading cause of cancer deaths. The majority of colorectal cancer cases are sporadic, and the average age of presentation is above 60 years. About 20% of patients have a family history of colorectal neoplasia. The most notable inherited syndromes are familial adenomatous polyposis (FAP) and hereditary nonpolyposis colorectal cancer (HNPCC), diseases for which the age of presentation is 15 to 20 years younger than for sporadic colorectal cancer.

For individuals with average risk, colorectal cancer screening typically starts at age 50, with the aim of detecting premalignant lesions. Colonoscopy is the most commonly recommended screening modality, as it allows access to the entire colon and permits the removal of premalignant lesions. This study should be performed every 10 years, beginning at age 50 for average risk individuals, and at age 40 for those with a family history of colorectal neoplasia (or 10 years younger than the affected family member should that family member be less than 50 years of age). Those with inflammatory bowel disease (IBD) and those with a family history of FAP or HNPCC should begin screening at a younger age. CT colonography with air insufflation represents a more recent and not yet completely established modality. The disadvantage of this test is that a colonoscopy is necessary for biopsy or polyp removal if neoplasia is identified.

In the treatment of colorectal cancer, the main goals are control of local disease and prevention of systemic disease. While there are several staging classifications for colon and rectal cancer, the American Joint Committee on Cancer and International Union against Cancer (AJCC/UICC) system, based on the TNM Classification of malignant tumors, is generally used. T refers to depth of invasion, N to nodal status, and M to the presence or absence of metastatic disease (Table 1).

Stage 0 describes carcinoma in situ, in which malignant cells are limited to the mucosa. Stage I tumors are early neoplasms that invade the submucosa (T1N0M0) or muscularis propria (T2N0M0) and are without lymph node (N0) or distant metastasis (M0). Stage II tumors more deeply penetrate the wall of the colon and rectum and are also without lymph node or distant metastases (T3N0M0 and T4N0M0). Stage III tumors are characterized by lymph node metastases. Stage IV represents patients with distant metastases (T_{any}, N_{any}, M1).

The Surveillance, Epidemiology and End Results (SEER) Program registry has allowed meaningful colorectal cancer survival studies. While individual studies differ, 5-year survival rates range from 90% for stage I disease to 40% for stage IIIB, and less than 10% for stage IV.[51]

Preoperative preparation for potentially curative surgery includes colonoscopic examination of the entire large bowel, determination of carcinoembryonic antigen (CEA) levels, and CT imaging of the chest, abdomen, and pelvis. Preoperative bowel preparation is controversial, but utilized by many. The Michigan Surgical Quality Collaborative (MSQC) data recommend oral antibiotics following the mechanical bowel preparation. Intravenous antibiotics are given within 30 minutes of incision. Our antibiotic options are Cefozolin and Metronidazole for those without penicillin allergies, and Ciprofloxacin and Metronidazole for those patients with penicillin allergies. These options are also based on MSQC data. Resection of colonic malignancies should be performed with appropriate intestinal and tangential margins to include the draining lymph node (LN) basins. Harvesting of at least 12 LNs has been shown to improve staging quality and is dependent on patient, surgeon, and pathologist. Postoperatively, chemotherapy is routinely administered to patients with stage III disease and in selected cases of stage II disease with high-risk features such as perforation or obstruction.

Rectal cancers represent about 25% to 30% of colorectal malignancies. As with colon cancer, preoperative evaluations include CEA levels, full colonoscopy when possible to exclude synchronous neoplasms, and CT imaging of the chest, abdomen, and pelvis to assess the possibility of metastatic disease. For local staging purposes, endorectal ultrasonography or pelvic MRI with endo-anal coils is employed to determine the depth of invasion of the rectal wall. Small T1 lesions may be

Table 1. TNM Classification and Staging of Colon Cancer*

Primary tumor staging (T)

T0	No evidence of primary tumor
Tis	Carcinoma in situ
T1	Tumor invades submucosa
T2	Tumor invades muscularis propria
T3	Tumor invades through the muscularis propria into the pericolonic tissue
T4a	Tumor penetrates to the surface of the visceral peritoneum (serosa)
T4b	Tumor invades and/or is adherent to other organs or structures

Regional lymph node staging (N)

N0	No regional lymph node metastasis
N1a	Metastasis in 1 regional lymph node
N1b	Metastasis in 2–3 regional lymph nodes
N1c	Tumor deposits in subserosa, mesentery, or nonperitonealized pericolic or perirectal tissues without regional nodal metastases
N2a	Metastasis in 4–6 regional lymph nodes
N2b	Metastasis in 7 or more regional lymph nodes

Distant metastasis staging (M)

M0	No distant metastasis
M1a	Metastasis confined to 1 organ or site
M1b	Metastasis in more than 1 organ/site or the peritoneum

Stage	T	N	M
0	Tis	N0	M0
I	1–2	N0	M0
IIA	T3	N0	M0
IIB	T4a	N0	M0
IIC	T4b	N0	M0
IIIA	T1-T2	N1–N1c	M0
	T1	N2a	M0
IIIB	T3–T4a	N1–N1c	M0
	T2–T3	N2a	M0
	T1–2	N2b	M0
IIIC	T4a	N2a	M0
	T3–T4a	N2b	M0
	T4b	N1–N2	M0
IVA	Any T	Any N	M1a
IVB	Any T	Any N	M1b

* Based on *AJCC,* 7th Ed., and Chang et al.[50]

amenable to transanal resection with standard techniques or, more recently, with trans-anal minimally invasive surgery (TAMIS), a laparoscopic transanal procedure. Larger (more than 3 to 4 cm) and higher stage rectal cancers require preoperative chemoradiation and radical excision, which may be LAR, coloproctectomy with coloanal anastomosis, or APR, any of which may be done with open, laparoscopic, or robotic approaches.

Radical excision by LAR, coloanal resection, or APR mandates resection of the neoplasm with appropriate intestinal and tangential margins. The tangential margin is key to the prevention of local recurrence and is optimized by utilizing the principle of TME. First described by Heald et al.,[52] this technique is characterized by resection of the rectum in a plane between the thin fascia propria of the rectum and presacral fascia posteriorly, and between the fascia propria and surrounding lymphovascular tissue anterior and laterally. The traditional distal intestinal margin is 2 cm, but outcomes with smaller margins may be acceptable for low rectal lesions with favorable histopathologic features, i.e., well differentiated malignancies without evidence of lymphovascular or perineural invasion.

Robot-Assisted Procedures

Robotic surgery may be considered "technologically advanced laparoscopic surgery." The three-dimensional image, stable camera platform, and third arm for fixed retraction have the potential to make robotic surgery on a floppy organ in multiple quadrants less challenging than the laparoscopic counterpart.

A well-organized and experienced operating team of circulating nurses, perioperative nurses, and anesthesia care providers is crucial for successful robotic surgery. Familiarity with the surgical robotic system and training to prepare and dock the robot are required to allow for efficient resource utilization and quick turnover times. Just as the novice laparoscopic surgeon is wise to start with less complex cases such as a right colectomy for benign disease, so too should the novice robotic surgeon.

Because many robotic colon and rectal surgeons have previous laparoscopic experience and because robotic surgery similarly involves the use of trocars, many robotic surgeons perform hybrid variations of laparoscopic-robotic surgery. For rectal cancer, some isolate the mesenteric vessels and mobilize the mesentery from the retroperitoneum laparoscopically. They then perform a TME with the robot. Others use the laparoscope to confirm the absence of prohibitive adhesions and then perform the entire procedure with the robot. Some robotic surgeons will dock the robot a second time when operating in two quadrants far removed (e.g., splenic flexure and pelvis), although we have found it very possible to perform an entire LAR, from splenic flexure to the levators, leaving the robot docked once over the left hip.

For the purposes of exploration and to verify the feasibility of the planned robotic approach, laparoscopy is performed at the beginning of every robotic procedure. More recently, we have used the robotic camera for laparoscopy during right colectomies, thereby sparing the cost of opening laparoscopic cameras, lenses, and instruments. There are a number of dedicated robotic instruments from which to choose.

We prefer switching between monopolar scissors, the Harmonic Scalpel® (Ethicon EndoSurgery, Cincinnati, OH), and a polymer clip (e.g., Hem-o-lok®) applier in robotic arm 1 (D1). The Intuitive Vessel Sealer has recently become available for use in robotic arm 1. This instrument coagulates vessels up to 7 mm in diameter and divides them. Bipolar graspers or Maryland graspers are used for gentle retraction of dissected tissues in arm 2 (D2 or D3), and an additional grasper is used as the third arm for fixed retraction (D2 or D3).

Specific Operative Techniques

Right Colectomy. Robotic right colectomies are performed with the robot docked over the patient's right side, slightly cephalad of the mid-abdomen. Ideal trocar placement is surgeon dependent. An example of this is shown in Figures 2a and 2b.

We prefer to have a camera port at the umbilicus, a dissecting port in the left lateral upper quadrant (D1), a fenestrated bipolar grasper in the suprapubic region (D2), an additional grasping retractor in the subcostal region just to the left of the midline (D3), and a 5 mm assistant port (Ast) in the left lower quadrant. This trocar scheme allows all instruments to point in the same direction and minimizes external and internal robotic arm collisions.

Prior to docking the robot, the patient is placed in moderate right-to-left rotation and slight Trendelenburg position. After docking the robot and positioning the instruments, the ileocolic vessels are identified and the mesentery is mobilized away from the retroperitoneum in a medial to lateral fashion, at which point the ureter is identified. Though we routinely perform medial to lateral dissection, other surgeons successfully employ lateral to medial dissection. Patient anatomy or body habitus may

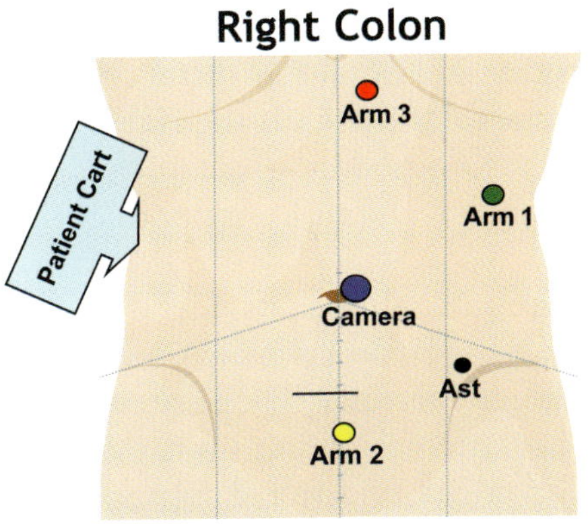

Figure 2a. Diagram of a right colectomy. Arm 1 = D1. Arm 2 = D2. Arm 3 = D3.

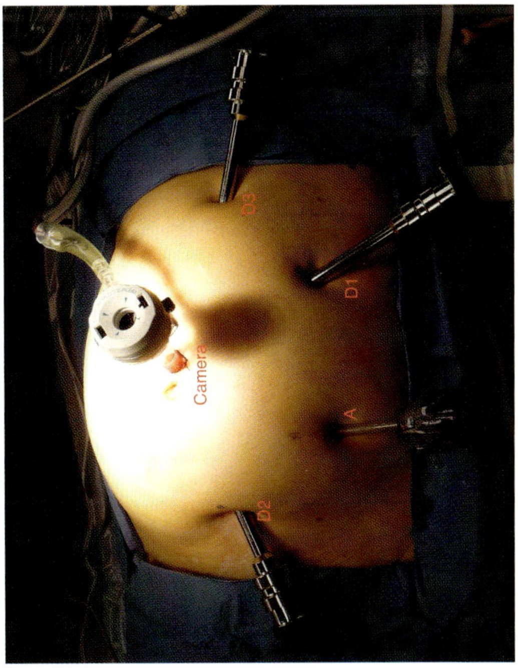

Figure 2b. Trocar placement and setup for right colectomy.

preclude safe medial to lateral dissection, in which case the alternative technique would be preferred.

The ileocolic vessels are then divided near their origin, either after application of polymer clips or by application of an energy device (Harmonic scalpel or Intuitive Vessel Sealer®), both of which are passed through the left upper quadrant port (D1). The right colic artery is then similarly transected near its origin. Lateral to medial dissection of the remaining retroperitoneal attachments, including those of the hepatic flexure, and dissection of the omentum from the proximal transverse colon and mesocolon conclude the mobilization process. All right colectomy specimens are resected, and the anastomosis is performed extracorporeally by enlarging the umbilical robotic camera port incision. An Alexis® wound protector is used for all cases. Fascia defects larger than 8 mm at any trocar site should be closed with sutures to prevent trocar site hernias.

If an intracorporeal anastomosis is performed, the extraction site incision may be in the Pfannenstiel location, by way of extending the suprapubic (D2) port site, or the specimen may be retrieved through the vagina.[28] Right colectomy is amenable to single port technology, in which case the only incision would be the umbilical midline incision.[53,54]

Robotic surgery may offer clear advantages over laparoscopic surgery for single port resection. The laparoscopic surgeon and assistant must compete for space at the patient's side. In addition, there is greater difficulty maintaining laparoscopic camera stability, visualization, and lens clarity. In contrast, the robotic surgeon console offers an unobstructed view and ample workspace.

Sigmoid Resection. Trocar placement for sigmoid resection is variable and is based on surgeon preference. Increased experience with robotic surgery often leads to better trocar placement, resulting in a minimum of external robotic arm and internal robotic instrument collisions. We prefer an arrangement including a camera trocar either at or just above and to the right of the umbilicus, a dissecting trocar in the right lower quadrant (D1), a bipolar grasping trocar in the subcostal region just to the right of the midline (D3), and a grasping trocar in the left lateral abdomen at the same craniocaudal level as the camera (D2). A suggested setup for robotic sigmoid resections is shown in Figures 3a and 3b.

A 12 mm assistant port (Ast) is placed in the right upper quadrant to accommodate an endoscopic stapler. Some prefer to pass the stapler through the right lower quadrant dissecting trocar, upgraded to 13 mm to accommodate the stapler. If this larger right lower quadrant port is utilized for the stapler, the right upper quadrant assistant port need only be 5 mm.

Prior to docking, the patient is placed in the Trendelenburg position with left-to-right rotation. The omentum and small bowel are laparoscopically placed in the right upper quadrant, out of the way of the target anatomy. The surgeon then positions her/himself on the right side of the table, thereby lining up the camera port with the left anterior superior iliac spine. The circulating nurse subsequently mobilizes the robot toward the left hip, while the surgeon demonstrates the line between the camera port, left hip, and robot.

The robotic arms are then attached to the trocars, the dedicated instruments are passed under direct vision, and the operating surgeon moves to the console.

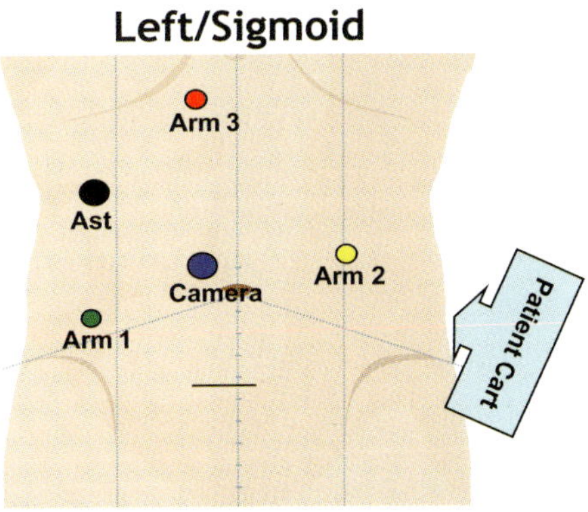

Figure 3a. Diagram of a sigmoid resection.

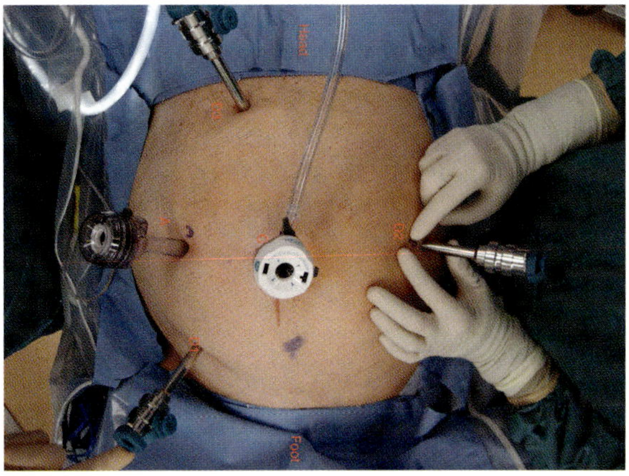

Figure 3b. Setup for robotic sigmoid resection.

The mesentery overlying the inferior mesenteric vessels is grasped with the third arm, allowing for visualization of the course of the inferior mesenteric artery (IMA) and providing clear access to its origin. Maintaining the small bowel in the upper right quadrant can be difficult, and fixed retraction with the third arm is especially helpful in situations such as this when visualization might otherwise be impossible (Figure 4).

The IMA is dissected from the surrounding retroperitoneal structures and sympathetic nerves, allowing the mesentery to be separated from the retroperitoneum and its origin to be identified. In obese individuals, identifying the origin of the IMA may be challenging. In these cases, it may be best to locate the superior hemorrhoidal artery near the sacral promontory and trace it back to the IMA. For benign disease, tracing the IMA to its origin may not be necessary. Subsequently, the IMA is divided after application of polymer clips or with the use of energy devices, all of which are passed through the dissecting robotic arm (D1). The left ureter should be identified prior to division of the IMA (Figure 5).

Lateral to medial dissection of the sigmoid and the descending colon follow the medial to lateral dissection of the sigmoid and descending colon mesentery. These steps allow for complete resection of the diseased segment and a tension-free anastomosis. The splenic flexure may or may not require mobilization, which may be done robotically or laparoscopically.

The mesorectum at the level of the upper rectum, where the taenia coli splay to form a longitudinal muscular coat, may be sequentially divided using an energy device or stapler. The upper rectum is then divided with a stapler placed through the 12 mm right upper quadrant assistant trocar, preferably with one application. After disconnecting the robotic arms from the trocars, the robot is then moved away from the patient. A Pfannenstiel or left lower quadrant incision is then made, and a wound protector placed. The end of the sigmoid is carefully retrieved through this incision, and the diseased segment is subsequently resected. A purse string suture is placed in the descending colon. A circular stapler is chosen, the anvil placed in the open end of the descending colon, and the purse string suture is tied. The descending colon is then returned to the abdominal cavity, and the pneumoperitoneum is

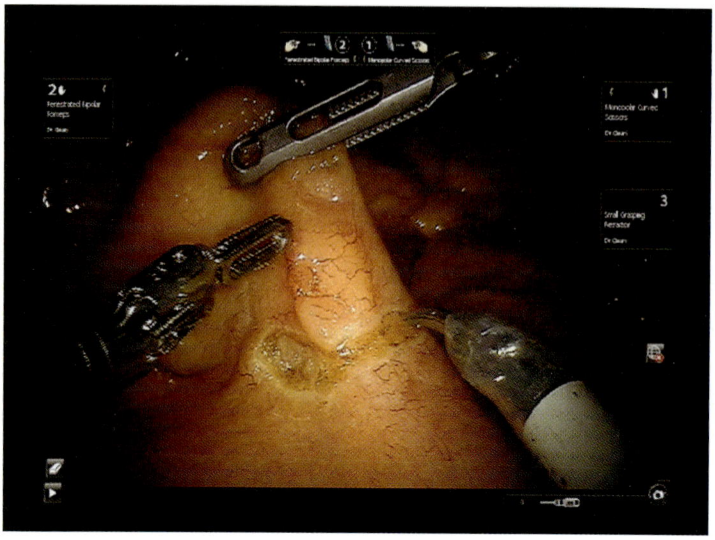

Figure 4. The third arm is ideal for retraction.

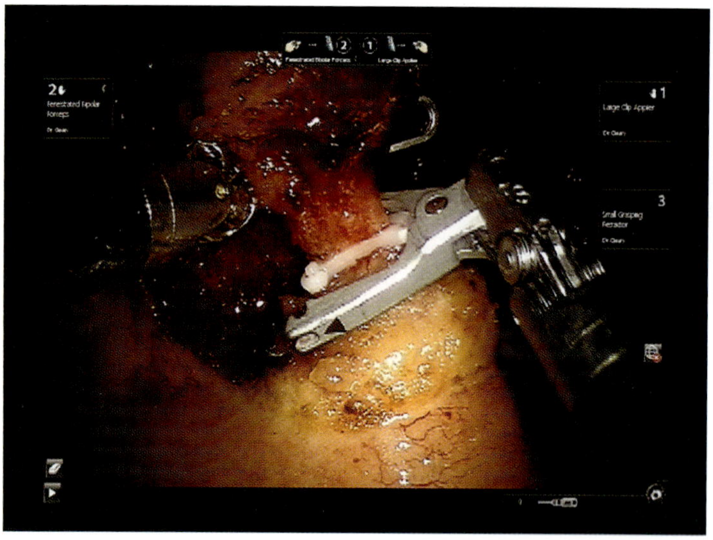

Figure 5. Wristed arm applying clip to IMA.

reestablished. Finally, the circular stapled anastomosis is performed, either under laparoscopic vision or after redocking the robot.

Low Anterior Resection. Trocar placement for LAR is variable and is based on surgeon preference. We prefer a setup similar to sigmoid resection, with an extra trocar placed in the left lower quadrant (Figure 6).

Dissection of the inferior mesenteric vessels, medial to lateral mobilization of the mesentery from the retroperitoneum, and lateral to medial dissection are performed

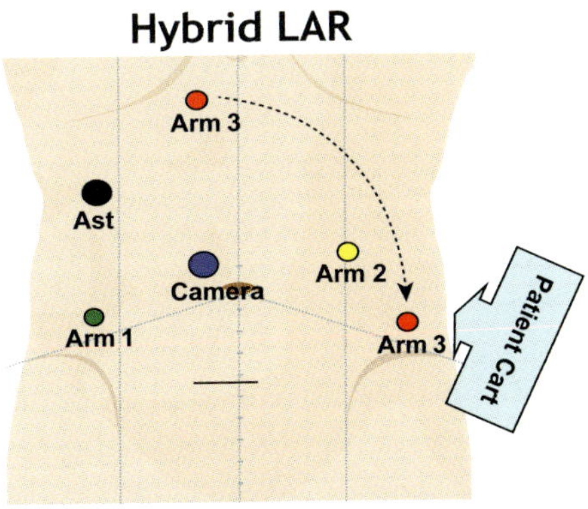

Figure 6. Diagram of a hybrid low anterior resection.

in the same fashion as for sigmoid resection. The IMA is ligated at its origin. Full mobilization of the mesentery from the retroperitoneum, to include mobilization of the splenic flexure, should be performed to ensure a tension-free anastomosis.

Following these maneuvers, when ready to start dissection in the presacral space, the subcostal da Vinci arm (D3) is rotated to the left lower quadrant. This results in a semicircular arrangement of the robotic arms directed toward the pelvis. In slender individuals, it is our preference to start the operation without the fourth left lower quadrant da Vinci trocar, as the subcostal instrument often reaches the pelvis, obviating the need for this additional port.

TME is then performed, taking care to stay in the plane between the fascia propria of the rectum and the presacral fascia. Because of the improved ability to visualize the depths of the pelvis, robotic surgery may have the greatest impact in patients with rectal cancer.[30,36] The lower rectum is divided, with a stapler placed either through a 12 mm right upper quadrant assistant port or a 13 mm right lower quadrant port, by upgrading the existing 8 mm da Vinci port at that location. After disconnecting the robotic arms from the trocars, the robot is then moved away from the patient.

A Pfannenstiel or left lower quadrant incision is then made, and a wound protector placed. The proximal end of the divided rectum is carefully retrieved through this incision, and the diseased segment is subsequently resected. A purse string suture is placed in the descending colon. A circular stapler is chosen. The anvil is placed in the open end of the descending colon, and the purse string suture is tied. The descending colon is then returned to the abdominal cavity and the pneumoperitoneum reestablished. The circular stapled anastomosis is then performed, either under laparoscopic vision or after redocking the robot. Anastomotic integrity is tested by proctoscopic air insufflation of the distal colorectum with saline in the pelvis.

Since we prefer to perform LAR without redocking the robot, it may be necessary to rotate the subcostal robotic arm (D3) to the fourth robotic trocar in the left lower quadrant prior to performing the TME.[39,55,56] Some surgeons find external robotic arm collisions to be problematic with this arrangement and prefer to mobilize the splenic flexure and left colon with the robot docked over the left shoulder. They then redock the robot between the legs for the pelvic part of the operation.[26,57]

There are many hybrid laparoscopic-robotic variations. Most involve starting the operation by conventional laparoscopic techniques, taking the inferior mesenteric vessels, mobilizing the mesentery from the retroperitoneum, mobilizing the splenic flexure, and then performing the pelvic part of the operation with the robot.[31] Park et al. described a reverse-hybrid technique for rectal cancer, whereby the IMA is ligated at its origin, the sigmoid colon is mobilized from the retroperitoneum, and TME is then performed.[58] This is all done with the robot docked between the legs and is followed by laparoscopic dissection of the descending colon, splenic flexure mobilization, and construction of the anastomosis.

Abdominoperineal Resection. The robot offers a distinct advantage over laparoscopic dissection for LAR and for this procedure. Because of the strategic position of the robotic camera on a stable platform with less lens soiling, the pelvic structures can be more clearly visualized. The nervi erigentes, which provide the parasympathetic innervation to the bladder and sexual organs, may be better visualized and preserved, potentially leading to fewer occurrences of postoperative sexual dysfunction. The levator muscles may be better visualized and divided after mobilizing the rectum through the abdominal approach, allowing for a cylindrical specimen to be obtained that may decrease the incidence of local recurrence in cases of rectal cancer. Trocar placement, dissection of the inferior mesenteric vessels, mobilization of the mesentery from the retroperitoneum, and lateral to medial dissection are analogous to robotic LAR.

The splenic flexure may not require mobilization. After division of the levator muscles, and after dividing the descending colon at the site marked for the end stoma, a perineal incision is made through which the specimen is retrieved. The perineal wound is then closed. The end of the descending colon is brought through the abdominal wall at the previously chosen stoma site, and the end colostomy matured per surgeon preference.

We prefer to start this operation with a perineal incision, with the patient in the prone jack-knife position. Much of the operation is performed using this perineal approach, including division of the anococcygeal ligament and levator muscles and mobilization of the rectum between the fascia propria of the rectum and presacral fascia. These maneuvers provide a cylindrical specimen that has not been coned down at the anorectal waist. After performing as much dissection as possible through this perineal approach, the resulting wound is closed. If small enough, the specimen can be retrieved through the stoma incision with a wound protector in place. Alternatively, the specimen can be retrieved through the perineal wound, or through a separate Pfannenstiel incision, depending on the patient's body habitus and the surgeon's personal preference and comfort level.

Resection Rectopexy for Rectal Prolapse. For patients with full thickness rectal prolapse, rectopexy with or without sigmoid resection is the most commonly employed procedure. Patients with a history of constipation may be offered a concomitant sigmoid resection, and in very rare cases of patients with colonic inertia, a subtotal colectomy and ileorectal anastomosis may be considered. Patients without a history of constipation are usually offered rectopexy without sigmoid resection. During this operation, the rectum is fully mobilized to the levators posteriorly between the fascia propria of the rectum and presacral fascia. Literature to date is controversial regarding lateral and anterior mobilization. As a result, this decision is based on surgeon preference and interpretation of existing data.

For trocar placement we prefer the same arrangement as that used for LAR (Figure 7). Similarly, the fourth left lower quadrant da Vinci trocar may not be necessary in aesthenic individuals. Pelvic mobilization of the rectum is usually performed prior

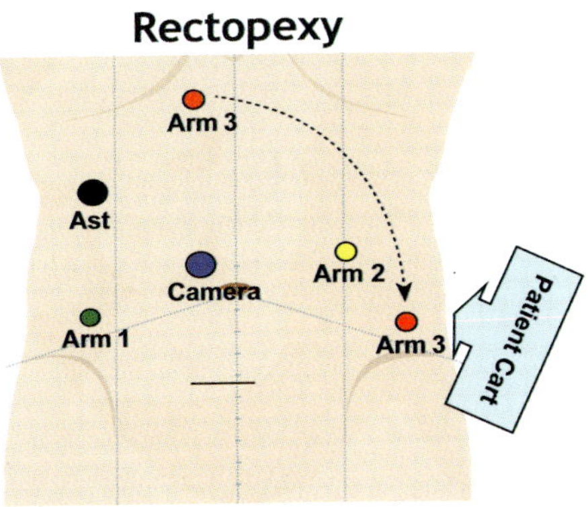

Figure 7. Diagram of a rectopexy.

to sigmoid resection. Because these patients are typically women and have standard features of prolapse (deep cul-de-sac, increased space between mesorectum and presacral fascia), this part of the operation may be technically facile. If a sigmoid resection is performed, it is done as described above. The rectopexy is done with nonabsorbable sutures, thereby fixing the mesorectum and peritoneum to the presacral fascia near the sacral promontory. Robotic suturing is typically a straightforward maneuver compared to the laparoscopic version, due to the wristed movements afforded by the dedicated robotic instruments.

Conclusion

Robotic surgical systems in colon and rectal surgery have tremendous potential to advance operative techniques and improve patient outcomes. At this time, the feasibility and safety of robotic colon and rectal surgery have been demonstrated in several smaller studies. Larger randomized controlled trials are in progress. These may more definitively confirm the improved outcomes compared to conventional or hand-assisted laparoscopic surgery as demonstrated in the smaller studies. The greatest beneficial impact of robotic surgery is likely to be in pelvic operations, where laparoscopic visualization and assistance are particularly challenging, and where robotic surgery systems allow for superior visualization and more precise dissection. The robot may also be ideal for single port surgery, where space at the operating table is at a premium and camera control is difficult to maintain (Figure 8).

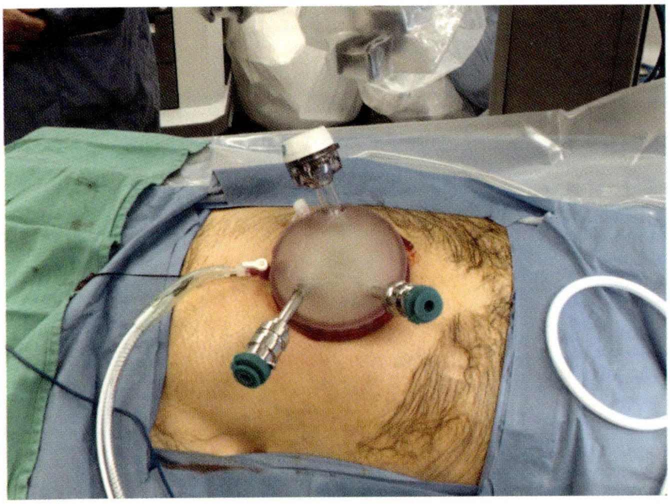

Figure 8. Setup for single port colectomy.

References

1. Graney MJ, Graney CM. Colorectal surgery from antiquity to the modern era. *Dis Colon Rectum.* 1980;23:432–41.

2. Semm K. Endoscopic appendectomy. *Endoscopy.* 1983;15:59–64.

3. Muhe E. [Laparoscopic cholecystectomy]. *Zeitschrift fur Gastroenterologie Verhandlungsband.* 1991;26:204–6.

4. Reynolds W Jr. The first laparoscopic cholecystectomy. *JSLS.* 2001;5:89–94.

5. Jacobs M, Verdeja JC, Goldstein HS. Minimally invasive colon resection (laparoscopic colectomy). *Surg Laparosc Endosc.* 1991;1:144–50.

6. Kennedy GD, Heise C, Rajamanickam V, Harms B, Foley EF. Laparoscopy decreases postoperative complication rates after abdominal colectomy: results from the national surgical quality improvement program. *Ann Surg.* 2009;249:596–601.

7. Fox J, Gross CP, Longo W, Reddy V. Laparoscopic colectomy for the treatment of cancer has been widely adopted in the United States. *Dis Colon Rectum.* 2012;55:501–8.

8. Nelson H, Sargent D, Wieland H; The Clinical Outcomes of Surgical Therapy Study Group. A comparison of laparoscopically assisted and open colectomy for colon cancer. *N Engl J Med.* 2004;350:2050–2059.

9. Fleshman J, Sargent DJ, Green E, et al. Laparoscopic colectomy for cancer is not inferior to open surgery based on 5-year data from the COST Study Group trial. *Ann Surg.* 2007;246:655–62; discussion 62–4.

10. Bonjer HJ, Hop WC, Nelson H, et al. Laparoscopically assisted vs. open colectomy for colon cancer: a meta-analysis. *Arch Surg.* 2007;142:298–303.

11. Colon Cancer Lapraoscopic or Open Resection Study Group; Buunen M, Veldkamp R, Hop WC, et al. Survival after laparoscopic surgery versus open surgery for colon cancer: long-term outcome of a randomised clinical trial. *Lancet Oncol.* 2009;10:44–52.

12. Delaney CP, Marcello PW, Sonoda T, Wise P, Bauer J, Techner L. Gastrointestinal recovery after laparoscopic colectomy: results of a prospective, observational, multicenter study. *Surg Endosc.* 2010;24:653–61.

13. Franklin ME, Kazantsev GB, Abrego D, Diaz EJ, Balli J, Glass JL. Laparoscopic surgery for stage III colon cancer: long-term follow-up. *Surg Endosc.* 2000;14:612–6.

14. Guillou PJ, Quirke P, Thorpe H, et al. Short-term endpoints of conventional versus laparoscopic-assisted surgery in patients with colorectal cancer (MRC CLASICC trial): multicentre, randomised controlled trial. *Lancet.* 2005;365:1718–26.

15. Hewett PJ, Allardyce RA, Bagshaw PF, et al. Short-term outcomes of the Australasian randomized clinical study comparing laparoscopic and conventional open surgical treatments for colon cancer: the ALCCaS trial. *Ann Surg.* 2008;248:728–38.

16. Jayne DG, Guillou PJ, Thorpe H, et al. Randomized trial of laparoscopic-assisted resection of colorectal carcinoma: 3-year results of the UK MRC CLASICC Trial Group. *J Clin Oncol.* 2007;25:3061–8.

17. Lacy AM, Garcia-Valdecasas JC, Delgado S, et al. Laparoscopy-assisted colectomy versus open colectomy for treatment of non-metastatic colon cancer: a randomised trial. *Lancet.* 2002;359:2224–9.

18. Milsom JW, Bohm B, Hammerhofer KA, Fazio V, Steiger E, Elson P. A prospective, randomized trial comparing laparoscopic versus conventional techniques in colorectal cancer surgery: a preliminary report. *J Am Coll Surg.* 1998;187:46–54; discussion 54–55.

19. Ramos JM, Beart RW Jr, Goes R, Ortega AE, Schlinkert RT. Role of laparoscopy in colorectal surgery. A prospective evaluation of 200 cases. *Dis Colon Rectum.* 1995; 38:494–501.

20. Schwenk W, Bohm B, Muller JM. Postoperative pain and fatigue after laparoscopic or conventional colorectal resections. A prospective randomized trial. *Surg Endosc.* 1998; 12:1131–6.

21. Senagore AJ, Luchtefeld MA, Mackeigan JM, Mazier WP. Open colectomy versus laparoscopic colectomy: are there differences? *Am Surg.* 1993;59:549–53; discussion 53–4.

22. Veldkamp R, Kuhry E, Hop WC, et al. Laparoscopic surgery versus open surgery for colon cancer: short-term outcomes of a randomised trial. *Lancet Oncol.* 2005;6:477–84.

23. Weber PA, Merola S, Wasielewski A, Ballantyne GH. Telerobotic-assisted laparoscopic right and sigmoid colectomies for benign disease. *Dis Colon Rectum.* 2002;45:1689–94; discussion 95–6.

24. Antoniou SA, Antoniou GA, Koch OO, Pointner R, Granderath FA. Robot assisted laparoscopic surgery of the colon and rectum. *Surg Endosc.* 2012;26:1–11.

25. Pigazzi A, Luca F, Patriti A, et al. Multicentric study on robotic tumor-specific mesorectal excision for the treatment of rectal cancer. *Ann Surg Oncol.* 2010;17:1614–20.

26. Kwon DS, Chang GJ. The role of minimally invasive surgery and outcomes in colorectal cancer. *Perm J.* 2011;15:61–6.

27. Pigazzi A, Ellenhorn JD, Ballantyne GH, Paz IB. Robotic-assisted laparoscopic low anterior resection with total mesorectal excision for rectal cancer. *Surg Endosc.* 2006; 20:1521–5.

28. Huettner F, Pacheco PE, Doubet JL, Ryan MJ, Dynda DI, Crawford DL. One hundred and two consecutive robotic-assisted minimally invasive colectomies—an outcome and technical update. *J Gastrointest Surg.* 2011;15:1195–204.

29. Spinoglio G, Summa M, Priora F, Quarati R, Testa S. Robotic colorectal surgery: first 50 cases experience. *Dis Colon Rectum.* 2008;51:1627–32.

30. Baik SH, Kwon HY, Kim JS, et al. Robotic versus laparoscopic low anterior resection of rectal cancer: short-term outcome of a prospective comparative study. *Ann Surg Oncol.* 2009;16:1480–7.

31. Patel CB, Ragupathi M, Ramos-Valadez DI, Haas EM. A three-arm (laparoscopic, hand-assisted, and robotic) matched-case analysis of intraoperative and postoperative outcomes in minimally invasive colorectal surgery. *Dis Colon Rectum.* 2011;54:144–50.

32. Baik SH, Ko YT, Kang CM, et al. Robotic tumor-specific mesorectal excision of rectal cancer: short-term outcome of a pilot randomized trial. *Surg Endosc.* 2008;22:1601–8.

33. Leong QM, Kim SH. Robot-assisted rectal surgery for malignancy: a review of current literature. *Ann Acad Med Singapore.* 2011;40:460–6.

34. Luca F, Cenciarelli S, Valvo M, et al. Full robotic left colon and rectal cancer resection: technique and early outcome. *Ann Surg Oncol.* 2009;16:1274–8.

35. Patriti A, Ceccarelli G, Bartoli A, Spaziani A, Biancafarina A, Casciola L. Short- and medium-term outcome of robot-assisted and traditional laparoscopic rectal resection. *JSLS.* 2009;13:176–83.

36. Bianchi PP, Ceriani C, Locatelli A, et al. Robotic versus laparoscopic total mesorectal excision for rectal cancer: a comparative analysis of oncological safety and short-term outcomes. *Surg Endosc.* 2010;24:2888–94.

37. Kwak JM, Kim SH, Kim J, Son DN, Baek SJ, Cho JS. Robotic vs laparoscopic resection of rectal cancer: short-term outcomes of a case-control study. *Dis Colon Rectum.* 2011;54:151–6.

38. Park JS, Choi GS, Lim KH, Jang YS, Jun SH. S052: a comparison of robot-assisted, laparoscopic, and open surgery in the treatment of rectal cancer. *Surg Endosc.* 2011;25:240–8.

39. Hellan M, Stein H, Pigazzi A. Totally robotic low anterior resection with total mesorectal excision and splenic flexure mobilization. *Surg Endosc.* 2009;23:447–51.

40. Hellan M, Anderson C, Ellenhorn JD, Paz B, Pigazzi A. Short-term outcomes after robotic-assisted total mesorectal excision for rectal cancer. *Ann Surg Oncol.* 2007; 14:3168–73.

41. Baek JH, McKenzie S, Garcia-Aguilar J, Pigazzi A. Oncologic outcomes of robotic-assisted total mesorectal excision for the treatment of rectal cancer. *Ann Surg.* 2010; 251:882–6.

42. deSouza AL, Prasad LM, Marecik SJ, et al. Total mesorectal excision for rectal cancer: the potential advantage of robotic assistance. *Dis Colon Rectum.* 2010;53:1611–7.

43. Collinson FJ, Jayne DG, Pigazzi A, et al. An international, multicentre, prospective, randomised, controlled, unblinded, parallel-group trial of robotic-assisted versus standard laparoscopic surgery for the curative treatment of rectal cancer. *Int J Colorectal Dis.* 2012;27:233–41.

44. Deutsch GB, Sathyanarayana SA, Gunabushanam V, et al. Robotic vs. laparoscopic colorectal surgery: an institutional experience. *Surg Endosc.* 2012;26:956–63.

45. Kanji A, Gill RS, Shi X, Birch DW, Karmali S. Robotic-assisted colon and rectal surgery: a systematic review. *Int J Med Robot.* 2011;7:401–7.

46. Turchetti G, Palla I, Pierotti F, Cuschieri A. Economic evaluation of da Vinci-assisted robotic surgery: a systematic review. *Surg Endosc.* 2012;26:598–606.

47. Klarenbeek BR, Coupe VM, van der Peet DL, Cuesta MA. The cost effectiveness of elective laparoscopic sigmoid resection for symptomatic diverticular disease: financial outcome of the randomized control Sigma trial. *Surg Endosc.* 2011;25:776–83.

48. Senagore AJ, Duepree HJ, Delaney CP, Dissanaike S, Brady KM, Fazio VW. Cost structure of laparoscopic and open sigmoid colectomy for diverticular disease: similarities and differences. *Dis Colon Rectum.* 2002;45:485–90.

49. Bertani E, Chiappa A, Biffi R, et al. Assessing appropriateness for elective colorectal cancer surgery: clinical, oncological, and quality-of-life short-term outcomes employing different treatment approaches. *Int J Colorectal Dis.* 2011;26:1317–27.

50. Chang GJ, Kaiser AM, Mills S, Rafferty JF, Buie WD. Practice parameters for the management of colon cancer. *Dis Colon Rectum.* 2012;55:831–43.

51. O'Connell JB, Maggard MA, Ko CY. Colon cancer survival rates with the new American Joint Committee on Cancer sixth edition staging. *J Natl Cancer Inst.* 2004; 96:1420–5.

52. Heald RJ, Moran BJ, Ryall RD, Sexton R, MacFarlane JK. Rectal cancer: the Basingstoke experience of total mesorectal excision, 1978–1997. *Arch Surg.* 1998;133:894–9.

53. Joseph RA, Goh AC, Cuevas SP, et al. "Chopstick" surgery: a novel technique improves surgeon performance and eliminates arm collision in robotic single-incision laparoscopic surgery. *Surg Endosc.* 2010;24:1331–5.

54. Singh J, Podolsky ER, Castellanos AE, Stein DE. Optimizing single port surgery: a case report and review of technique in colon resection. *Int J Med Robot.* 2011;7:127–30.

55. Choi DJ, Kim SH, Lee PJ, Kim J, Woo SU. Single-stage totally robotic dissection for rectal cancer surgery: technique and short-term outcome in 50 consecutive patients. *Dis Colon Rectum.* 2009;52:1824–30.

56. Koh DC, Tsang CB, Kim SH. A new application of the four-arm standard da Vinci® surgical system: totally robotic-assisted left-sided colon or rectal resection. *Surg Endosc.* 2011;25:1945–52.

57. Zimmern A, Prasad L, Desouza A, Marecik S, Park J, Abcarian H. Robotic colon and rectal surgery: a series of 131 cases. *World J Surg*. 2010;34:1954–8.

58. Park IJ, You YN, Schlette E, et al. Reverse-hybrid robotic mesorectal excision for rectal cancer. *Dis Colon Rectum*. 2012;55:228–33.

Chapter Twelve

Fibroid Surgery

Rajiv J. Deenadayalu, MD; Brandy N. Michaels, MD; JoLyn M. Seitz, MD

Surgical Approach

Once the decision has been made to proceed with surgical intervention via an abdominal approach, the surgeon must carefully assess whether the appropriate method of procedure is via laparoscopy or laparotomy. Many factors can play a role in this decision-making process, including the size and location of the fibroids, the size of the patient, and the patient's previous surgical history.

Equally important is the comfort level of the surgeon with a laparoscopic approach. The learning curve is much steeper with this method and that can lead to a laparotomy as the default choice. Traditionally, laparoscopic myomectomy posed certain challenges, such as difficulty with dissecting the plane between fibroid and myometrium, enucleation of the fibroid body, and difficulty with effective suturing techniques to close the cavity left by the evacuated fibroid. In addition, the linear, unidirectional instrument movements, combined with a two-dimensional image, made this option less desirable.

With the introduction of the robotic platform into gynecologic surgery, laparoscopic myomectomy became much more feasible. Some of the advantages with robotic myomectomy include enhanced visualization with the InSite Vision System (Intuitive Surgical), which provides true three-dimensional viewing through a 12-mm binocular camera. More recent improvements in technology have allowed for the creation of smaller camera sizes. Robotic instrumentation also offers improved mobility and dexterity, allowing for much more precise dissection and suturing capability. The manipulation offered by the 7 degrees of movement of the tips of the robotic instrument allows for replication of the full range of motion of the surgeon's hands, all while being controlled from the surgical console. As such, patients with fibroids previously thought too difficult to approach laparoscopically can be ideal candidates, putting both the surgeon and the patient more at ease.

From an ergonomic perspective, the comfort of being seated at a console that can be adjusted to custom fit the surgeon's preferences has distinct advantages over traditional laparoscopic surgery, which requires constant attention to keeping the camera steady. Avoiding the unnatural positioning of the surgeon's arms and back that is sometimes required to reach certain intra-abdominal locations during traditional laparoscopic surgery is also a benefit enjoyed with robotic surgery (Figure 1).

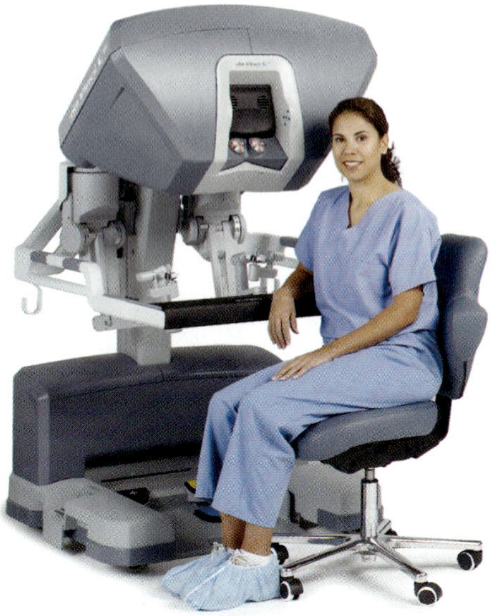

Figure 1. Surgeon seated at the da Vinci console. Credit: © 2013 Intuitive Surgical, Inc.

Operative Setup

When initially introduced, the robotic setup was viewed as time consuming and cumbersome. As newer, smaller, more easily moveable models have evolved, the time required from room entry to beginning the operation has decreased. Particular attention should be paid to the steps involved in surgical setup and patient positioning, as the prudent surgeon will develop a system that can be reproduced from case to case.

The patient is wheeled into the operating room, and after all the appropriate consents and time-outs have been reviewed, a general anesthetic is induced and a prophylactic antibiotic is usually administered. At this point, the surgical team prepares the patient by positioning the arms and legs. Typically, Allen stirrups are used to maneuver the legs in a dorsal lithotomy position, with careful attention paid to the heels resting comfortably in the boots of the stirrups. There should be no compression on the fibular head in order to avoid peroneal nerve injury. The surgeon should be able to place a finger with ease between the top of the boot and the patient's gastrocnemius muscle.

A number of appropriate means are available to secure the arms of the patient laterally along the side of the body. Before the creation of vacuum devices such as the Hug-u-Vac, the simple application of egg-crate foam around the ventral and dorsal surfaces of the forearm served to protect the elbow and wrists from unnecessary tension or compression during surgery. A draw sheet placed on the OR table prior to moving the patient from her preoperative stretcher also allows the surgeon to wrap the sheet around the patient's arms and surrounding egg-crate

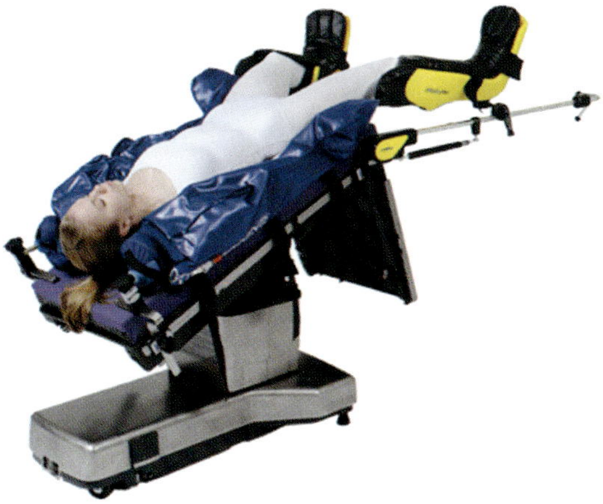

Figure 2: Patient positioned on OR table using Hug-u-Vac system.

foam, thereby allowing an additional layer of security to prevent the arms from abduction during surgery.

The Hug-u-Vac system also allows for secure positioning of the patient's arms once the air is removed from the device, thereby allowing it to harden and mold around the patient laterally. It is generally felt that some protection, such as the egg-crate foam or simply a towel around the lateral aspect of the patient's arm, is needed to buffer against the firmness of the Hug-u-Vac. After arm positioning is complete, it is imperative that the surgeon assesses the intravenous (IV) line to verify the line is flowing smoothly. Improper positioning of the arm can affect the patency of the IV, something that should be discovered prior to starting the operation (Figure 2).

Securing the shoulders can also be accomplished with either method. If the egg-crate foam is used, the surgeon tapes the foam in place along the bottom of the side of the OR table, and then the foam is placed across the chest to the opposite shoulder, thereby forming an "X" across the patient's upper chest. Both sides of the foam are taped to the OR table, which keeps the patient stable despite the steep Trendelenburg that is necessary for robotic surgery.

Similarly, the Hug-u-Vac can also be molded around the patient's shoulders to provide stabilization for OR table positioning. It is often useful to place a towel or foam around the shoulders for the same reasons mentioned earlier.

Once the surgeon is satisfied that the arms and legs are secure, there are no pressure points on any of the extremities, and the IV line is flowing without difficulty, it is time to test the patient's tolerance of steep Trendelenburg. If the patient has been secured properly, there will be little movement (if any) cephalad as the head of the bed is tilted to its maximal position. Once this has been tested, there is very little likelihood that the patient will move up the table once the robot is docked.

Vaginal Instrumentation

Once the patient has been prepped and draped, an exam under anesthesia (EUA) is performed to assess the size and mobility of the uterus and the location of the fibroids. The exam performed on a patient under general anesthesia provides a true assessment of pelvic pathology and allows the surgeon a much clearer mental picture of the pelvic anatomy about to be encountered. Once the EUA is completed, a bivalve speculum is placed vaginally and a single tooth tenaculum can be used to grasp the anterior lip of the cervix, allowing the surgeon to sound the uterus and dilate the cervix to place a uterine manipulator.

There are a number of different manipulators from which to choose. Typically the selection of one over another is due to surgeon preference. The key to any device is its utility in allowing the surgeon to elevate and rotate the uterus in all directions to better assess the size and location of the fibroid(s) and also to allow for the optimal angles to suture the cavity once the fibroid is removed. Once the uterine manipulator is in place, the remaining vaginal instruments are removed and a Foley catheter is placed for accurate recording of urine output during the case.

The KOH ring, which is paramount in a laparoscopic hysterectomy, does not need to be placed during a myomectomy unless the patient and surgeon are in agreement that an unsuccessful myomectomy would likely result in a hysterectomy during the same procedure. The selection and placement of the KOH ring are reviewed in chapter 13 covering setup for a hysterectomy.

Abdominal Instrumentation

Once the vaginal setup is complete, attention is turned to the patient's abdomen. The patient is taken out of any Trendelenburg that may have been required for vaginal instrumentation, and the umbilical skin is elevated. Typically, the Veress needle is inserted after a small incision is made centrally in the umbilicus. It is helpful to utilize local anesthetic prior to any skin incisions being made, as this often can help mark the location of the skin incision as well as to provide some additional level of pain relief postoperatively. Careful preoperative review of the patient's previous surgical history may alter the approach to primary entry into the abdomen, but for the purposes of this chapter, the assumption is made that the patient's past history would not necessitate deviation from the standard approach.

Once adequate pneumoperitoneum has been achieved, the supraumbilical incision is made. A good rule to follow allows for a hands-breadth (approx. 10–12 cm) above the highest level of the fundus of the uterus when it is maximally elevated with the uterine manipulator. This can help identify the proposed location of the supraumbilical incision, and the surgeon must safeguard from any uncertainty in thinking that the incision may be too cephalad. If possible, it is always better to err on the side of being too high with the supraumbilical incision rather than being too close to the umbilicus.

Once the supraumbilical or camera trocar has been inserted, the da Vinci camera is then passed through the trocar and an initial inspection is performed to assess for any injuries from trocar entry. Elevation of the uterus via the uterine manipulator will allow the surgeon to identify the exact location of the fibroid(s) and can help in planning the approach to myomectomy.

The placement of the additional da Vinci trocars will vary from surgeon to surgeon. In general, they are placed approximately 10–12 cm lateral and 2 cm down from the level of the supraumbilical trocar placement. A good rule of thumb is the right and left da Vinci trocars, once placed, are located at approximately the level of the umbilicus. The auxiliary port is typically placed on the right side between the right da Vinci arm and the camera trocar, forming the equidistant apex of a triangle that would connect the three instruments (Figure 3). Alternately, the auxiliary

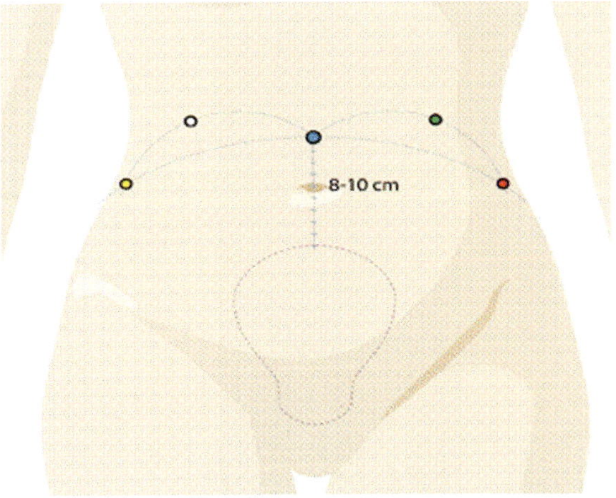

Figure 3. Da Vinci trocar placement.
Credit: © 2013 Intuitive Surgical, Inc.

port, either a 5 mm or 10 mm sized trocar, can be placed on the left side at the discretion of the surgeon as indicated in the figure.

The use of the third arm can be crucial to the success of both myomectomy and hysterectomy, allowing the surgeon much better exposure without compromising the distribution of the trocars in the abdomen. If the third robotic arm is to be utilized, the surgeon will generally place the left-sided da Vinci trocar just 10–12 cm (and not the additional 2 cm inferior to the level of the camera trocar) lateral to the supraumbilical trocar. The trocar for the third arm is then inserted in a location that is approximately 5 cm superior to the left anterior superior iliac spine.

Once the trocar placement has been completed, the circulating nurse is ready to wheel the robot into place. The surgeon directs the orientation of robotic docking, and the machine can either be driven to a location between the legs of the patient or, more commonly, come in at a side angle (also known as side docking) with the left base leg of the robot located directly adjacent to the inner aspect of the left base of the operating table.

There are many advantages afforded by a decision to utilize a side docking methodology. Access to the patient vaginally is maximized and can aid in manipulation of the uterus with either a hysterectomy or myomectomy. More importantly, there is greater flexibility in regard to ease of robotic arm docking as well as maneuverability with the robotic arms, especially if the third arm is utilized. Prior to docking the robot, the patient is placed in steep Trendelenburg and the docking is finalized. This provides another opportunity for the surgeon to make sure the patient is secure on the operating room table. Once the robotic arms are docked, the instruments are placed through the trocars and the surgeon is ready to start the operation.

Operative Technique

One of the theories about why fibroids grow in size is that they are parasitic in nature and thereby feed off of the adjacent vessels that supply blood to the uterine musculature. Since there is no effective way to slow blood flow to the uterus during a laparoscopic myomectomy, vasopressive agents can be utilized to assist in controlling blood loss as the dissection plane of the fibroid is identified.

The use of vasopressin should be discussed with your anesthesia colleagues to make sure the patient has no contraindications for use. To minimize the cardiac side effects of this medication, a dilution of 20 units of vasopressin in 100 mL of

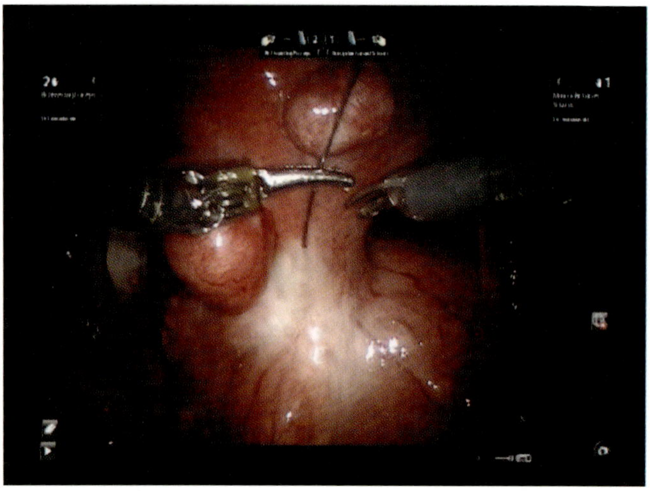

Figure 4. Vasopressin injection via spinal needle passed through the abdominal wall into the surface of the fibroid. Note the blanching effect of the vasopressin.

saline is utilized and is generally well tolerated by our young, healthy patient population. The bedside assistant places a 22-gauge, seven-inch spinal needle directly through the abdominal wall. The entry point of needle insertion can be determined by where the fibroid is located when maximal uterine elevation is achieved via the uterine manipulator. Once the optimal site of entry is determined for the injection, the operating surgeon can grasp the tip of the needle with one of the robotic instruments and then guide placement of the spinal needle (Figure 4).

Depending on the body habitus of the patient and location of the fibroids in question, introduction of the spinal needle through the abdominal wall can sometimes prove to be challenging. The operating surgeon can determine the introduction point of spinal needle insertion based on where the fibroid is located once the uterus is elevated.

Once this location has been determined, the surgeon can carefully place the tip of the needle under the uterine serosa and the bedside assistant can then inject the diluted vasopressin solution directly into the line of the planned dissection plane and the surrounding tissue. Immediate blanching of the surface of the serosa is observed, and a wheal is created indicating appropriate vasoconstriction as well as appropriate depth of injection.

The monopolar scissors are a very effective tool for creating the initial dissection plane. Once this linear incision has been made into the uterine serosa directly overlying the fibroid, the robotic Gyrus instrument can be utilized to dissect the fibroid plane. The bedside assistant can aid in traction of the fibroid by grasping it with a single tooth tenaculum that can be passed through the 10 mm auxiliary port. This facilitates easier dissection of the fibroid-uterine junction, and elevation of the fibroid can also allow for identification of vasculature that can be cauterized prior to transection. This technique allows for effective enucleation of the fibroid body, facilitating an easier dissection.

Once the fibroid has been dissected out, it is typically placed in the posterior cul-de-sac until morcellation can be undertaken. When there are multiple myomas to be removed, the surgeon has to decide whether to suture the fibroid cavity first rather than enucleating additional fibroids. Because the base of the evacuated fibroid does not achieve effective hemostasis due to lack of penetration of the initial injection of the vasopressin, the surgeon must diligently and expeditiously undertake closure of the fibroid cavity if bleeding is identified. At that point, additional fibroids can be resected.

There are various methods of closure that can be used. Surgeon comfort and preference generally guide the choice of method for type of closure. The goal in closing the uterine defect left by the extirpated fibroid should be to bring the myometrial tissue planes together as symmetrically as possible. A multilayer closure is generally thought to achieve the best closure mimicking what is done at the time of an open myomectomy.

This closure can be accomplished successfully by the use of interrupted figure-of-eight sutures of 0-polyglactin on a CT-2 needle. As mentioned earlier, a double layer closure typically results in effective hemostasis and, because individual sutures are placed, the cavity is more closely approximated. The serosal layer is typically closed with a running baseball stitch of 3-0 polyglactin on an SH needle.

Although this method of closure is extremely effective in closing the space left by the fibroid as well as achieving excellent hemostasis, the major drawback involves the difficult learning curve that may be present in trying to become proficient in intracorporeal knot tying, even with the enhanced mobility afforded by the robotic platform. The length of time spent in the OR, combined with the additional costs of a lengthened case, has been described as a detriment to the laparoscopic approach. Once the surgeon is proficient in suturing techniques, closure can be performed efficiently with little increase in operative morbidity to the patient.

More recently, the use of a barbed suture has been introduced into gynecologic surgical procedures. The obvious advantage to the use of a unidirectional barbed suture is that it overcomes the time necessary to become proficient in tying of intracorporeal knots. This reduces the time required for cavity closure and also decreases the time spent under general anesthesia. Alessandri et al. performed a randomized trial comparing unidirectional barbed suture closure with a continuous suture and concluded that the barbed sutures reduced the time required to close the uterine wall defect as well as decreasing intraoperative blood loss.[1]

One of the disadvantages of this approach is that a surgeon may become too dependent on the barbed suture, thereby allowing the skills required for individual knot tying to erode. In addition, if the surgeon is not happy with a particular suture placement, there is no way to release the previous stitch. The surgeon is then either forced to cut the suture and re-start or find a way to correct the problem created by the original placement. While a barbed suture can be utilized for myometrial closure, it has been theorized that the barbs, when exposed on a serosal closure, could be potential sites for adhesion formation. Therefore, it is generally recommended to avoid this type of suture for closure of the uterine serosa.

Once effective uterine closure is performed, morcellation of the myoma is ready to be undertaken. Morcellation of a fibroid allows the surgeon to cut the fibroid into thin, tube-like pieces that can then be removed through the morcellating trocar. The surgeon must be fastidious in visualizing the rotating cutting tip of the morcellator at all times and also must make every attempt to remove as many of the fibroid fragments as possible.

Postoperative Management

One of the obvious advantages to laparoscopic myomectomy is the shortened length of stay and quicker return to normal activity experienced by patients postoperatively compared to abdominal myomectomy. The smaller laparoscopic incisions allow for increased activity after surgery, quicker transition to oral narcotics, and, until adequate per oral (PO) intake can be achieved, patients often require nothing more than intermittent doses of parenteral narcotics. They typically are started on a regular diet on the evening of the surgery or on postoperative day one and most often are discharged within 24–36 hours from the initial surgery.

Febrile morbidity associated with myomectomy is common. The elevation in temperature is rarely infectious in origin but rather related to accumulation of blood in the resection site, as well as the tissue inflammatory mediators related to being immediately postoperative. The use of postsurgical antibiotic prophylaxis is not recommended unless there is a specific concern for development of postoperative infection.

Adhesion Formation

One of the most significant morbidities associated with myomectomy is the formation of postoperative adhesions, estimated to be 30–40%.[2] These adhesions can form at the site of fibroid resection and subsequent suturing and can involve the omentum, bladder, adnexa, or intestinal organs. Various studies have looked at the number of fibroids removed, the locations of the fibroids, and the appearance of the wound post-repair as independent risk factors for adhesion formation.

A surgeon operating subsequent to the initial myomectomy may encounter adhesions that can significantly increase the complexity of the case and can sometimes require the assistance of a general surgeon. As there are often multiple fibroids that may need myomectomy, the wound status left from myometrial cavity closure and suturing might influence the development of postoperative adhesions despite the use of adhesion-preventing agents.[3]

Different methods of adhesion prevention have been employed, with two of the more common agents being the oxidized regenerated cellulose (Gynecare Interceed, Ethicon, Inc., Somerville, NJ, USA) and a bio-resorbable adhesion barrier composed of hyaluronic acid and carboxymethylcellulose (Seprafilm, Genzyme Corp.).

Many authors have looked at the use of adhesion barriers aimed primarily at reducing the potential for postoperative adhesion formation. Kumakiri et al. investigated 108 patients who underwent second-look laparoscopy after an initial laparoscopic myomectomy to assess the formation of postoperative adhesion formation.

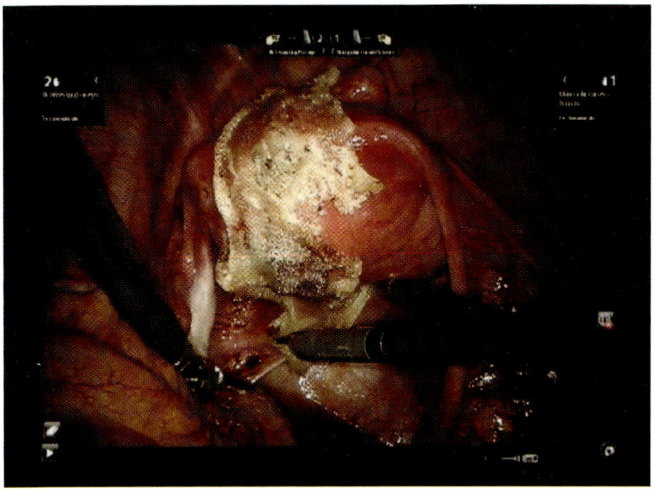

Figure 5. Placement of an adhesion barrier over the myomectomy site.

They found that the diameter of the largest enucleated myoma, the number of enucleated myomas, and the number of suture layers were significantly higher in wounds with protrusion. Furthermore, the condition of the wound (protruding similar to that found in a subserosal wound repair) that had been formed at the initial surgery was closely associated with adhesion formation.[3]

The choice of one adhesion barrier over the other is generally related to surgeon preference, and both are easy to apply. Interceed is directly placed over the site of surgical wound closure and is moistened for better contact on the tissue surface (Figure 5).

Seprafilm is typically cut into thin strips and must be mixed with saline early in the operation so that it has sufficient time to form into a gel-like solution that can then be directly applied to the wound. This direct application of this adhesion barrier to the fibroid bed is accomplished via a red Robinson catheter introduced directly into the abdomen through the accessory port (Figure 6).

The bedside assistant fills a 60 cc syringe and attaches it to the end of the catheter, and with gentle pressure the Seprafilm "slurry" can be placed over the fresh wound site. Because of its viscosity, the film solution has a tendency to adhere to the myomectomy site, which is one of the theories as to why it can be effective in helping to reduce postoperative adhesions. As you can see in Figure 6, the uterus is elevated, and the Seprafilm does have a tendency to collect in the posterior cul-de-sac, which is the location of the uterus in its natural state, thereby bathing the back of the uterine surface in this image in the accumulated Seprafilm for additional adhesion reduction.

Pregnancy after Myomectomy

Myomectomy is often performed for the preservation of the uterus for future childbearing. The presence of fibroids is felt to contribute to pelvic pressure, pain,

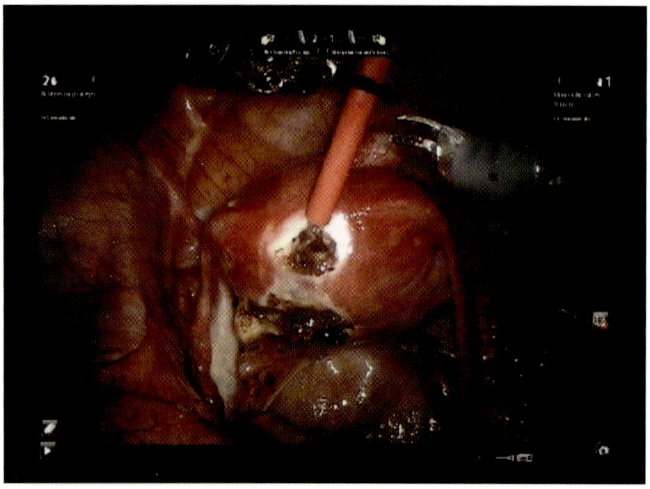

Figure 6. Seprafilm slurry placed through a red Robinson catheter over suture line to decrease adhesion formation.

discomfort with intercourse, and also bleeding disorders. In addition, the fibroids themselves may be a primary factor in a woman's inability to spontaneously conceive. Since fibroids are estimated to exist in 20–30% of all reproductive-aged women, these smooth muscular growths can impact a significant number of patients.

It has long been thought that the size of the enucleated fibroid as well as the locations of the myomectomy incision contributes to the potential for uterine rupture with a subsequent pregnancy. Although uterine rupture is a rare event in patients with a previous myomectomy, the exact rate of occurrence is unknown. Independent risk factors proposed as causative agents include excessive tissue coagulation, use of smaller caliber suture material (i.e., 3-0, 4-0 sutures for myometrial re-approximation), and development of myometrial hematomas.[4]

Furthermore, there are no good studies that analyze the differences in uterine rupture rates if the enucleated fibroid cavity is repaired by interrupted figure-of-eight sutures or a unidirectional barbed suture closure.

Financial Considerations

Critics of the da Vinci robotic platform will often cite the substantial upfront costs associated with acquiring a robot and setting up a robotic surgery program. In many instances, these upfront costs may not be fully recuperated if the surgeons who intend to utilize the technology do not make a concerted effort to learn the skills necessary for success. Because operating times can be substantially higher, the benefits to the patient may initially be outweighed by the frustration level of the individual surgeon, an independent factor that can make adoption of a robotic skill set beyond the patience of the surgeon.

Once the surgeon feels comfortable with the skills required to perform a robotic surgery proficiently, the additional patient benefits of smaller incisions, decreased blood loss, decrease in operative time, and decrease length of stay postoperatively all become clear advantages to robotic surgery. In an era where cost containment on inpatient hospitalization is going to be at a premium, this type of surgical approach can significantly improve a hospital's bottom line by reducing length of stay time.

Advincula et al. performed a retrospective case-matched analysis comparing 29 women who underwent abdominal myomectomy and 29 women who underwent robotic-assisted myomectomy. The study compared short-term surgical outcomes relative to the immediate costs associated with the surgery. As expected, initial upfront hospital charges and professional reimbursement rates were higher in the robotic group, but when costs attributed to depreciation of the equipment per case were factored in, the authors' conclusion was that the robotic myomectomy may be the lower-cost option for hospitals over time due to the significantly lower complication rates, length of stay, and subsequent nursing costs.[5]

Therefore, it is reasonable to conclude that, in addition to the myriad of patient benefits, the long-term benefits for both surgeon and medical institution may be significant as well.

Myomectomy Surgical Outcomes

In an attempt to report the surgical outcomes of robotic gynecologic surgery at St. Joseph Mercy Hospital, a chart review was completed in concordance with IRB approval, using ICD-9 codes for myomectomy (Table 1). The inclusion criterion for chart review was any case completed between January 1, 2007, and December 31, 2011, in which the da Vinci Robotic System was attempted. Once an eligible chart was identified, data were abstracted from operative reports, pathology reports, and daily progress notes. The information was then de-identified before further analysis.

Table 1. Five-Year Outcomes for Robotic-Assisted Myomectomy—SJMH

	2007	2008	2009	2010	2011	Total/ Mean
Cases attempted	0	0	7	4	6	17
Inability to complete	—	—	1	—	—	1
EBL (mL)	—	—	196	203	218	205
Operative time (h)	—	—	*	3.7	3	3.25
LOS (h)	—	—	38	34	38	37
IOC		—	—	—		0
POC		—	—	—		0
ER visit	—	—	—	—	3	3
Readmit	—	—	—	—		0

*Operative time not available in medical records prior to October 19, 2009.

Abbreviations: SJMH, St. Joseph Mercy Hospital–Ann Arbor; EBL, estimated blood loss; LOS, length of stay; IOC, intraoperative complication; POC, postoperative complication; ER, emergency room.

From January 2007 to December 2011, there were 17 da Vinci assisted myomectomies attempted at St. Joseph Mercy Hospital. Sixteen of the seventeen were completed with the da Vinci system. One case was unable to be completed using the robotic system due to poor planes around the leiomyoma and bleeding. The mean blood loss was 205 mL, with a range from 10 to 1000 mL. The mean operative time was 3.25 hours, with a range from 2 to 5.5 hours. Of note, operative times were not available in medical records for cases before mid-October 2009. The mean length of stay was 37 hours with a range of 25 to 72 hours. Twelve of the sixteen patients were discharged home on postoperative day 1. Three patients had emergency room visits within the first 6 postoperative weeks: one for uncontrolled nausea, one for calf pain with a negative evaluation, and one for dizziness with a negative workup. There were no readmissions.

References

1. Alessandri F, Remorgida V, Venturini PL, Ferrero S. Unidirectional barbed suture versus continuous suture with intracorporeal knots in laparoscopic myomectomy: a randomized study. *J Minim Invasiv Gynecol.* 2010;17:725–29.

2. Hurst BS, Matthews ML, Marshburn PB. Laparoscopic myomectomy for symptomatic uterine myomas. *Fertil Steril.* 2005;83:1–23.

3. Kumakiri J, Kikuchi I, Kitade M, Matsuoka S, Kono A, Ozaki R, Takeda S. Association between uterine repair at laparoscopic myomectomy and postoperative adhesions. *Acta Obstet Gynecol Scand.* 2012;91:331–37.

4. Sizzi O, Rossetti A, Malzoni M, et al. Italian multicenter study on complications of laparoscopic myomectomy. *J Minim Invasiv Gynecol.* 2007;14:453–62.

5. Advincula A, Xu X, Goudeau S, Ransom S. Robot-assisted laparoscopic myomectomy versus abdominal myomectomy: a comparison of short-term surgical outcomes and immediate costs. *J Minim Invasiv Gynecol.* 2007;14:698–705.

Chapter Thirteen

Uterine Surgery

Lisa H. Morris, MD; Gayle S. Moyer, MD; Martha M. Walsh, MD; Rajiv J. Deenadayalu, MD; Brandy N. Michaels, MD; JoLyn M. Seitz, MD; Susanne L. Archer, MD

History of Hysterectomy

Hysterectomy is the most common non-obstetrical surgical procedure performed on women, with approximately 600,000 performed annually in the United States. The term *hysterectomy* is an English word from the Greek root *hyster*, meaning "womb," and ectomy, deriving from the Greek root *ektome*, which means "to cut out." It is estimated that by the age of 45, a woman's calculated incidence of undergoing a hysterectomy is approximately 40%, which emphasizes how common the procedure is.

This procedure involves removal of the uterus and cervix, also called a total hysterectomy. If the cervix is retained, the procedure is often referred to as a partial hysterectomy or, more precisely, a supracervical hysterectomy. Depending on the patient's clinical condition and associated symptoms, the Fallopian tubes and ovaries may also be removed concurrently.

Hysterectomy can be used to treat cancerous conditions, but the vast majority of these surgeries are used to improve the quality of life for patients. Symptoms such as pain, excessive bleeding, fullness or pressure from fibroids, and pelvic organ prolapse can all be treated with surgical intervention, which should be utilized mainly in a setting where other, less invasive options have already been attempted.

The origins of hysterectomy can be traced back to the second century, when Soranus of Ephesus was credited with performing the first vaginal hysterectomy. In the earliest days, hysterectomies were exclusively a vaginal procedure performed without anesthetic or attention to aseptic techniques. Most often, vaginal hysterectomies were performed due to inversion of the uterus following childbirth and the patients rarely survived, succumbing to factors including hemorrhage, peritonitis, and exhaustion. Early practices involved leaving a ligature drain in the pelvis to allow for drainage of pus. However, this technique also increased the risk of subsequent infection and was often the leading cause of death postoperatively.

Thomas Keith, a physician from Scotland, recognized the dangers of leaving a drain in place and employed the practice of cauterization of the cervical stump at the time of inversion to control bleeding. He would then allow the cervix to revert back

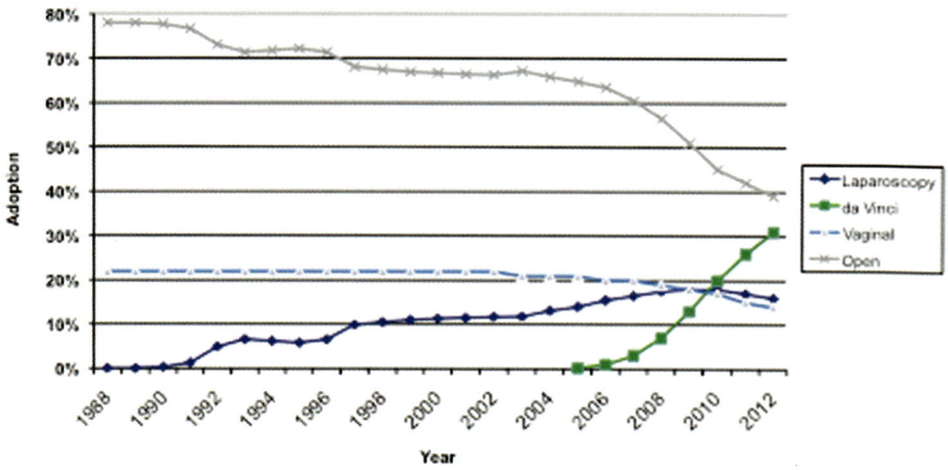

Figure 1. Rates of Hysterectomy by Modality.

to its natural internal positioning in lieu of removal of the uterus. The initiation of this practice caused an abrupt drop in the mortality rate, down to approximately 10%.

Charles Clay, a physician in Manchester, England, performed the first abdominal hysterectomy in November 1843. However, the patient died in the immediate post-operative period. Because he had the wrong diagnosis and treatment for his patient, the significance of his accomplishment was diminished.

By the 1930s, Richardson refined the techniques of total abdominal hysterectomy, and concurrent advances in surgical techniques, anesthesia, and attention to aseptic protocols, combined with the use of antibiotics, helped advance survival rates following hysterectomy. In the years since, there were few changes in the techniques of abdominal and vaginal hysterectomy until the initiation of endoscopic surgery in the 1980s.

Harry Reich, a gynecologist from Pennsylvania, performed the first laparoscopic hysterectomy in 1988, thus beginning the era of endoscopic gynecologic surgery as it exists presently. Today, the use of laparoscopic techniques has contributed greatly to enhanced recovery times, diminished length of stay in the hospital postoperatively, less pain after the procedure, and a faster return to normal activities.

Since 2002, the number of open hysterectomies has decreased by half, while da Vinci hysterectomies have increased by a factor of thirty over the last 7 years (Figure 1). It is no wonder that the number of abdominal hysterectomies has begun to decrease significantly as more gynecologists begin to realize the benefits from laparoscopic hysterectomy and as they take the time to learn the skills required to become proficient laparoscopic surgeons. Moving forward, the advantages offered with the da Vinci surgical approach will likely make this type of surgery a popular choice.

Preoperative Evaluation

Most patients who undergo a hysterectomy are generally healthy individuals. There are some recommendations for preoperative testing, but most literature shows that healthy individuals undergoing an intermediate risk surgery, like a hysterectomy, do not need advance testing.[1]

Prior to a robotic hysterectomy, it is recommended that consideration be given for the patient to have a preoperative ultrasound or an MRI for evaluation of the pelvis. An MRI is important; first, because it will be less likely an unexpected pathology will be found at the time of the hysterectomy; and second, so the appropriate route of hysterectomy may be planned. When patients have a large fibroid uterus, an MRI can be important to identify patients who could undergo a minimally invasive approach versus those who would be better served with a laparotomy.

Laboratory evaluation of patients should be kept to a minimum. Several studies have shown that there is no difference in perioperative complications in patients with indicated preoperative testing versus those who had no testing.[2,3,4,5] This has brought into question how much preoperative testing needs to be done. It is recommended that any patient having a surgery with a risk of significant blood loss have a preoperative hemoglobin evaluation. Also, since an elevated serum creatinine is an independent risk factor for surgical morbidity and mortality, it is recommended that patients over 50 years old have a preoperative serum creatinine level test. If either of these tests has been done in the last 4 months, it is unnecessary to repeat them. Lastly, it is recommended by the American Society of Anesthesiologists that any woman of childbearing age have a preoperative urine pregnancy test.[6] Other laboratory testing should be done only on the basis of patient disease or current medications.

The American College of Cardiology/American Heart Association 2007 Guidelines on Perioperative Cardiovascular Evaluation state that any asymptomatic patient without a history of coronary artery disease undergoing an intermediate risk surgery (hysterectomy) needs no further cardiovascular evaluation. If a patient has symptoms of heart disease or at least one risk factor for cardiovascular disease, noninvasive testing should be considered prior to their scheduled surgery. These risk factors include ischemic heart disease, compensated or prior heart failure, cerebrovascular disease, diabetes, and renal insufficiency. A 12-lead EKG should also be done on any patient undergoing intermediate risk surgery with known cardiovascular disease, peripheral artery disease, or cerebrovascular disease.[7]

Chest X-rays have minimal value in preoperative diagnosis. Only patients with known cardiopulmonary disease need to have a preoperative chest X-ray. This test should also be considered for any patient with current symptoms or findings on a physical exam that would warrant a chest X-ray.

Finally, any patient with a known medical disease that has been unstable recently should obtain a clearance from their medical doctor treating them for that disease.

Candidates for Robotic Hysterectomy

Indications for a robotic hysterectomy are the same indications for any type of hysterectomy, including menorrhagia, dysmenorrhea, symptomatic fibroid uterus, uterine prolapse, pelvic pain, endometriosis, and gynecologic cancers. There are very few contraindications to a robotic approach to hysterectomy. These include inability to undergo general anesthesia, obesity precluding steep Trendelenburg position, other medical problems that would not allow either steep Trendelenburg or pneumoperitoneum, and adhesions significant enough that visualization with laparoscopy is not possible.

Each patient should be evaluated on an individual basis for the type of hysterectomy that would be best suited. When comparing laparoscopic hysterectomy to a vaginal hysterectomy, the two procedures have similar blood loss, intraoperative injury, postoperative complications, length of hospital stay, and length of time to return to work.[8,9] Both have been shown to be superior to a laparotomy approach in most of these parameters. The advantages of a vaginal approach are decreased operating time, no abdominal incisions, and decreased cost. The advantages of a laparoscopic approach are better visualization of intra-abdominal organs, the ability to lyse adhesions and treat endometriosis, and the ability to remove a larger uterus laparoscopically.

When evaluating a patient for the best type of hysterectomy, consideration should first be given to the attempt to use a minimally invasive approach, including vaginal or laparoscopic. One of the most important considerations in this decision should be the experience of the operator. Training and experience should certainly be considered in order to give the patient the best operative outcome. Many surgeons have better training in either vaginal surgery or laparoscopic and robotic surgery. Several studies have shown that the more experienced a surgeon is at laparoscopic hysterectomy, the lower the complication rate.[10,11]

A second consideration of the type of approach used should be the size of the uterus. Most uteri can be removed laparoscopically. However, there are a small number of very large uteri that cannot be safely removed laparoscopically. One of the advantages of a robotic approach over a straight laparoscopic hysterectomy is that you have better visualization and better mobility to get around a large uterus and remove it safely. In order to be able to remove a uterus laparoscopically, you need to have the space to safely place all of the ports, to get around to the broad ligaments to ligate the blood supply, and to move and see adequately to remove the uterus safely. There is no specific weight of a uterus that would guide this decision. Instead, it should be based on the location and size of the fibroids.

If on exam the patient has significant lateral spread of the fibroids, it will be difficult to get around to the blood supply on each side, and this patient likely is not a good candidate for a robotic approach. If the patient's uterus is significantly higher than the umbilicus, you will likely not be able to get sufficient visualization to do the hysterectomy robotically. When placing the camera port, you need to place it a hands-breadth above the top of the uterus. If the uterus is too large, you will not have the space to place this port without running into the sternum. If, upon exam, there is a concern that the uterus is too large or the configuration of the fibroids would preclude a robotic approach, but there is some uncertainty, it is reasonable to first look in the abdomen with a laparoscope to evaluate the area further. If the visualization is not adequate, it is then reasonable to convert to a laparotomy.

Another consideration in deciding the approach to a hysterectomy should be previous abdominal surgeries and risk of adhesions. If a patient has had a number of previous abdominal surgeries, they may have significant adhesions that would make it difficult to remove the uterus vaginally. Intra-abdominal adhesions can also increase the risk of injury at the time of the hysterectomy. Using a robotic approach, you get to visualize the adhesions from above and can lyse them prior to starting the hysterectomy, in order to decrease risk of injury. If a patient has had a previous C-section, it can be very difficult to take the bladder flap off the lower uterine segment and cervix. Another advantage of the robotic approach is that it allows for greater magnification and mobility than with straight laparoscopy, which enables the surgeon to take the bladder down safely. If a patient has had several previous abdominal surgeries and there are concerns about adhesions, it is reasonable to make a small incision in the left upper quadrant and put a 5 mm laparoscope through this port to visualize the rest of the abdomen. The left upper quadrant is typically the place least likely to have adhesions from previous surgeries and, therefore, the safest place to evaluate the rest of the abdomen.

Patients who are having their hysterectomy for known endometriosis are also good candidates for using a robotic approach to the hysterectomy. With endometriosis, there can be adhesions, thickened tissue, difficult tissue planes to dissect, and anatomic distortion. With the magnification, 3-D images, and mobilization afforded by the robotic approach, it is much easier to visualize the ureters, dissect out the endometriosis, and safely remove the uterus.

One other specific advantage of the laparoscopic approach to a hysterectomy is the increased ability to diagnose previously unknown pathology. Laparoscopy has a distinct advantage at diagnosis and treatment of findings, such as ovarian pathology, endometriosis, and fibroids previously unknown at the time of the surgery. This advantage is specifically established over the vaginal approach.[12]

The majority of patients are candidates for a laparoscopic approach to a hysterectomy. The advantage of the use of the robot is superior magnification, 3-D view, and ease of movement about the abdomen. All of these things should be considered when deciding candidates for this approach to a hysterectomy.[13]

When a hysterectomy is planned, it is important to have a conversation with the patient about the option to retain or remove her cervix and also the option to retain or remove her ovaries. When discussing a supracervical hysterectomy or a total hysterectomy, it is important that the patient first have a recent normal Papanicolaou smear. If the patient has a recent history of cervical dysplasia, it is recommended that she have the cervix removed at the time of hysterectomy.[14] Several recent trials randomizing women to either a supracervical hysterectomy or a total abdominal hysterectomy done either by laparotomy or laparoscopy have shown that there is no difference in procedural-related morbidity, quality of life scores, or sexual functioning.[15,16,17]

It is important to also let the patient know about the possibility of cyclic vaginal bleeding when the cervix is retained. This occurs in approximately 20% of women who have had a supracervical hysterectomy. Several of these women will ultimately go through a procedure to have the cervix removed. It is important to inform the patient of all these possibilities, and then the decision to retain or remove the cervix should ultimately be the patient's decision.

It is also essential to have a discussion with the patient about whether they would like to retain or have their ovaries removed at the time of the hysterectomy. The main advantages of removing the ovaries are decreased risk of ovarian cancer and risk of reoperation to remove the ovaries. Any patient with a genetically increased risk of ovarian cancer, including those with BRCA1, BRCA2, and Lynch syndrome, should have their ovaries removed at the time of their hysterectomy. In patients without this increased risk, the decision to remove their ovaries is not as clear. The risk of ovarian cancer in the general population is quoted to be around 1/70–1/90. This is a small risk, and the age of the patient needs to be considered when making this decision. If a woman does decide to retain her ovaries, the risk of reoperation for ovarian pathology is between 3% and 5%.[19,20] It is important to consider the disease for which the hysterectomy is being done in deciding the risk of reoperation. If the patient has adhesive disease, endometriosis, or pelvic inflammatory disease (PID), the risk of reoperation would be increased, and the surgical difficulty of the subsequent case would also increase.

The surgeon should also discuss with the patient the disadvantages of having their ovaries removed. First of all, if the patient is premenopausal, she will go through a surgical menopause and typically have vasomotor symptoms associated with this. Second, it is important to consider the impact of a bilateral salpingo-oophorectomy (BSO) on overall health. In 2005, Parker et al. did a Markov decision model to determine whether a woman should have her ovaries removed at the time of her hysterectomy. They found that there was no survival benefit to a BSO at any age and that there was a significant survival advantage to retaining the ovaries up until age 65.[21] It has been shown in several observational studies, including the Women's Health Initiative and the Nurses' Health Study, that women who had their ovaries removed had a significantly increased risk of cardiovascular disease as well as osteoporotic fractures. It is important to go over the positives and negatives of a prophylactic BSO and to let the patient make this decision as well.

Surgical Approach

With the introduction of the robotic platform into gynecologic surgery, laparoscopic hysterectomy has become much more feasible. Some of the advantages of robotic laparoscopic hysterectomy over standard laparoscopy include enhanced imaging, superior dexterity and precision, and improved ergonomics for the surgeon.

The da Vinci Robotic System uses two wide-angle lenses producing a 3-D image. Improved imaging enhances precision. The EndoWrist instruments allow seven degrees of movement. This enables the surgeon to replicate the full range of wrist motion. Enhanced articulation facilitates dissection and enables the surgeon to successfully accomplish more complex benign gynecologic procedures laparoscopically. From an ergonomic perspective, the comfort of being seated at a console that can be adjusted to custom fit the surgeon's preferences has distinct advantages over traditional laparoscopic surgery, which requires constant attention to keep the camera steady. Avoiding the unnatural positioning of the surgeon's arms and back

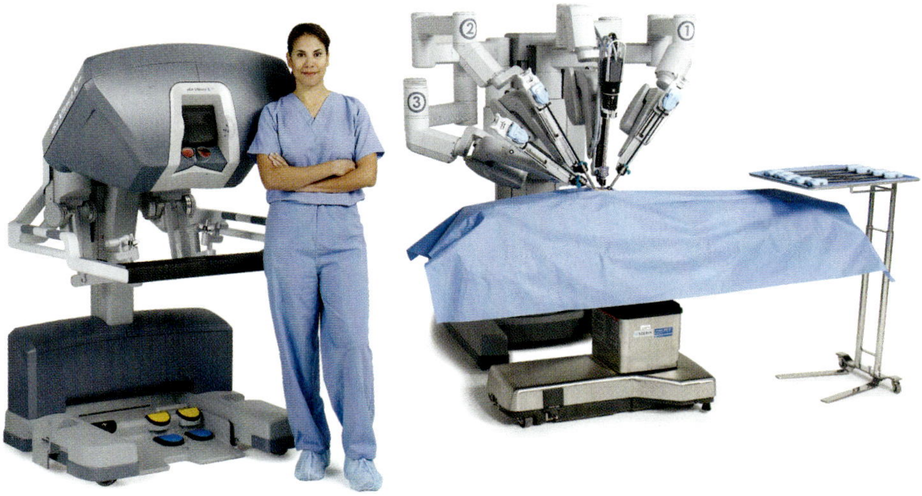

Figure 2. The surgeon console.
Credit: © 2013 Intuitive Surgery, Inc.

that is sometimes required to reach certain intra-abdominal locations during traditional laparoscopic surgery is also a benefit.

These advantages have helped surgeons overcome the surgical limitations of standard laparoscopy and to enhance their skills for more complex cases laparoscopically. The number of patients and cases that can be accomplished laparoscopically rather than using open techniques via a laparotomy incision has increased. Patients with fibroids, scar tissue, previous surgery, in particular cesarean sections, and adhesions who were once thought to be too difficult to approach laparoscopically can now be ideal candidates for laparoscopic surgery. This puts both the surgeon and the patient more at ease.

The da Vinci Robotic System is a laparoscopic assistive device with three major components: the vision system, the surgeon console, and the robotic platform. The vision system is comprised of an endoscope with 3-D imaging. The surgeon console is remote from the patient (Figure 2). It enables the surgeon to sit at the console and control the robot via assisted instruments. The robotic platform includes 3 to 4 robotic arms. The 12 mm endoscope is in one robotic arm. The additional 2 to 3 arms hold various 8 mm EndoWrist instruments. There are various EndoWrist instruments that can be interchanged among the various robotic arms, including needle drivers, scissors, and PK dissecting forceps.

Operative Setup

When initially introduced, the robotic setup was viewed as time consuming and cumbersome. As newer, smaller, more easily moveable models have evolved, the time required from room entry to beginning the operation has decreased. Particular attention should be paid to the steps involved in surgical setup and patient positioning. The prudent surgeon will develop a system that can be reproduced from case to case.

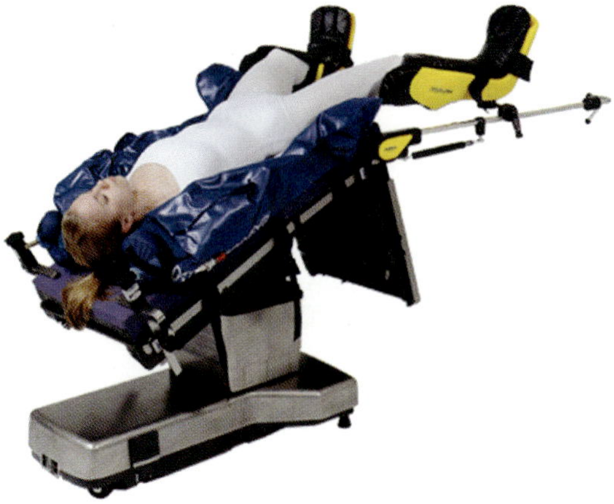

Figure 3. The Hug-u-Vac.

The patient is wheeled into the operating room, and after all the appropriate consents and time-outs have been reviewed, a general anesthetic is induced and a prophylactic antibiotic is administered. The patient is then placed in the dorsal lithotomy position and eventually is placed in steep Trendelenburg. Consideration has to be given to preventing sliding on the operating room table. Several options are available. A drawsheet and egg-crate foam may be placed on the OR table prior to moving the patient from her preoperative stretcher to the bed. The arms are padded and tucked to the patient's side with the drawsheet. A simple application of egg-crate foam around the ventral and dorsal surfaces of the forearm serves to protect the elbow and wrists from unnecessary tension or compression during surgery. Another option is a vacuum beanbag, a Hug-u-Vac (Figure 3).

The Hug-u-Vac system also allows for secure positioning of the patient's arms once the air is removed from the device, thereby allowing it to harden and mold around the patient laterally. It is generally felt that some protection, such as the egg-crate foam or simply a towel around the lateral aspect of the patient's arm, buffers against the firmness of the Hug-u-Vac.

After arm positioning is complete, it is imperative that the surgeon assess the intravenous (IV) line to insure it is flowing without any hesitation. Improper positioning of the arm can affect the patency of the IV, something that should be discovered and corrected prior to starting the operation.

It is also important to reevaluate the positioning of hands, wrists, and elbows to ensure they are anatomically positioned and pressure points are avoided. We are able to successfully secure the patient without shoulder stops; therefore, we do not use them in order to avoid the risk of shoulder nerve injury associated with their use. Legs are placed in low stirrups manufactured for gynecologic surgery. We use Allen stirrups. Careful attention is paid to ensure the heels rest comfortably in the boots of the stirrups. There should be no compression on the fibular head in order to avoid peroneal nerve injury. The surgeon should be able to place a finger with ease between the top of the boot and the patient's gastrocnemius muscle.

Either method can also be used for securing the shoulders. If the egg-crate foam is to be used, the surgeon tapes the foam in place along the bottom side of the OR table. Then the foam is placed across the chest to the opposite shoulder, thereby forming an *X* across the patient's torso. Both sides of the foam are taped to the OR table, and this keeps the patient stable despite the steep Trendelenburg that is necessary for robotic surgery.

Similarly, the Hug-u-Vac can also be molded around the patient's shoulders to provide stabilization for OR table positioning. It is often useful to place a towel or foam around the shoulders for the same reasons mentioned earlier.

Once the surgeon is satisfied that the arms and legs are secure, there are no pressure points on any of the extremities, and the IV line is flowing without difficulty, it is time to test the patient's tolerance of steep Trendelenburg. This enables evaluation of ventilatory performance and security of positioning. If the patient has been secured properly, there will be little movement (if any) up the table, as the head of the bed is tilted to its maximal position. Once this has been tested, there is very little likelihood that the patient will move up the table once the robot is docked.

Vaginal Instrumentation

Once the patient has been prepped and draped, an exam under anesthesia (EUA) is performed to assess the size and mobility of the uterus and the location of the fibroids. The exam performed on a patient under a general anesthesia provides a true assessment of pelvic pathology and allows the surgeon a much clearer mental picture of the pelvic anatomy about to be encountered. At this time, the surgeon can assess trocar placement with the uterus elevated vaginally. With large uteri, the trocars need to be placed further cephalad. The surgeon will also assess delivery options for the uterus vaginally versus morcellation. The surgeon will also decide on the need for a fourth robotic arm. Once the EUA is completed, a bivalved speculum is placed vaginally, and a single tooth tenaculum can be used to grasp the anterior lip of the cervix, allowing the surgeon to sound the uterus and dilate the cervix to place a uterine manipulator.

At this point, the uterine manipulator, KOH colpotomy ring (Cooper-Surgical) and vaginal occluder balloon are placed. There are a number of different manipulators from which to choose, and typically the selection of one over another is due to surgeon preference. The key to any device is its utility in allowing the surgeon to elevate and rotate the uterus in all directions to better assess the size and location of the fibroid(s) and also to allow for the optimal angles to suture the cavity once the fibroid is removed. Adequate uterine manipulation improves safety and efficiency of the procedure.

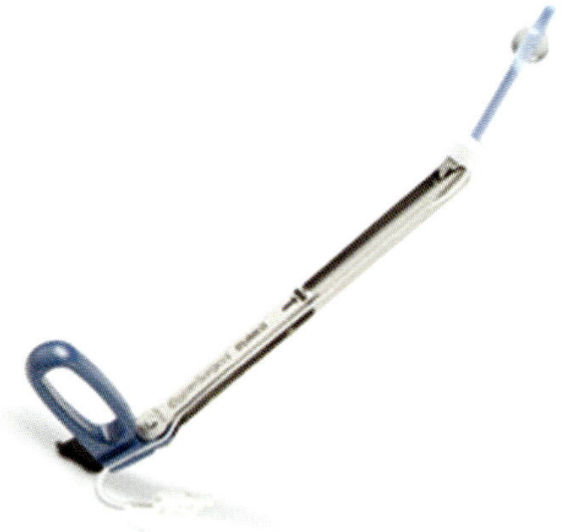

Figure 4. RUMI II uterine manipulator.

One option is the RUMI II uterine manipulator. One of the advantages of this instrument is that the manipulator length is variable and can be tailored to the uterine size. This provides increased mobility of the uterus and vaginal KOH ring during the surgery (Figure 4).

The KOH colpotomy ring (Cooper-Surgical) is paramount in a laparoscopic hysterectomy. The proper KOH colpotomy ring size is selected to fit the cervix. You want to select the appropriate size so that the KOH colpotomy ring will fit high in the vaginal fornix to prevent shortening the vagina at the time of the colpotomy. The KOH colpotomy ring is used as a landmark at the time of the colpotomy, as well as improving safety by laterally displacing the ureters. The da Vinci lacks tactile feedback. Therefore, you can use it as a visual reference point. The plastic KOH colpotomy ring decreases lateral thermal spread during cauterization of the uterine vessels and during the colpotomy.

Once the uterine manipulator is in place, the remaining vaginal instruments are removed. A Foley catheter is placed for accurate recording of urine output during the case, and the stomach is emptied with the nasogastric tube. Preoperatively, we have the patients undergo a mechanical bowel prep. This can improve visualization by decompressing the distal colon and rectosigmoid.

Abdominal Instrumentation

Once the vaginal setup is complete, attention is turned to the patient's abdomen. The patient is taken out of any Trendelenburg that may have been required for vaginal instrumentation, and the umbilical skin is elevated. Typically, the Veress needle is inserted after a small incision is made centrally in the umbilicus. It is helpful to utilize local anesthetic prior to any skin incisions being made, as this can often help to mark the location of the skin incision as well as to provide some additional level of pain relief postoperatively. Careful preoperative review of the patient's previous surgical history may alter the approach to primary entry into the abdomen, but for the purposes of this chapter, the assumption is made that the patient's past history would not necessitate deviation from the standard approach.

Once adequate pneumoperitoneum to 15 mmHg has been achieved, port placement sites are marked. Each port site is injected with 0.5% Marcaine for post-operative pain control. The sites are injected under direct visualization to aid in port placement. The supra-umbilical incision is assessed. A 12 mm trocar is used. This trocar is used to house the da Vinci camera. A zero-degree camera is used for most cases. A good rule to follow allows for a hands-breadth (approximately 10–12 cm) above the highest level of the fundus of the uterus when it is maximally elevated from the uterine manipulator. This can help identify the proposed location of the supra-umbilical incision. The surgeon must safeguard from any uncertainty in thinking that the incision may be too cephalad. If possible, it is always better to err on the side of being too high with the supra-umbilical incision rather than being too close to the umbilicus. You want to provide adequate working space between the endoscope and the uterus.

During placement of this first trocar, you want to be very careful to direct the trocar toward the anterior cul-de-sac, while controlling speed and not using excessive pressure. You want to try to avoid injury to iliac vessels and surrounding structures. It can be helpful to maximize the pneumoperitoneum in order to

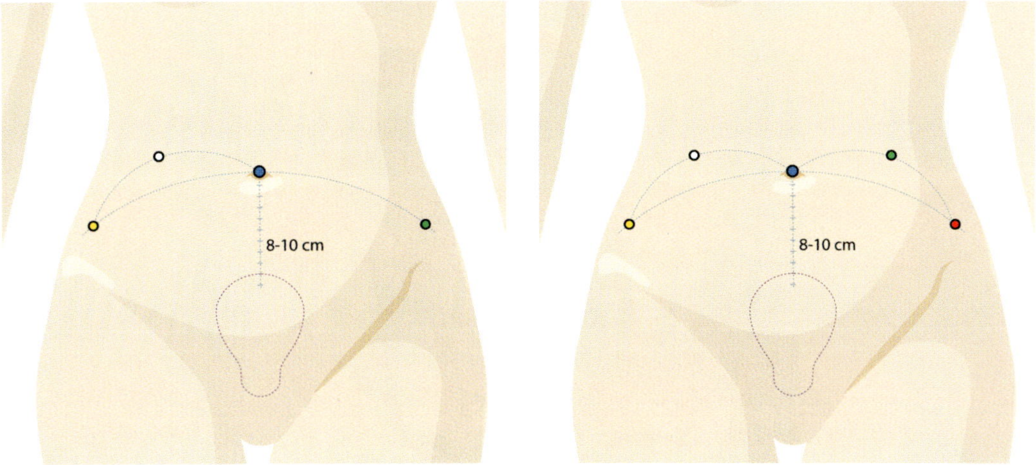

Figure 5. (left) *Three-arm port placement.* (right) *Four-arm port placement.*
Credit: © 2013 Intuitive Surgery, Inc.

increase counterpressure and increase the amount of air and distance between the underlying structures and the entry point of the trocar.

Once the supra-umbilical or camera trocar has been inserted, the da Vinci camera is then passed through the trocar and an initial inspection is performed to assess for any injuries from the trocar entry. Elevation of the uterus via the uterine manipulator will allow the surgeon to evaluate the pelvis and assess the feasibility of the intended procedure.

The additional trocars should be placed under direct visualization. Care should be taken to avoid the inferior epigastric vessels that pass lateral to the umbilical ligament. Remember that if the uterus is larger, the ports need to be placed higher to provide enough space between the instruments and the pathology to adequately manipulate the instruments. The instruments are typically placed 8–10 cm above the elevated uterus (Figure 5).

Two mm da Vinci trocars are placed in the right and left lower quadrants. These trocars are directly attached to the robotic platform and house the EndoWrist instruments. In general, they are placed approximately 10–12 cm lateral and 2 cm down from the level of the supra-umbilical trocar.

The auxiliary port is typically placed on the right side between the right da Vinci arm and the camera trocar, forming the equidistant apex of a triangle that would connect the three instruments. You want to make sure that there is at least 10–12 cm distance between all ports. This trocar is not attached to the da Vinci platform. It is used to provide bedside assistance using graspers, manipulators, and irrigation. A 5 or 12 mm trocar can be used for the auxiliary port. The selection is determined by the requirements of the case. For example, if an Endo Catch bag is necessary, a 12 mm trocar will be placed. The smallest trocar possible is preferred to decrease hernia formation. This results in less postoperative pain. The bedside assistant is placed on the side of the auxiliary port.

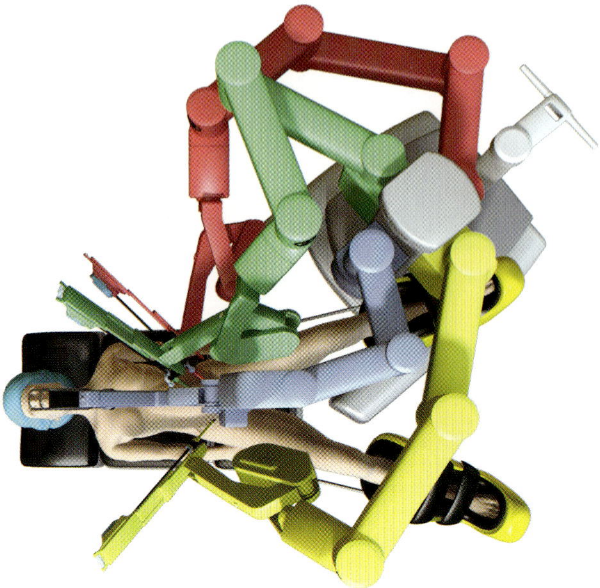

Figure 6. Side docking of the da Vinci Robotic System.
Credit: © 2013 Intuitive Surgery, Inc.

The use of the third da Vinci arm attached to the da Vinci platform can be crucial to the success of hysterectomy, allowing the surgeon much better exposure and uterine manipulation. The third arm can also improve the efficiency and safety of the case. If the third robotic arm is utilized, the surgeon will generally place the left sided da Vinci trocar just 10–12 cm (and not the additional 2 cm inferior to the level of the camera trocar) lateral to the supra-umbilical trocar and then insert the trocar for the third arm in a location approximately 5 cm superior to the left anterior superior iliac spine.

Once the trocar placement has been completed, the circulating nurse is ready to wheel the robot into place. The surgeon directs the orientation of robotic docking. The machine can either be driven to a location between the legs of the patient or, more commonly, come in at a side angle (also known as side docking), with the left base of the robot located directly adjacent to the inner aspect of the left base of the operating table (Figure 6).

There are many advantages afforded by a decision to utilize a side docking methodology. Access to the patient vaginally is maximized and can aid in manipulation of the uterus. More importantly, there is more flexibility in regard to ease of the robotic arm docking as well as maneuverability with the robotic arms, especially if the third arm is utilized.

Key principles of setup include:

- Bring the side cart in at a 45-degree angle to the axis of the patient on the operating room table. There are no sweet spots when side docking.
- Orient the column (also known as the spine of the robot) in line to the contralateral shoulder.

- Prior to docking the robot, the patient is placed in a steep Trendelenburg (>20%) and the bed is lowered. This provides another opportunity for the surgeon to make sure the patient is secure on the operating room table.
- The arms are then docked. Arm one is docked first. The arm is oriented laterally. Straighten proximal joint. This provides open access to the vagina. The number on the arm should be facing toward the contralateral wall. The camera is then docked and should be in line with the vagina.
- Arm 2 is docked next. To optimize placement, the proximal joint is folded in toward the patient-side cart column. The number on the arm should be facing the contralateral wall and can be slightly caudal.
- Arm 3 is then docked. The proximal joint again is folded back toward the patient-side cart column, similar to arm 2.
- All numbers on the arms should be facing laterally toward the contralateral wall. The arm can be lateral and a bit caudal.
- Once the robotic arms are docked, the instruments are placed through the trocars, and the surgeon is ready to start the operation.

The operative assistant is on the side of the auxiliary port. The assistant is responsible for the EndoWrist instrument exchanges on the da Vinci robot arms, support with the auxiliary port with graspers suction, and managing the uterine manipulator.

Operative Technique

A variety of EndoWrist instruments are available—the PK dissecting forceps (bipolar), Hot Shears (monopolar curved scissors), Mega needle driver, fenestrated forceps (bipolar), and the Cobra Grasper.

The PK dissecting forceps utilize active tissue impedance feedback control. This results in a lower thermal spread than the prior bipolar instruments and an improved seal of the vascular pedicles. It is important to maintain good surgical technique by skeletonizing the vessels. This enables sealing and cauterizing smaller pedicles, allowing better application of the PK dissecting forceps to the tissue and less thermal spread. It is important to remember that the PK dissection forceps requires tension-free application to the tissue.

The monopolar Hot Shears use high cutting current. These cut tissue very effectively and coagulate small vessels. The radio-frequency energy uses the path of least resistance. Therefore, caution is necessary.

At the beginning of the procedure, the surgical assistant places the PK dissecting forceps in the left arm and the monopolar Hot Shears in the right arm. If a fourth arm is used, a Cobra Grasper or a tenaculum is advanced for cephalad and lateral traction of the uterus.

Throughout the case, basic surgical principles of open hysterectomy are incorporated in the laparoscopic hysterectomy. These include development of avascular planes and skeletonization of vascular pedicles.

The ureters should be identified, if possible. This is the most common organ injured in a hysterectomy. The ureter runs 1 cm lateral to the cervix. The second location of possible ureteral injury is at the infundibulopelvic ligament. This sometimes occurs at the time of the oophorectomy. Therefore, it is important at the beginning of the case to identify the ureteral location and their course to the bladder. If necessary, it can be dissected to ensure the location. In a case that is anticipated to have a significant amount of scarring and adhesions, consideration could be given to placing lighted ureteral stents preoperatively.

In both a total laparoscopic hysterectomy with or without removal of the ovaries, the adnexa are transected from the uterus. This provides better visualization of the broad ligament and skeletonization of the uterine artery. At the time of the removal of the ovaries, the ovaries are grasped and held medially, opening a plane of dissection and improved visualization of the infundibulopelvic ligament. This provides a plane of dissection away from the pelvic sidewall, decreasing the risk of ureter injury.

The Fallopian tube and utero-ovarian ligaments are then identified. The bipolar PK dissecting forceps coagulate and seal the pedicles. The pedicles are then transected with "cold" monopolar Hot Shears. The use of energized cutting can disrupt the seal of the vessels with the PK dissecting forceps and result in bleeding.

The round ligament is then identified, coagulated, sealed, and divided. The posterior leaf of the broad ligament is incised. The ureter runs in the posterior leaf of the broad ligament. This releases the ureter laterally and decreases the risk of ureteral injury. The anterior leaf of the broad ligament is incised. This dissection is continued anterior to the bladder flap. The bladder flap is developed by dissecting below the vesicouterine reflection. Both instruments are used to create the reflection.

The uterine artery is then skeletonized. Once again, the principles of an open hysterectomy are replicated in a laparoscopic hysterectomy—dissection of avascular planes and skeletonization of the vessels. This enables better application of the PK dissecting forceps and decreases the risk of lateral thermal spread, thus decreasing risk of injury to surrounding tissue and organs, in particular to the bladder and ureter. The dissection is assisted by cephalad movement of the uterus. This can be done by the assistant applying cephalad pressure on the uterine manipulator or upward traction of the uterus with the fourth arm. A Cobra Grasper or tenaculum forceps is used to grasp the uterus with the fourth arm for upward traction of the uterus. This opens the tissue planes and allows improved dissection of the uterine artery pedicles. In addition, the counter-traction helps displace the ureter laterally, decreasing the risk of ureteral injury. The bladder flap is reevaluated to ensure that it is well developed and away from the uterine artery pedicle. The PK dissecting forceps are then applied to the uterine artery with a tension-free application. The uterine artery is then coagulated and sealed with the bipolar PK dissecting forceps and transected with the Hot Shears using "cold" transection.

If a supracervical hysterectomy is going to be performed, the uterus is transected from the cervix. The junction of the cervix and the lower uterine segment is identified. The bladder flap is reevaluated to ensure that it is well developed down and away from the intended transection. The uterine artery pedicle is again identified to ensure that it is away from the intended transection. The uterus is then transected from the cervix using monopolar Hot Shears at the level of the internal os. The

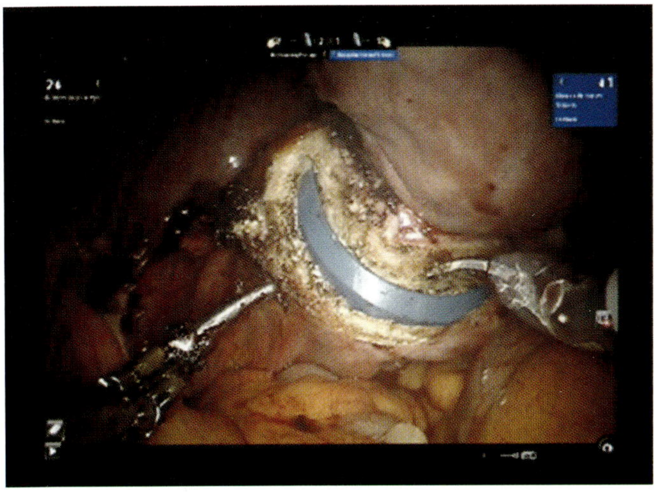

Figure 7. Blue KOH ring at time of colpotomy.

canal of the cervix is cauterized to decrease incidence of cyclic vaginal spotting. Hemostasis of the cervix is confirmed. Cauterization is used if necessary. The cervix can also be over-sewn with 0-Vicryl suture on a CT-1 or CT-2 needle.

The uterus requires morcellation and extraction through the abdominal ports. This can be accomplished using the assistance of the da Vinci or it can be done after the da Vinci has been undocked. There are several types of morcellating devices on the market. We typically undock the left lower trocar (depending on the number of da Vinci arms used, this will be arm number two or three) and replace it with the morcellator trocar. This requires extension of the incision. This trocar is placed under direct visualization.

If the morcellation is done with the assistance of the da Vinci, a tenaculum forceps or Cobra Grasper is placed in arm number one. The surgical assistant morcellates the uterus under direct visualization. The surgeon at the console assists by grasping the uterus and delivering to the morcellator. It is important to ensure that the uterine morcellator is not near any organs or vessels. We find it safest to morcellate the uterus in the deep pelvis near the cervix, under direct visualization.

The morcellation also can be done after undocking the da Vinci. Once the da Vinci is undocked, a 5 mm camera is used at the bedside. The surgical assistant operates the camera and the tenaculum. The surgeon morcellates the uterus under direct visualization.

When a total hysterectomy is performed, the cardinal and uterosacral ligament complexes bilaterally are divided with Hot Shears monopolar scissors. The pneumoperitoneum will be maintained by the Colpo-Pneumo Occluder. If the vaginal insufflation balloon has not already been insufflated, it should be insufflated at this time. The surgical assistant provides upward uterine traction to facilitate identification of the KOH ring (Figure 7). The upward traction of the uterus also helps displace the ureter laterally and decrease the risk of shortening the vagina or injuring the bladder.

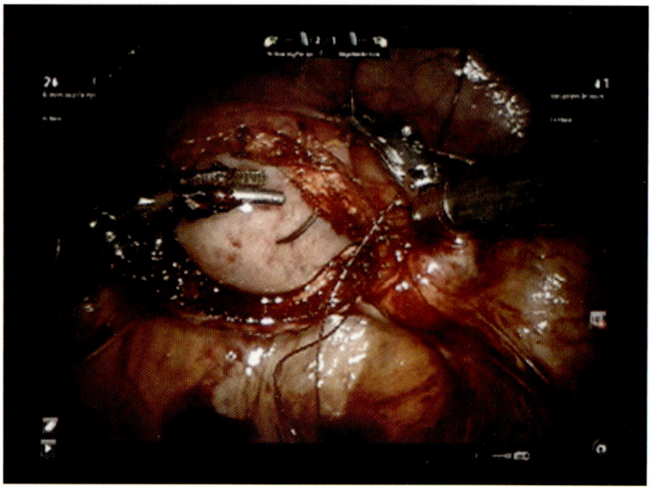

Figure 8. Vaginal cuff closure using 2-0 V-lock suture. Uterus in vagina to maintain pneumoperitoneum.

The course of the ureters should be identified prior to the colpotomy. The monopolar Hot Shears are used to perform the colpotomy. Minimize the amount of electrosurgery applied to the vaginal cuff to decrease tissue damage and increase the risk of postoperative cuff dehiscence. The uterus can then be delivered into the vagina. The uterus can be used to maintain the pneumoperitoneum. The Colpo-Pneumo Occluder can be replaced if the uterus is inadequate. A sterile glove stuffed with Ray-Tech sponges can also be used to maintain a pneumoperitoneum. If the uterus is too large to deliver through the vagina, it can be morcellated as described above.

If a bilateral salpingo-oophorectomy is planned, this can be done at this time. The adnexa are identified. The ureter is identified in the retroperitoneum. The infundibulopelvic should be skeletonized. The adnexa should be grasped and held medially to open the spaces for dissection and identification of the structures. The PK dissecting forceps are used to coagulate and seal the vessels. The monopolar Hot Shears are used for cold transection of the pedicle. The ovaries are then placed in the vagina. These can be retrieved by the surgical assistant with a ring forceps and delivered through the vagina.

The vaginal cuff is closed with suture with a running stitch. Several options for closure are possible. One option is to close with 0-Vicryl suture on a CT-2 needle. You can close using two needles with 6-inch long sutures and close from each cuff angle. Alternatively, you can use one 11-inch long suture and close with a single running stitch. The ends need to be tied intra-corporeally or you can use Lapra-Ty, is a reusable device used to anchor and secure a suture with an absorbable suture clip.

Another option is to use a 2-0 or 0 V-lock suture (Figure 8). The advantage to this suture is that the unidirectional barbs grasp the tissue at numerous points and distribute the tension across the wound. This suture also provides an efficient closure, eliminating the need to tie knots. Regardless of which suture method you use for closing, it is very important to take adequate bites back from the cauterized tissue and incorporate the vaginal mucosa. This is done to decrease the risk of post-operative vaginal cuff dehiscence. The instruments used are PK dissecting forceps or fenestrated bipolar forceps in the left robotic arm and a needle driver in the right arm. The needles can be placed into the pelvis through the 12 mm camera port, or the auxiliary port if it is a 12 mm port.

At the conclusion of the case, all pedicles and pelvis are irrigated with normal saline. The pressure is dropped to 5 mmHg to ensure hemostasis. The instruments are removed under direct visualization from each port. The da Vinci is undocked. The pneumoperitoneum is released. The incisions are injected with 0.5% Marcaine without epinephrine and closed.

Hysterectomy Surgical Outcomes

In an attempt to report the surgical outcomes of robotic gynecologic surgery at St. Joseph Mercy Hospital, a chart review was completed in concordance with IRB approval, using ICD-9 codes for laparoscopic total hysterectomy and laparoscopic supracervical hysterectomy. The inclusion criterion for chart review was any case completed between January 1, 2007, and December 31, 2011, in which the da Vinci robotic system was attempted. Patient charts were excluded if the indication for surgery was malignancy. Once an eligible chart was identified, data were abstracted from operative reports, pathology reports, and daily progress notes. The information was then de-identified before further analysis.

After review, with the above inclusion and exclusion criteria, 290 da Vinci assisted hysterectomies were attempted at St. Joseph Mercy Hospital (Table 1). Of these attempted cases, 212 were total hysterectomies and 78 were supracervical

Table 1. Five-Year Outcomes for Robotic-Assisted Hysterectomy—SJMH

	2007	2008	2009	2010	2011	Total/ Mean
Cases attempted	8	26	62	78	116	290
Inability to complete	1	1	1	1	1	5
EBL (mL)	38	84	106	90	61	81
Uterine weight (g)	197	197	219	218	264	234
Operative time (h)	*	*	2.97*	2.81	2.68	2.75
LOS (h)	34	40	33	37	35	35.5
IOC	—	—	—	1	4	5
POC	—	—	2	4	5	11
ER visit	1	—	1	4	11	17
Readmit	—	1	3	3	4	11

*Operative time not available in medical records prior to October 19, 2009.

Abbreviations: SJMH, St. Joseph Mercy Hospital–Ann Arbor; EBL, estimated blood loss; LOS, length of stay; IOC, intraoperative complication; POC, postoperative complication; ER, emergency room.

hysterectomies. Many of these procedures were also completed with concomitant unilateral or bilateral salpingectomy and/or cystoscopy. Of the 290 attempted cases, 5 were unable to be completed using the da Vinci Robotic System (1.7% of cases). Two of the hysterectomies were converted to laparotomy due to the inability to ventilate the patient in the Trendelenburg position and the inability to achieve adequate visualization. Three of the hysterectomies were converted to traditional laparoscopy for reasons including the inability to ventilate the patient in a steep Trendelenburg position, the inability to place a supra-umbilical camera port, and a recurring malfunction of "recoverable fault" of the da Vinci system. The mean estimated blood loss was 81 mL with a range from 10 to 1300 mL. The mean weight of the uterus was 234 grams, with a range from 32 to 1710 grams. The mean operative time was 2.75 hours. Of note, the operative times were not available in medical records for cases before mid-October 2009. The mean length of stay was 35.5 hours.

Complications of surgery were evaluated and divided into three time periods—intraoperative, postoperative or occurring at the time of same admission, and emergency department visits and/or readmissions within 6 weeks of surgery. Five patients (1.7%) had intraoperative complications including 1 cystotomy, 2 partial cystotomies, 1 deserosalization of bowel, and 1 false urethral tract made at the time of cystoscopy.

Eleven patients (3.8%) were found to have postoperative complications including:

- pulseless code blue on postoperative day zero that responded to Narcan with a negative cardiology evaluation;
- two patients with ileus that required prolonged hospitalization (80 hours and 81.75 hours), both resolved with conservative management;
- one postoperative fever with a diagnosed UTI;
- one patient with significant right shoulder pain who was later evaluated at an emergency department visit and underwent extensive outpatient imaging until the diagnosis of an acute brachial neuropathy from compression of brachial plexus was made;
- one patient with pneumatosis intestinalis requiring observation for 72.5 hours;
- one patient with urinary retention secondary to transobturator sling placed by urology at time of hysterectomy;
- one patient with symptomatic anemia who required transfusion of 2 units PRBCs;
- one patient with a prolonged admission for inadequate pain control; and
- one patient with unexplained thrombocytopenia that resolved spontaneously.

Eleven patients (11.8%) had hospital readmissions within the 6 week postoperative period. Indications for readmission included:

- two patients with abdominal pain and CT findings of pelvic fluid collections that were expectantly managed;
- ileus managed with bowel rest and concurrent UTI treated with oral antibiotic course;

- vaginal bleeding requiring return to operating room for exploratory laparotomy showing a ruptured corpus luteum cyst and bowel adhesions to vaginal cuff;
- two vaginal cuff abscesses treated with IV antibiotics;
- ileus and extended spectrum beta lactamase abdominal abscess requiring drainage by interventional radiology and prolonged antibiotics with PICC line;
- abdominal pain leading to exploratory laparotomy and removal of pelvic hematoma;
- vaginal cuff dehiscence requiring exploratory laparotomy: interval abdominal packing with subsequent removal of packing in OR and abdominal closure;
- vaginal cuff dehiscence requiring reoperation (this complication occurred at approximately 8 weeks postop);
- and ileus managed with bowel rest.

Seventeen patients (5.9%) presented to the emergency department for evaluation within the 6 weeks postoperative period.

- Four patients presented with the complaint of shoulder and chest pain; three of these patients ultimately were diagnosed with retained abdominal air and one, as mentioned above, was diagnosed with a brachial plexus compression injury.
- Three patients presented with the complaint of pelvic pain with negative evaluations.
- Three patients presented with concerns regarding incision, and all three incisions were documented as well healing, intact, and without evidence of infection.
- Two evaluations were completed with negative workup for dyspnea. Negative evaluations were also completed for the chief complaints of vaginal bleeding, thigh pain, and dizziness.
- One patient was seen and treated for dehydration and urinary tract infection.
- One additional patient presented to the emergency department within the 6-week period for acute alcohol intoxication.
- Of note, eight patients were also seen in the office for the complaint of dysuria, only one of whom had a positive urine culture.

After evaluation of the past five years of robotic hysterectomies that have been attempted at our institution, several observations can be made. First, the overall attempted da Vinci assisted hysterectomy rate increased by 1450%, while the number of cases that were unable to be completed remained static at 1 per year, with the conversion rate decreasing from 12.5% to <1%.

Second, the average uterine weight increased by 67 grams, with the average weight for 2011 being 264 grams. This is pertinent because traditionally uteri with weight greater than 250 grams are associated with longer operative times and greater blood loss.[22] It is observed that, at our institution, the increasing uterine weight was actually inversely correlated to operative time, with a nearly 20 minute decrease in operative time from 2009 to 2011 (again noting that operative times were not available prior to October 19, 2009).

Third, there appeared to be an initial increase in estimated blood loss from 2007 to 2009. However, the trend from 2009 to 2011 shows a decrease of 45 mL or a 42% reduction. Once again, this decrease is present despite the increasing uterine weight.

Finally, the length of stay has remained stable, with the average hospital admission being 35.5 hours, with most patients being discharged to home on postoperative day number one. In conclusion, the data suggest that both operative time and estimated blood loss are decreasing, while the number of cases being completed by the da Vinci is increasing each year, as is the ability to perform da Vinci hysterectomy on larger uteri.

References

1. Smetana G. Preoperative medical evaluation of the healthy patient. In: *UpToDate*, Rose BD (Ed), UpToDate, Waltham, MA, 2012.

2. Gerges F, Kanazi G, Jabbour-khoury S. Anesthesia for laparoscopy: a review. *J Clin Anesth*. 2006 Feb;18(1):67–78.

3. Narr B, Hansen T, Warner M. Preoperative laboratory screening in healthy Mayo patients: cost-effective elimination of tests and unchanged outcomes. *Mayo Clin Proc*. 1991 Feb;66(2):155–159.

4. Kaplan EB, Sheiner LB, Boeckmann AJ, et al. The usefulness of preoperative laboratory screening. *JAMA*. 1985 June 28;253(24):3576–81.

5. Chung F, Hongbo Y, Yin L, et al. Elimination of preoperative testing in ambulatory surgery. *Anesth Analg*. 2009 Feb;108(2):467–475.

6. Lamont T, Coates T, Mathew D, et al. Checking for pregnancy before surgery: summary of a safety report from the National Patient Safety Agency. *BMJ*. 2010;341.

7. ACC/AHA 2007 guidelines on perioperative cardiovascular evaluation and care for noncardiac surgery. *Circulation*. 2007;116:e418–e500.

8. Nieboer TE, Johnson N, Lethaby A, et al. Surgical approach to hysterectomy for benign gynaecological disease. *Cochrane Database Syst Rev*. 2009 Jul 8;(3): CD003677. doi: 10.1002/14651858.CD003677.pub4.

9. ACOG Committee Opinion No. 444: Choosing the route of hysterectomy for benign disease. *Obstet Gynecol*. 2009 Nov;114(5):1156–8.

10. Chang WC, Li TC, Lin CC. The effect of physician experience on costs and clinical outcomes of a laparoscopic-assisted vaginal hysterectomy: a multivariate analysis. *J Am Assoc Gynecol Laparosc*. 2003 Aug;10(3):356–359.

11. Twijnstra AR, Blikkendaal MD, van Zwet EW, et al. Predictors of successful surgical outcome in laparoscopic hysterectomy. *Obstet Gynecol*. 2012 Apr;119(4): 700–708.

12. Garry R, Fountain J, Mason S, et al. The eVALuate study: two parallel randomized trials, one comparing laparoscopic with abdominal hysterectomy, the other comparing laparoscopic with vaginal hysterectomy. *BMJ*. 2004;328:129.

13. Lyons T. Laparoscopic approach to hysterectomy. In: *UpToDate*, Rose BD (Ed), UpToDate, Waltham, MA, 2012.

14. Falcone T. Overview of hysterectomy. In: *UpToDate*, Rose BD (Ed), UpToDate, Waltham, MA, 2012.

15. ACOG Committee Opinion No. 388: Supracervical hysterectomy. 2007 Nov; 110(5):1215–7.

16. Gimbel H, Zobbe V, Andersen BM, et al. Randomised controlled trial of total compared with subtotal hysterectomy with one-year follow up results. *BJOG.* 2003 Dec; 110(12):1088–1098.

17. Einarsson J, Suzuki Y, Vellinga T, et al. Prospective evaluation of quality of life in total versus supracervical laparoscopic hysterectomy. *J Minim Invasive Gynecol.* 2011; 18(5):617–621.

18. Kuppermann M, Summit RL, Varner RE, et al. Sexual functioning after total compared with supracervical hysterectomy: a randomized trial. *Obstet Gynecol.* 2005 Jun; 105(6): 1309–18.

19. Valea F, Mann WJ. Oophorectomy and ovarian cystectomy. In: *UpToDate,* Rose BD (Ed), UpToDate, Waltham, MA, 2012.

20. Hickey M, Ambekar M, Hammond I. Should the ovaries be removed or retained at the time of hysterectomy for benign disease? *Human Reprod Update.* 2010 Mar–Apr; 16(2):131–141.

21. Parker WH, Broder M, Liu Z, et al. Ovarian conservation at the time of hysterectomy for benign disease. *Obstet Gynecol.* 2005 Aug;106(2): 219–226.

22. O'Hanlan KA, McCutcheon SP, McCutcheon JG. Laparoscopic hysterectomy: impact of uterine size. *J Minim Invasive Gynecol.* 2011 Jan–Feb;18(1):85–91.

Chapter Fourteen

Surgery for Sleep Apnea

Paul T. Hoff, MD, MS; Matthew E. Spector, MD

Introduction

Obstructive sleep apnea (OSA) is a significant health-care problem in the United States, given the well-known association of OSA to cardiopulmonary and neurologic sequelae. The increasing incidence of OSA has gone hand in hand with the obesity epidemic, with more than one-third of Americans now considered obese, and the number considered morbidly obese increasing 5-fold.[1] It is likely that the prevalence of obesity and obstructive sleep apnea will continue to increase, making expansion of treatment options for these patients critical. Since the description of a patient with obesity-associated hypoventilation syndrome (Pickwickian syndrome) was first outlined, the lack of effective interventions to minimize morbidity has also been recognized.[2] Currently, the incidence of obstructive sleep apnea with morbid obesity is increasing, although this may be due to the increased ability to detect this disease process and its sequelae.

The surgical management of OSA has always had appeal to both patients and providers as a single intervention that could limit health-care costs and avoid the use of continuous positive airway pressure (CPAP). While CPAP is extremely effective in the treatment of OSA, the tolerability of CPAP, adherence to its use, and the social stigma make it difficult for many patients. Previous procedures have focused on individual sub-sites of obstruction and have had variability in their effectiveness. Procedures such as tonsillectomy and uvulopalatopharyngoplasty (UPPP) have been used to address the oropharynx and, with careful patient selection, have been effective.[3] Oral appliances and tongue advancement prostheses, as well as mandibular advancement devices, have also had efficacy in hypopharyngeal obstruction.[4] Bimaxillary advancement is a viable alternative for patients with skeletal abnormalities. Tracheotomy has been used to bypass the pharyngeal obstruction completely, although patients typically wish to avoid this intervention.[5] Bariatric surgery has also been considered, although this too has high complication rates and is not always effective as previously thought.[5] Despite the multiple available procedures, current treatments continue to rely on careful patient selection and appropriate application of surgical interventions. By defining new surgical treatments, there may be an opportunity to improve outcomes in OSA.

Obstructive Sleep Apnea and Polysomnography Definitions

Obstructive sleep apnea syndrome is defined as the cessation of airflow or reduction of airflow during the respiratory cycle while sleeping, accompanied by other symptoms, typically daytime sleepiness. Mild OSA is defined as 5–14 events per hour, moderate OSA with 15–29 events per hour, and severe OSA with ≥30 events per hour. While obese patients (BMI >30 kg/m^2) have a higher prevalence of OSA, there are patients who are not obese who will have the disease. There is also an increasing prevalence based on age, gender (male > female), and certain ethnicities.[6] Comorbidities such as HTN, stroke, myocardial infarction, diabetes mellitus, and arrhythmias are more common in this population.[6,7,8]

The gold standard for the diagnosis of obstructive sleep apnea and other sleep disorders is polysomnography (PSG). A variety of sleep studies are available, including Type 1 attended polysomnography, in which multiple measurements are collected. These measurements include EEG, ECG, EMG, oxygen saturation, airflow monitoring, chest movement, blood pressure, and positioning during sleep. Type 2 studies are unattended and measure at least 7 of these parameters. Type 3 and 4 studies are unattended and measure a minimum of 4 and 3 channels, respectively. There are portable (Types 2–4) monitoring systems available, and these are used in many countries, such as Italy, where formal PSG is reserved for high-risk patients. The sleep study report includes the apnea/hypopnea index (AHI), or the number of apneas and hypopneas that occur per hour. Other measurements include sleep latency and duration, sleep efficiency, and snoring. The respiratory disturbance index (RDI) includes all events (not only apneas and hypopneas) that occur per hour. Taken together, the PSG defines the severity of OSA and can help guide the clinician to identify patients who may be successful with surgical interventions.

Preoperative Evaluation and Anatomic Considerations

Preoperative evaluation of patients for sleep apnea surgical procedures, such as transoral robotic surgery (TORS), includes a thorough office examination followed by diagnostic, drug-induced sleep endoscopy (DISE). Figure 1 shows our intake questionnaire documenting physical exam findings at the St. Joseph Multidisciplinary Sleep Disorders Center. Patients referred for TORS are advised that a polysomnogram must be obtained prior to evaluation. Patients with moderate to severe OSA (AHI >20) are potential candidates for TORS; AHI <20 is often amenable to other treatments, including oral appliance or tonsillectomy and UPPP/lateral expansion pharyngoplasty with or without thyro-hyoidopexy.[9]

The application of TORS to the treatment of OSA is new, and the effect on the growing tongue base and supraglottis has not been studied. Therefore, TORS should not be performed on patients under 18 years of age, nor is it approved by the FDA for this indication. Table 1 lists ideal preoperative criteria for TORS.

Vicini et al.[10] have shown TORS to have an efficacy of 75% at 6 months in patients with a BMI under 30 kg/m^2. As BMI increases, the results of TORS fall to 55%. The obesity epidemic in North America has likewise increased the prevalence

St. Joseph Multidisciplinary Sleep Disorders Center

Patient Name:
Date:
Examiner:

Height (cm)
Weight (kg)
BMI (m2/kg)
Collar size (cm)

Physical Examination:

Tonsil size

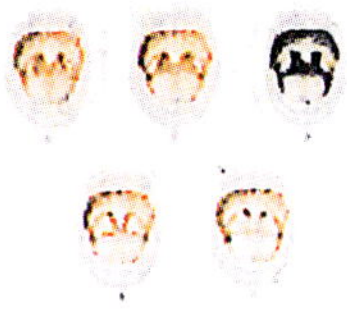

Tongue position

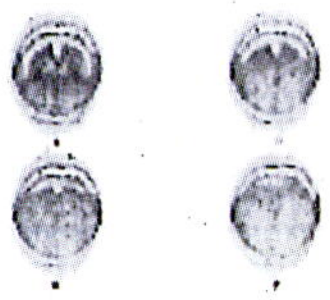

Post Airway/Chin

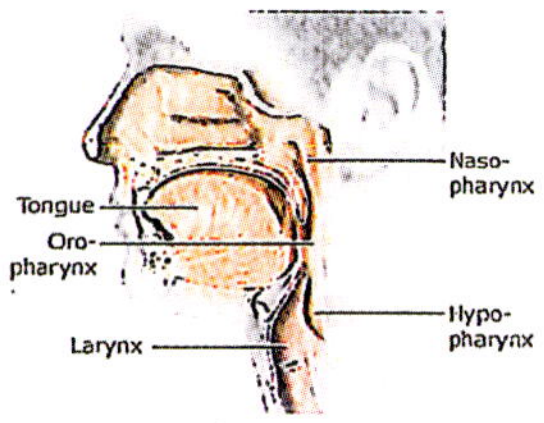

Cormack and Lehane Laryngoscopy view

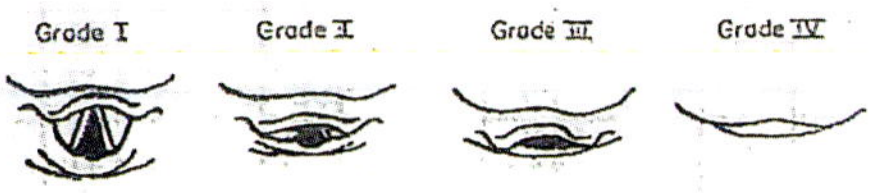

Sino-nasal tract

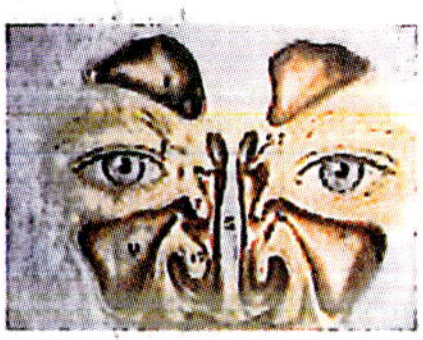

Uvula

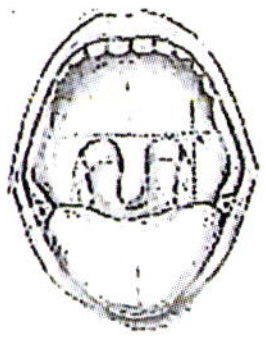

Sleep study data:

Home study: Y N Monitored study: Y N
AHI:_____
Min SaO2:_____
Hypopnea index: _____
Apnea index:______
CPAP: Y N
Prior CPAP: Y N
Epworth scale: ____
Thornton scale: ____
Other:

Physical Exam:

Ears
Nose
Oral cavity
Oropharynx
Larynx
Neck
Neuro

Comorbidities:

Hypertension CAD Obesity
Diabetes Stroke Other:

Impression :

Plan:

Figure 1. St. Joseph Mercy Hospital Multidisciplinary Sleep Disorders Center Intake Form showing preoperative data points important for treatment decision making.

of OSA. Lopez et al.[11] find the incidence of OSA in severely obese patients to be as follows: BMI 35–39 kg/m^2 (71%), 40–49 kg/m^2 (74%), 49–59 kg/m^2 (79%), and >60 kg/m^2 (95%).

Table 1. Ideal Preoperative Criteria for TORS

1. Moderate to severe OSA (AHI >20)
2. Age >18 years
3. BMI <30 kg/m^2
4. Failed trial of PAP
5. Failed surgery
6. DISE

Surgeons offering TORS as an option for their patients with OSA must proceed judiciously and not raise unrealistic expectations for success in obese patients; despite ideal anatomic criteria for TORS, cure of OSA in obese patients remains elusive. It is advisable to encourage obese patients to enter a medical weight loss program while using CPAP. Many comprehensive sleep labs will offer CPAP clinics to improve compliance. Bariatric surgery may also be an option for these patients. Bariatric surgery is a very effective tool for the treatment of OSA, with a success rate of 70% in a meta-analysis of 12 studies of patients with moderate to severe OSA.[12] Many patients will find that their OSA resolves with weight loss. Repeat polysomnography should be performed after targeted weight loss has been achieved.

Subjective measures of sleepiness and snoring have been developed and are commonly used as a measure of treatment success. The Epworth sleepiness scale is a 24-point scale measuring subjective sleepiness in 8 different scenarios. Figure 2 shows our snoring and sleepiness subjective questionnaires. The Thornton snoring scale is a similar scale in which the patient evaluates the effect of disruptive snoring on his or her relationship in different scenarios. Both should be measured before and after treatment.

Physical findings that are critical to successful TORS are identified in the clinic (Table 2). Severe nasal obstruction due to septal deformity may preclude trans-nasal intubation. Any nasal deformity (deviated septum, inferior turbinate hypertrophy, adenoid hypertrophy) should be addressed at the time of DISE. Radio-frequency ablation of the inferior turbinates can be done as an office procedure or added to DISE without the need for general anesthesia.

Careful assessment of inter-incisor distance and dentition will prevent surprises in the operating room. Patients with trismus or retrognathia (Angle's class II) will pose a problem with accessibility during placement of the robotic arms and camera. Most patients have an inter-incisal distance greater than 4 cm; less than 2 cm will preclude successful TORS. If there is marginal accessibility, it is recommended that the Davis-Meyer mouth gag and the robotic arms be positioned at the time of DISE to confirm candidacy for TORS.

Tongue position and tonsil size have become the mainstay of the Friedman staging system.[3] Tongue position (Grade 1–4) is based on a modification of the Mallampati grade used by the anesthesiologist in assessing tongue position. The modification classifies tongue position in the resting position (not protruded) with the mouth wide open. Tonsil size is graded 1–4. Based on tongue position, tonsil size, and BMI, a staging system was developed with the goal of predicting surgical success in patients with OSA.

Table 2. Physical Exam Findings

1. Nasal obstruction
2. Trismus
3. Dentition
4. Angle class
5. Friedman tongue position
6. Tonsil size
7. Modified Cormack-Lehane view
8. Lingual tonsil size

SNORING QUESTIONNAIRE

If you snore, you are very familiar with the impact lack of sleep has on your quality of life. Snoring not only disrupts sleep, it may also be a sign of a serious condition called Obstructive Sleep Apnea (OSA). To find out if you should be concerned about your snoring, choose a number from the scale below that best describes your snoring in each situation.

0 = Never
1 = Infrequently (1 night per week)
2= Frequently (2-3 nights per week)
3 = Most of the time (4 or more nights per week)

SITUATION	YOUR SCORE
My snoring affects my relationship with my partner	________
My snoring causes my partner to be irritable or tired	________
My snoring requires us to sleep in separate rooms	________
My snoring is loud	________
My snoring affects other people when I am sleeping away from home (hotel, camping, etc.)	________

TOTAL SCORE ________

If you scored a 5 or greater, please show these results to your physician.

Your physician can discuss available treatment options.

Address Label

*Adapted from the Thornton Snoring Scale

SLEEPINESS QUESTIONNAIRE

In contrast to just feeling tired, how likely are you to doze off or fall asleep in the following situations? Use the scale below to choose the most appropriate number for each situation:

0 = Would never doze
1 = Slight chance of dozing
2= Moderate chance of dozing
3 = High chance of dozing

SITUATION	YOUR SCORE
Sitting and reading	________
Watching television	________
Sitting inactive in a public place (movie theater)	________
As a car passenger for an hour without a break	________
Lying down to rest in the afternoon	________
Sitting and talking to someone	________
Sitting quietly after lunch without alcohol	________
In a car while stopped for a few minutes in traffic	________

TOTAL SCORE ________

If you scored a 6 or greater, please show these results to your physician.

Your physician can discuss available treatment options.

Address Label

*Adapted from the Epworth Sleepiness Scale

Figure 2. Adapted Epworth and Thornton scales used to evaluate subjective symptoms in patients with obstructive sleep apnea.

Figure 3 shows the Friedman staging system as it pertains to relevant oropharyngeal anatomy.

Modified Cormack-Lehane view is, in the authors' opinion, the most important clinical tool in assessing patient candidacy for TORS. The Cormack-Lehane classification (Figure 4) was developed as a tool for anesthesiologists as they described the view of the larynx during direct laryngoscopy. A modification has been created using a flexible nasopharyngoscope that gives the observer a physiologic view of the retropalatal and retrolingual anatomy during the awake state.

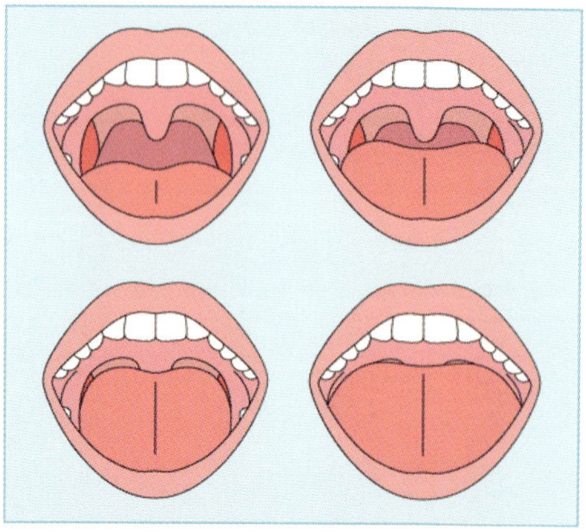

Figure 3. Adapted Friedman staging system as it pertains to relevant oropharyngeal anatomy. Credit: C. Vicini.

Grading the size of the lingual tonsil is important in assessing candidacy for surgery, as well as comparing results across observers. To grade lingual tonsils, the tongue should be in the resting position, with the mouth closed as occurs in sleep. The patient should be in the supine position. Comparison of awake and sedated lingual tonsil size can be done during DISE; however, the final grade should be assessed with the patient awake and supine. Lingual tonsils are given a grade of 1–4 (Figure 5): grade 1 not visible or absent; grade 2 partial fills vallecula; grade 3 fills vallecula but does not displace epiglottis; grade 4 fills vallecula and causes secondary prolapse of epiglottis. While we are currently validating this sizing criteria, patients with grade 3 or 4 lingual tonsils are considered good surgical candidates.

The best candidates for TORS have discrete areas of lingual tonsil hypertrophy low in the vallecula and/or secondary collapse of the epiglottis due to direct contact with enlarged lingual tonsils (Figure 6a). Patients with a large, muscular tongue (Friedman class 3 or 4) and minimal lingual tonsil tissue are typically poor candidates for TORS (Figure 6b). Many of the latter patients also have a BMI >30 kg/m^2; a large tongue is often due to fatty infiltration in obese patients.

Preoperative imaging including MRI, CT, and cephalometrics is not essential and, in some cases, may not be a covered insurance benefit. The role of preoperative imaging is under investigation.

Drug-Induced Sleep Endoscopy

Drug-induced sleep endoscopy (DISE) was first described in 1991 by Croft and Pringle.[13] DISE allows the treating physician to observe areas of physical obstruction that occur during induced sleep. These observations have led to a better understanding of the multilevel obstruction that characterizes obstructive episodes. As the population of OSA patients grows, the use of DISE is gaining widespread acceptance. Many of these patients are young and active and are not willing to use PAP. DISE gives treating physicians a better understanding of the pathophysiology

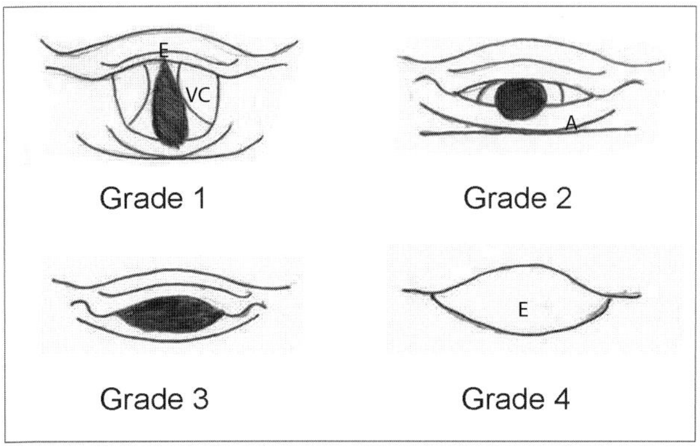

Figure 4. Adapted Cormack-Lehane classification of laryngeal viewing during nasopharyngoscopy. E = epiglottis; VC = vocal chord; A = arytenoid.

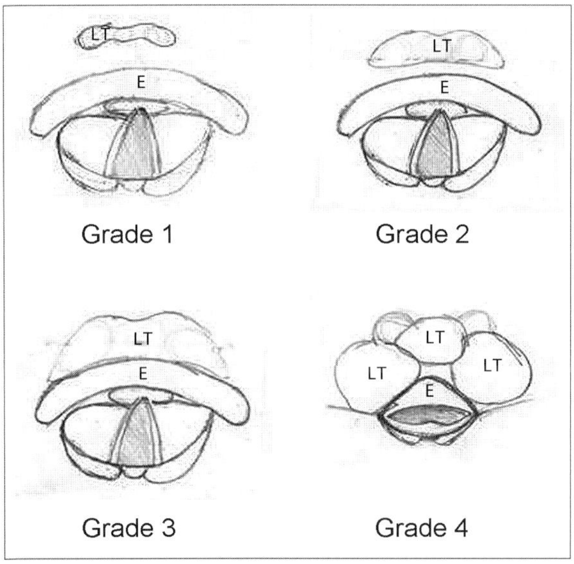

Figure 5. Lingual tonsil grading system from a direct/indirect laryngoscopic view. LT = lingual tonsil; E = epiglottis.

by identifying site(s) of obstruction that may be amenable to surgical treatment, including TORS.

The examination takes place in the operating room with an anesthesiologist and surgical technician present. The patient is placed in the supine position in preparation for both awake and sedated examination of the airway. A flexible nasopharyngoscope is attached to a high-definition camera, and the examination is recorded for future review. The scope is lubricated and the nose may be topicalized with decongestant (oxymetazoline) and anesthetic (2% lidocaine). To decrease oral secretions, glycopyrolate (0.1 mg, IV dose) may also be used. Other investigators believe that one should avoid topical agents and drying agents as they tend to

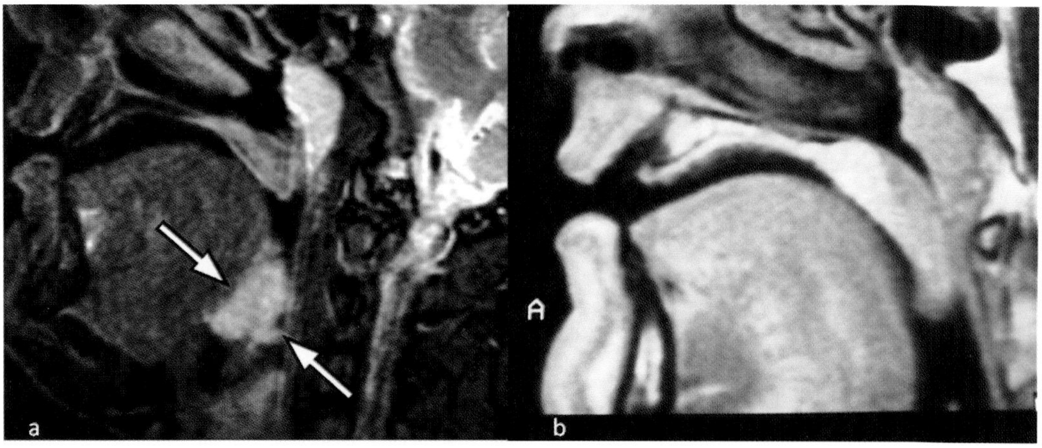

Figure 6. Parasagittal Magnetic Resonance Images showing examples of different tongue base anatomy. Figure 6a shows prominent lingual tonsils (arrows) that would make a good surgical candidate. Figure 6b shows a large muscular tongue that would make a poor surgical candidate. Credit: C. Vicini.

alter the physiologic secretions that may contribute to obstruction (Vicini, personal communication).

The examiner stands at the head of the bed; this gives an anatomically correct view from a surgical perspective (Figure 7). The epiglottis is viewed anterior and can be seen to fall posterior with variable obstruction of the larynx. Figure 8 illustrates the importance of sleep endoscopy in differing tongue positions. Figure 8a shows a supine, awake patient with prominent lingual tonsils, while Figure 8b shows a patient undergoing DISE. Note the increasing collapse of the lingual tonsils and epiglottis.

Several authors have described their techniques for sleep endoscopy.[14,15] The current technique utilizes IV propofol sedation. Propofol can be given as a bolus or as constant infusion. Bispectral index (BIS) monitoring has been helpful, with a target response between 40 and 60; others rely on a target level of anesthesia similar to the modified Ramsay score of 5—arousable to loud verbal stimuli. Recent studies suggest the use of target-controlled anesthesia may give the most consistent results in DISE.[10] The use of analgesics (fentanyl) and anxiolytics (versed) should be avoided. Supplemental oxygen is on standby but is not used throughout the procedure.

The examiner evaluates the airway in a very methodical fashion as described by Vicini et al.[15] The NOHL (nasopharynx, oropharynx, hypopharynx, and larynx) classification is demonstrated anatomically in Figure 9. This is a two-stage process: awake and sedated. The sites examined include the nasopharynx, oropharynx (retropalatal), hypopharynx (retrolingual), and larynx (a = supraglottic, b = glottic). For each site, the degree (grade) of obstruction (<25% grade I, 25–50% grade II, 50–75% grade III, and >75% grade IV), the pattern (c = concentric, ap = anterior posterior, l = lateral), and mechanics (vibration, collapse) are recorded (Table 3). The examiner should pay close attention to the differences between the awake and sedated exam, as Campanini et al.[16] found an overall discordance of 35%. The

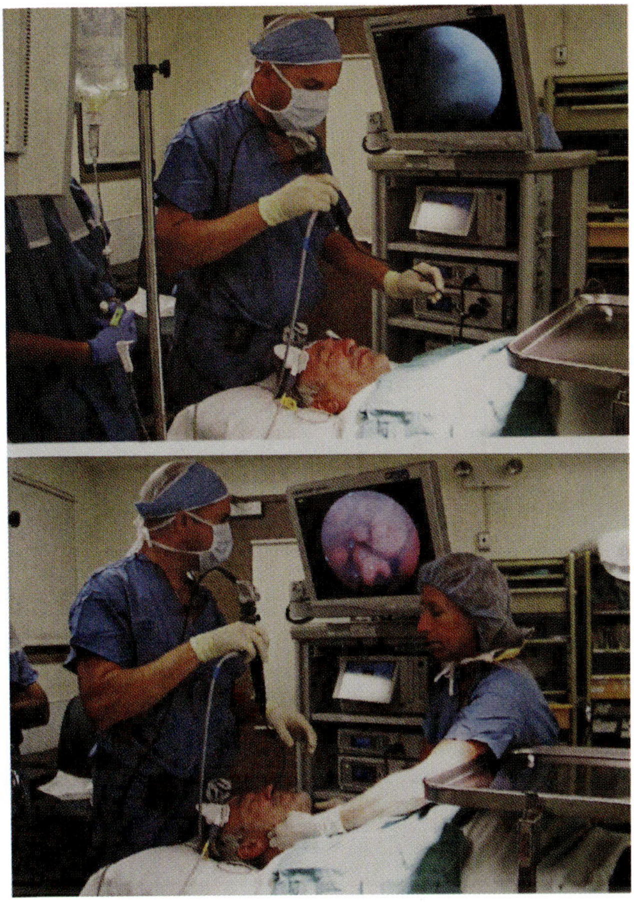

Figure 7. Proper positioning during sleep endoscopy.

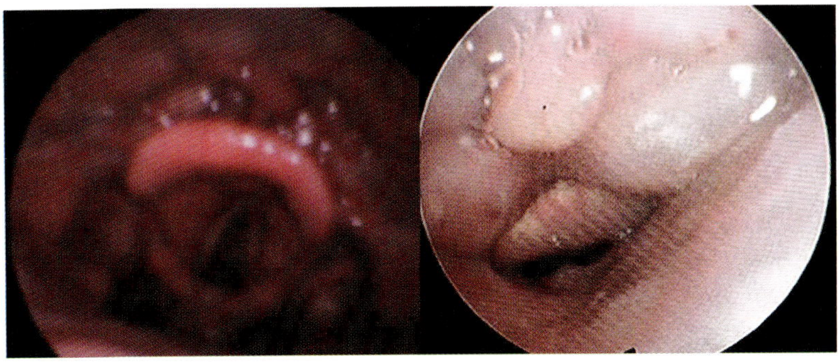

Figure 8. Examples of differing tongue positions during sleep endoscopy. (left) *A supine, awake patient with prominent lingual tonsils;* (right) *A sedated patient undergoing DISE. Note the increasing collapse of the lingual tonsils and epiglottis.*

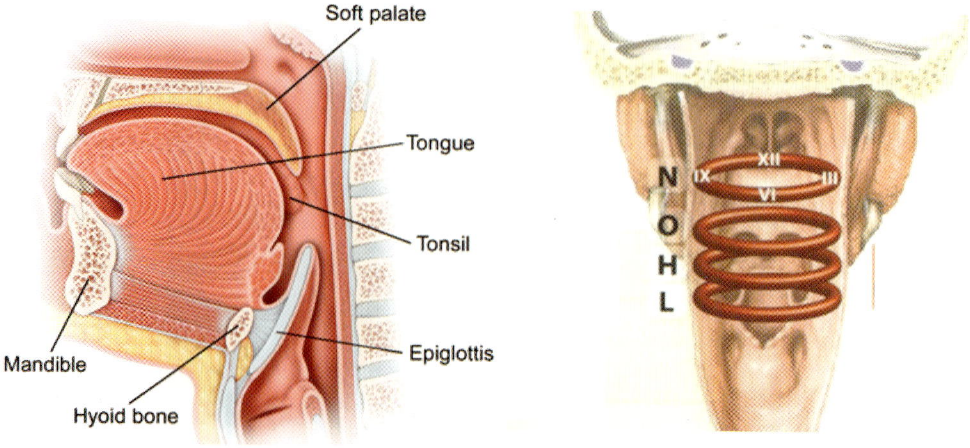

Figure 9. NOHL classification used to measure level and degree of obstruction.[15] *The sites examined include the nasopharynx, oropharynx (retropalatal), hypopharynx (retrolingual), and larynx (a = supraglottic, b = glottic). Credit: C. Vicini.*

primary areas of discordance were the oropharynx (33%), hypopharynx (50%), and larynx (33%). Figure 10 shows examples of different levels of collapse using the NOHL classification.

Indications for DISE have been described by Vicini et al. (Table 4) and have been expanding. In pediatric patients with OSA and normal size tonsils and adenoids, DISE can reveal undiagnosed laryngomalacia, lingual tonsil hypertrophy, or hypopharyngeal neoplasm. For adults with mild to moderate OSA undergoing evaluation for a mandibular advancement device (MAD), the use of DISE with an adjustable MAD can optimize fit and efficacy.[18]

Patients who are being considered for DISE are most often undergoing evaluation for surgical treatment. These patients present to the treating physician with a long history of frustrating and failed PAP trials. Most patients will present with documented OSA, bringing either a monitored polysomnogram or a home sleep study to the evaluation. It is the authors' opinion that the DISE should be done as a stand-alone procedure, apart from any major surgical intervention. The exception to this recommendation is corrective nasal surgery, including turbinate reduction and/or septoplasty, performed at the time of DISE; it is helpful to perform these procedures before TORS, which requires trans-nasal intubation.

DISE often reveals areas of obstruction that were not anticipated during office examination and may significantly change the surgical plan.[14] In addition, the patients appreciate the opportunity to review the findings during a separate office consultation, where the video is reviewed and the surgical plan is outlined. Based on

Table 3. Recording Schema for the NOHL Classification

Site	Grade	Pattern	Mechanics
N/O/H/La/Lb	1–4	c/ap/l	v/c

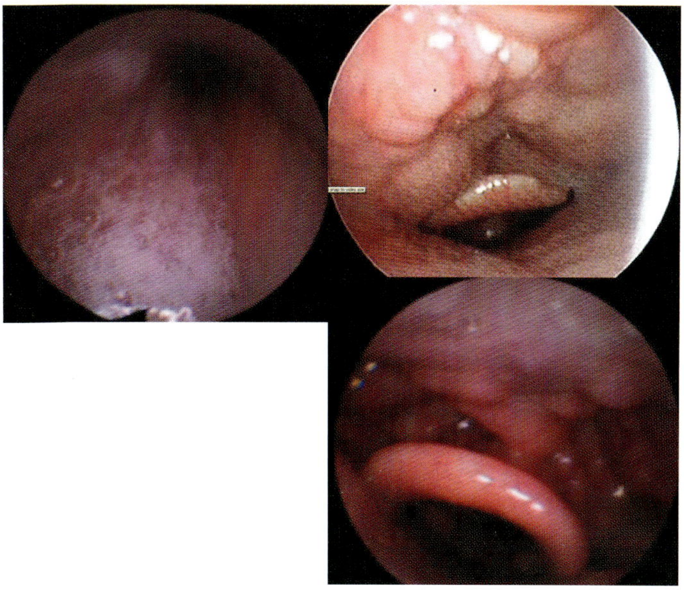

Figure 10. Examples of different sites of collapse during sleep endoscopy.

the findings during DISE, alternatives to TORS, such as the mandibular advancement device, bi-maxillary advancement, or weight loss, may be recommended. For those patients who are considered good surgical candidates, one cannot underestimate the confidence patients gain in their understanding of the disease process after review of their video with the treating physician.

DISE is brief when done as a stand-alone procedure. Operative time is typically 10–15 minutes and can be done in between cases during turn-over for TORS or other cases. Coding for DISE utilizes CPT code 31526. Patients are told they will need transportation to and from the appointment. Postoperative discomfort is minimal, and patients can resume normal activity within 24 hours of the procedure.

Drug-Induced Sleep Endoscopy Pre-op TORS Algorithm

Sleep study AHI >20
PAP trial failure
Prior UPPP/etc. failure
Comprehensive office evaluation (see sheet)
BMI <30 kg/m^2

↓

DISE (+/– nasal surgery)

↓

TORS

↓

Post-op PSG in 3 months

Transoral Robotic Surgery Basic Setup

Transoral robotic surgery requires organization and efficiency from a multispecialty team. The team includes the surgeon, a surgical technician who has dedicated time to train and scrub for robotics cases, and a consistent bedside assistant familiar with TORS. There is a basic instrument setup that is standard for TORS, and familiarity of the team with this setup is essential. The retractor typically used by this author is the Davis-Meyer, although the McGyver, Crow-Davis, Dingman, and F-K retractor can also be used. Figure 11 shows the Davis-Meyer Mouth Gag with the integrated blade and suction port.

Table 4. Indication for Drug-Induced Sleep Endoscopy (adapted from Vicini)

Severe OSA
Surgical failure
Discordant exam
Suspected stridor
Possible TORS

The basic setup of the operating room is shown in Figure 12. The main retractor used in the robotic instrumentation arm is the Maryland dissector. The second arm can either be used as a monopolar or two different laser options: the RevoLix LISA laser (thulium) or the OmniGuide CO_2 laser. The placement of the mouth gag with the arrangement of the TORS instruments in the mouth is shown in Figure 13. Table 5 and Figure 14 show optimal conditions for positioning of the robot. This takes practice, but with a consistent OR team can become effortless.

Scrub Nurse Setup

The scrub nurse is an integral part of the team and ideally will be assigned to TORS cases consistently. The instrument setup is designed to allow both the bedside assistant and the nurse efficient access to robotic instruments, alternative tongue blades, and hemostatic instruments.

The mouth gag can be supported by either a Storz instrument clamp or a Mayo stand. If a Mayo stand is used, a Dedo extension may be necessary for larger patients. The Mayo stand is a convenient place for the nurse to place additional

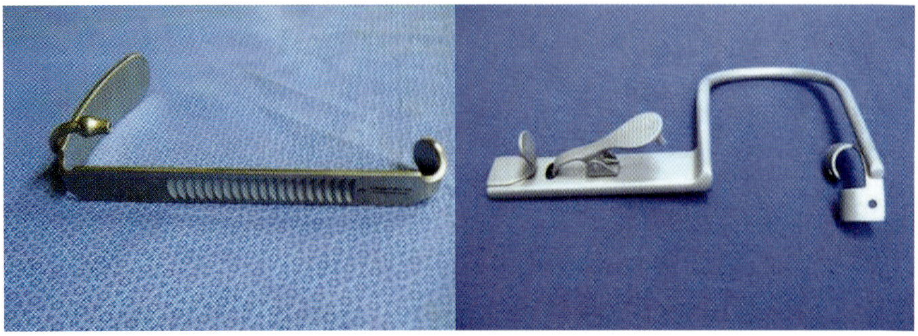

Figure 11. Davis-Meyer Mouth Gag used for exposure during transoral robotic surgery. Credit: © 2010 Intuitive Surgical, Inc.

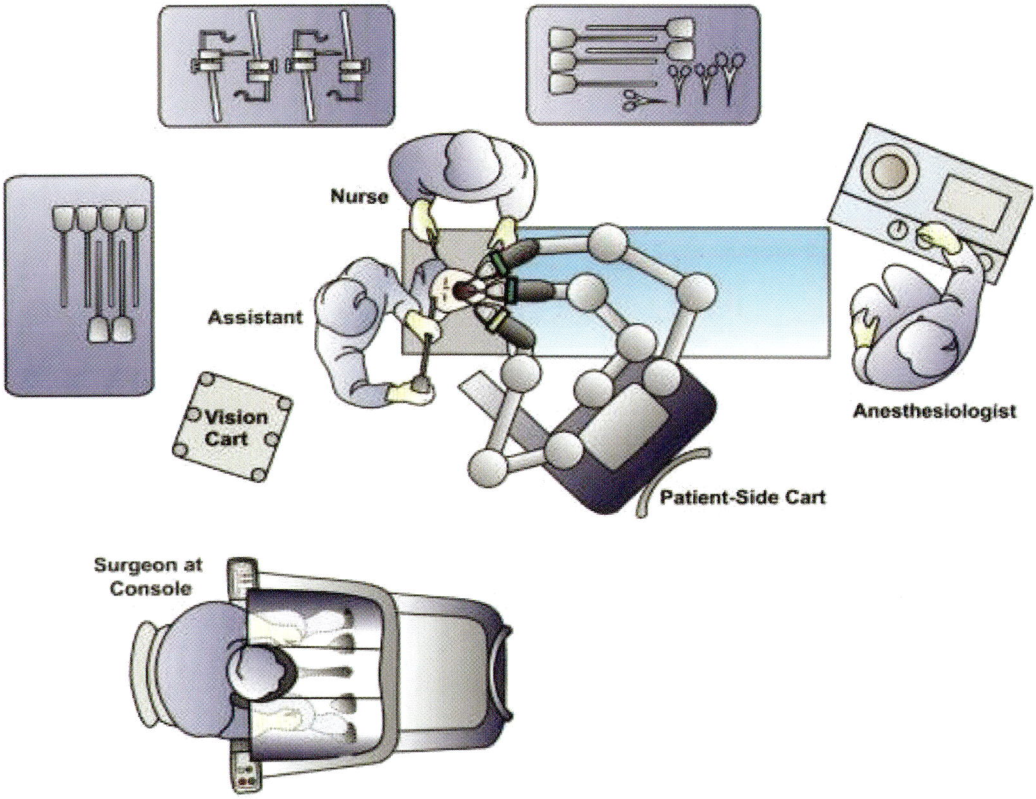

Figure 12. Operating room setup to maximize space utilization and room efficiency. Credit: © 2010 Intuitive Surgical, Inc.

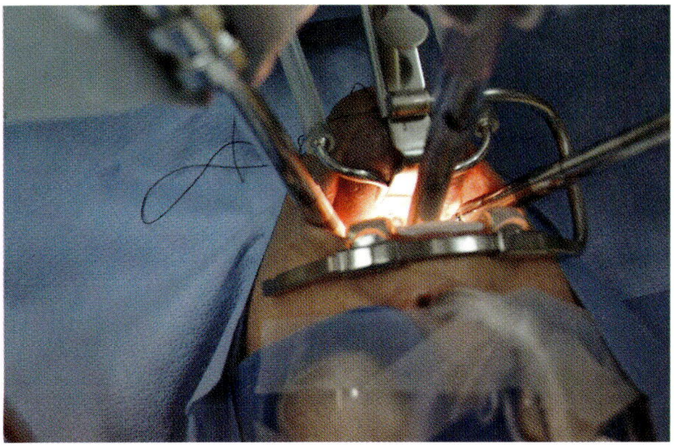

Figure 13. Proper placement of the mouth gag with the arrangement of the transoral robotic surgery instruments.

tongue blades, needle driver and 2-0 silk (tongue stitch), gauze (aids in pulling tongue forward), and FRED (fog reduction/elimination device).

Robotic instruments should be placed on a separate table within easy access of the bedside assistant to facilitate quick exchange. Most cases can be performed with

Table 5. Optimal Positioning of Robot

1. OR table to lowest level
2. 180 degree turn with patient's head at foot of bed
3. Robot foot at 30 degree angle from midline axis of bed
4. Drive medial foot of robot to midline axis of bed
5. Instrument cannula can touch oral commissure at fulcrum (thick black line)
6. Use 30 degree scope in up position for tongue base work

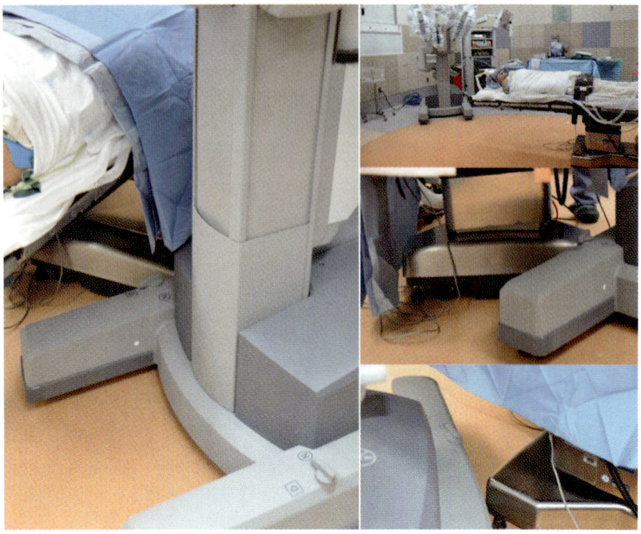

Figure 14. Optimal positioning of the robotic base to maximize movement of robotic arms.

the Maryland dissector and the monopolar cautery alone. However, it is useful to have a Schertel retractor and a needle driver available.

The back table can be used for organization of additional mouth gags (F-K and McGyver), a 0 degree camera, tonsil sponges, Floseal (Baxter), and the measuring device. The measuring device is comprised of a syringe (20–60 cc) half-filled with saline. The scrub nurse records the volume (mL) of saline displaced, which gives us the volume of tissue removed (Figure 15).

Role of Bedside Assistant

The bedside assistant plays a crucial role in the success of any robotic procedure. The following instruments are required for use by a successful assistant: two Bovie bags, two suctions (straight and baby oral), suction cautery, bipolar cautery, and hemoclips (medium). The successful bedside assistant needs to be able to anticipate and implement retraction and control bleeding with hemoclips and handheld suction cautery. The assistant can facilitate placement of a tongue stitch, assist in tongue retraction during gag placement, and should be facile with changing robot instruments and camera.

TORS Procedure: Lingual Tonsillectomy

Typically, access for lingual tonsillectomy is obtained using the Davis-Meyer mouth gag (typically blade 1 or 2). A tongue stitch is used to retract tongue during gag placement. The monopolar is set at 30 J and a Maryland dissector is placed in the opposite operating arm. The bedside assistant retracts with baby oral suction

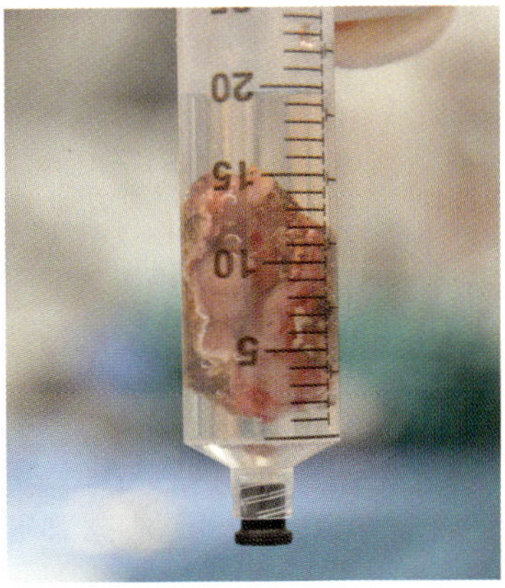
Figure 15. Measurement of tongue base tissue removed by water displacement.

and straight suction. Suction cautery and hemoclips are available to the bedside assistant.

The procedure begins with an initial horizontal cut with monopolar cautery just posterior to the distal end of the tongue blade. This will create an edge that can then be grasped by the Maryland retractor. The incision is subsequently deepened broadly and the plane of dissection should develop toward the vallecula. Many times it is helpful to divide the lingual tonsil mass vertically in the midline. This technique, described by Vicini et al.,[17] allows for better visualization as one approaches the epiglottis and vallecula. The right and left lingual tonsil specimens should be removed separately. A surgical technician measures the volume of tissue removed using displacement technique (Figure 15). Bleeding is typically minimal. As one enters the vallecula branches of the superior laryngeal artery course in the pharyngoepiglottic fold, branches of the dorsal lingual artery may enter near the hyoid and lateral tongue. Though uncommon, if these are encountered, they should be clipped 3 times proximally and 2 times distally. To ensure hemostasis, I often will place Floseal (Baxter) on the wound for 5 minutes and then carefully rinse away the excess before extubation.

In some cases, lingual tonsillectomy is followed by epiglottoplasty. The upper third of the suprahyoid epiglottis is removed using either monopolar cautery or laser (Figure 16).

The epiglottis is held with the Maryland retractor and divided vertically in the midline. A right angle cut is then made both to the right and left, removing the upper portion of the suprahyoid epiglottis. Caution should be exercised when working close to the endotracheal tube (ETT) with the monopolar or the laser. I do not use the laser in this area because there is not a laser-safe ETT that can be placed transnasally. Moist neuro ray pledgets are placed over the ETT and PaO_2 is run at <30% when working around the epiglottis. Troublesome bleeding from the superior laryngeal artery can be controlled with clips or cautery.

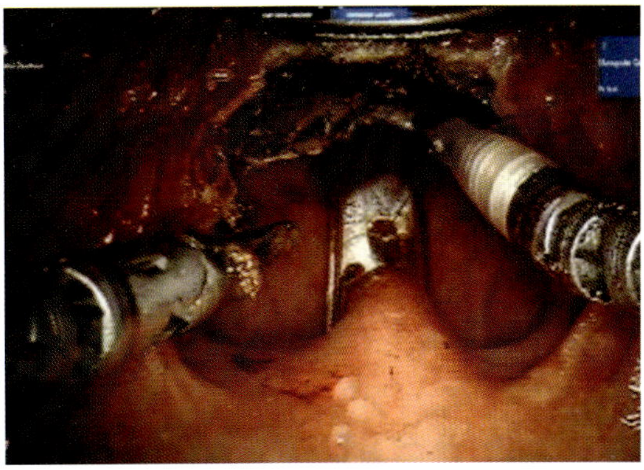
Figure 16. Removal of the upper third suprahyoid epiglottis.

Allow us to make a few comments and offer some advice about performing a successful lingual tonsillectomy. The volume of tissue required for success is of upmost importance. Vicini has determined that between 5 cc and 20 cc of tissue should be removed for success. Seven cubic centimeters is typically described as more than an adequate amount in the average patient.

Another important consideration is positioning of the instrument trocar fulcrum (wide black line) at the oral commissure (Figure 13). By retracting the oral commissure with the trocar, this will facilitate adequate exposure.

With the Davis-Meyer blade in the proper position, the epiglottis is typically hidden by a mound of hypertrophic lingual tonsil tissue. In some cases, the epiglottis can be initially visualized by lifting the lingual tonsil using oral suction.

It is also important to avoid mucosal excision in glosso-tonsillar sulcus as it transitions from lingual to palatine tonsils, as this can result in troublesome cicatricial webbing. Patients will experience dysphagia as food catches in this neo-sulcus.

Non-TORS Procedures Performed Concurrently

There has been some reluctance in the literature to combine multilevel surgery into one procedure due to concern about airway obstruction in the postoperative period. In our experience and in that of many others in the literature, the degree of airway compromise due to pharyngeal, tongue, or laryngeal edema has been negligible. To prevent untoward edema, all patients are treated with perioperative steroids and antibiotics. Multilevel surgery may include some or all of the following:

Nasal procedures:

1. Turbinate reduction (radio-frequency ablation (RFA))
2. Septoplasty

Oropharyngeal procedures:

1. Tonsillectomy
2. Uvulopalatopharyngoplasty (UPPP)
3. Lateral pharyngoplasty
4. TORS

Laryngeal procedure:

1. Epiglottoplasty

If inferior turbinates are enlarged or obstructive septal deviation is present, corrective procedures during DISE can be performed. If this was not done at the time of DISE, nasal procedures can be performed with the patient under monitored anesthesia care (MAC) just prior to intubation. RFA cannot be done safely or effectively with the ETT in the nose. It is preferable to perform oropharyngeal procedures after the TORS lingual tonsillectomy and epiglotoplasty are complete, unless massive palatine tonsils hinder access to the hypopharynx.

Airway Management

Airway management in TORS patients can be divided into intra-operative and postoperative management. Patients undergoing TORS all have moderate to severe OSA and the associated difficult airway. The primary concerns intra-operatively are establishing the airway and keeping the operative field clear to allow unobstructed access for the surgeon. Postoperative concerns are primarily airway edema, bleeding, and sedation that may precipitate an acute airway obstruction.

The decision to use oral or nasal intubation, and even tracheostomy, varies among surgeons. This author prefers trans-nasal (TN) intubation in virtually all cases involving base of tongue or supra-glottic larynx. By performing TN intubation, the endotracheal tube does not have to be manipulated by the bedside assistant, thereby decreasing exposure to inadvertent extubation or airway fire. If the use of laser (CO_2 or thulium) is anticipated, one can use TN intubation. However, there are no laser-safe TN tubes available. Should laser be used, careful placement of saline-soaked neuro ray paddies and coordination with anesthesia to keep inspired O_2 under 30% are necessary safety measures. Transoral intubation using a Laser-flex tube is an alternative. Laser is not necessary for lingual tonsillectomy or epiglottectomy in the authors' view. Tracheostomy is not necessary, but did allow early investigators the opportunity to advance TORS in the safest setting for the patient. If tracheostomy is performed, patients are typically decannulated within a week. To optimize the airway for extubation, all patients are given Decadron (8–10 mg IV) intra-operatively; this is continued every eight hours during their hospital stay.

The timing of extubation has evolved in our hands over the past 2 years. Initially all patients were kept intubated overnight and extubated the following morning after demonstrating a good cuff leak during expiration. We experienced one adverse event requiring re-intubation (suspected aspiration) following this protocol. After careful post-extubation assessments of the airway using fiberoptic laryngoscopy revealed no edema of the tongue base or epiglottis, we have now moved to extubation in the operating room immediately following surgery and have had no adverse events. Patients continue to be monitored overnight in the surgical intensive care unit (SICU) with continuous cardiopulmonary monitoring. Most are discharged to home on postoperative day one from the SICU.

Discharge Medications

At the time of discharge, patients are given the following medications:

1. Nystatin swish and swallow 100,000 units/cc 5 mL po qid 1 week
2. Roxicet 5/325 (5 mL po q4 prn)
3. Lortab elixir (15 mL po q4 prn)
4. Prednisone (20 mg po qd 1 week)
5. 2% viscous lidocaine (5 mL po q2 prn)
6. Amoxicillin suspension (500 mg po tid 1 week).

Deep Venous Thrombosis and Pulmonary Embolus Prevention

Prevention of deep venous thrombosis (DVT) and pulmonary embolus (PE) is critical. Patients with OSA are typically at moderate to high risk for DVT.[19] All of our patients receive both low subcutaneous heparin (5000 units) and sequential compression devices (SCDs) preoperatively and postoperatively until ready for discharge. As a result of this protocol, we have not had bleeding issues either intraoperatively or postoperatively. Patients requiring anticoagulation (warfarin) or antiplatelet medication clopidogrel (Plavix) must remain off their medication for two weeks after surgery to prevent bleeding complications. Cardiology recommendations may preclude some patients from undergoing TORS.

References

1. Freedman DS, Khan LK, Serdula MK, et al. Trends and correlates of class 3 obesity in the United States from 1990 through 2000. *JAMA.* 2002;288:1758–1761.

2. Burwell CS, Robin ED, Whaley RD, et al. Extreme obesity associated with alveolar hypoventilation: a Pickwickian syndrome. *Am J Med.* 1956;21:811–818.

3. Friedman M, Ibrahim H, Joseph NJ. Staging of obstructive sleep apnea/hypopnea syndrome: a guide to appropriate treatment. *Laryngoscope.* 2004 Mar;114(3):454–459.

4. Lim J, Lasserson TJ, Fleetham J, Wright J. Oral appliances for obstructive sleep apnoea. *Cochrane Database Syst Rev.* 2006 Jan 25;(1):CD004435.

5. Smith S, Lang C, Sullivan K, Warren J. Two new tools for assessing patients' knowledge and beliefs about obstructive sleep apnea and continuous positive airway pressure therapy. *Sleep Med.* 2004 Jul;5(4):359–367.

6. Peppard PE, et al. Prospective study of an association between SDB and HTN. *N Engl J Med.* 2000;342:1378–84.

7. Marin JM, et al. Long-term cardiovascular outcomes in men with OSAHS with or without treatment with CPAP—an observation study. *Lancet.* 2005;365:1046–53.

8. Yaggi HK, et al. OSA as a risk factor for stroke and death. *N Engl J Med.* 2005; 353:2034–41.

9. Pang KP, Woodson BT. Expansion sphincter pharyngoplasty: a new technique for the treatment of OSA. *Otolaryngol Head Neck Surg.* 2007 Jul;137(1):110–14.

10. Vicini C, Dallan I, Canzi P, et al. TORS of the TB in OSAHS: Anatomic considerations and clinical experience. *Head Neck.* 2012 Jan;34(1):15–22.

11. Lopez PP, Stefan B, Schulman CI, Byers PM. Prevalence of sleep apnea in morbidly obese patients who presented for weight loss surgery evaluation: more evidence for routine screening for obstructive sleep apnea before weight loss surgery. *Am Surg.* 2008 Sep;74(9):834–38.

12. Greenburg DL, Lettieri CJ, Eliasson AH. Effects of surgical weight loss on measures of obstructive sleep apnea: a meta-analysis. *Am J. Med.* 2009 Jun;122(6):535–42.

13. Croft CB, Pringle M. Sleep nasendoscopy: a technique of assessment in snoring and obstructive sleep apnoea. *Clin Otolaryngol Allied Sci.* 1991 Oct;16(5):504–9.

14. Kezirian EJ, Goldberg AN. Hypopharyngeal surgery in obstructive sleep apnea: an evidence-based medicine review. *Arch Otolaryngol Head Neck Surg.* 2006 Feb; 32(2):206.

15. Vicini C, De Vito A, Benazzo M, Frassineti S, Campanini A, Frasconi P, Mira E. The nose oropharynx hypopharynx and larynx (NOHL) classification: a new system of diagnostic standardized examination for OSAHS patients. *Eur Arch Otorhinolaryngol.* 2012 Apr;269(4):1297–300. Epub 2012 Feb 19.

16. Campanini A, Canzi P, De Vito A, Dallan I, Montevecchi F, Vicini C. Awake versus sleep endoscopy: personal experience in 250 OSAHS patients. *Acta Otorhinolaryngol Ital.* 2010 Apr;30(2):73–77.

17. Vicini C, Dallan I, Canzi P, et al. Transoral robotic surgery of the tongue base in obstructive sleep apnea-hypopnea syndrome: anatomic considerations and clinical experience. *Head Neck.* 2012 Jan;34(1):15–22. doi: 10.1002/hed.21691. Epub. 2011 Mar 11.

18. Rodriguez-Bruno K, Goldberg AN, McCulloch CE, Kezirian EJ. Test-retest reliability of drug-induced sleep endoscopy. *Otolaryngol Head Neck Surg.* 2009 May; 140(5):646–51.

19. Caprini JA, Arcelus JI, et al. State of the art thromboembolism prophylaxis. *Scope.* 2001;8:228–240.

Appendix: How to Get Started in a TORS Program

Identify a colleague with similar interest in robotic surgery. This colleague will provide an eager partner as you begin your training in robotic surgery. Early in your experience, you will find it very helpful to share cases with one partner acting as console surgeon and the other as bedside assistant. Both will learn room setup details and, more importantly, the intricacies of positioning the robot.

Attend robotics courses as recommended by your Intuitive representative. In the past, these courses have included a live pig lab at one of the Intuitive training sites, followed by a Masters level cadaver course typically hosted by high-profile TORS surgeons.

Studies have been done looking at outcomes in the training of successful TORS surgeons. The number of cases performed in the first months after training is predictive. Students with an active partner are more successful. Use Intuitive data.

Talk with OR administration and secure TORS block time.

In addition, you will need a surgical technician and/or nurse dedicated to lead a TORS team.

Begin to schedule sleep endoscopy on patients you are considering for TORS. There is a fair amount of education necessary for the anesthesia team to keep this consistent.

Your hospital will have its own credentialing protocol for robotic cases. Most hospitals will have ironed out this protocol with their urologists and ob/gyn surgeon. Most hospitals require surgeons to have three cases proctored before granting privileges. Proctors are identified by Intuitive and are available to facilitate this process. More information can be found on their web site http://www.intuitivesurgical.com.

I would highly recommend committing time early in your TORS career to visit other institutions to learn from your colleagues. Every surgeon has a different approach. You will be a better surgeon if you spend the time to amalgamate the shared experience of your fellow surgeons. You will find surgeons happy to share their experience with you as I have with my mentors (Drs. O'Malley, Weinstein, Magnusson, Vicini, and Montevecchi).

TORS surgeons are on the forefront of head and neck surgery. I would encourage all surgeons who are beginning TORS to consider becoming active in clinical research as we seek to establish the efficacy of these techniques among a broad population. (Clinical Trials at UAB, UPenn).

Marketing is an important component of building a TORS practice. For OSA, your relationship with local sleep labs is of paramount importance. With the acceptance of surgery by local pulmonologist/sleep specialists as an alternative to CPAP, you will steadily build your experience with both sleep endoscopy and TORS. As your experience and confidence grow, the hospital or your practice can explore television, radio, and print marketing. Mailings to referring doctors to introduce TORS as a viable new option for patients with OSA can be helpful. Direct marketing to patients is very effective, but can be expensive and is best developed as part of a robotics program at your hospital.

Chapter Fifteen

Head and Neck Cancer

Jan A. Akervall, MD

Introduction

Since the Veterans Affairs trial by Wolf and others,[1] the European Organization for Research and Treatment of Cancer (EORTC),[2] and RTOG 91-11[3] studies, primary concomitant chemoradiation has been the main treatment for head and neck cancer (HNC), especially in the anatomic subsites of the oropharynx, pharynx, and larynx. These three studies compared chemotherapeutic and radiation protocols with traditional open surgery followed by radiation. The studies showed better results with regards to organ preservation and similar outcomes with regards to overall survival. However, in none of these studies was minimally invasive surgery offered to patients, which is the surgical equivalent to organ preservation. Instead, traditional open, radical resections and neck dissections were offered, since that was considered the gold standard at the time.

Open approaches to head and neck cancers, e.g., via mandibular swing or through transcervical procedures, have been the only accepted surgical alternatives in HNC treatment until very recently. These procedures were followed by reconstructive efforts using regional flaps, e.g., pectoralis major and, more lately, free tissue transfer, predominantly radial forearm flaps. Open head and neck surgery, even though seen as a standard of care, carries significant downsides with regards to OR time; necessity for large, multidisciplinary teams; long rehabilitation; and often results in poor functional outcome.

Minimally invasive head and neck surgery, on the other hand, is faster and easier for the patient and the surgeon, and rehabilitation of swallowing and speech functions is much better. Traditional head and neck surgeons have argued that margins are compromised with minimally invasive surgery, but outcomes data now clearly show that this is not the case. In head and neck surgery, close proximity of the tumor to the carotid artery or the prevertebral fascia is often the limiting factor with respect to clear margins, but that does not differ whether the surgeon approaches the tumor through the neck or transorally.

As a surgeon, you can skeletonize these structures with both techniques. Transoral laser or robotic surgical techniques have now developed into a paradigm shift in head and neck surgery, and every progressive head and neck program in the country is currently adding transoral resections to their repertoire. For those of us who have been in the game for a long time, this comes as no surprise. When Professor Steiner, from Göttingen, Germany, first presented his outcomes data based on a large series of patients operated on with transoral laser resections, he was heavily criticized for compromising basic surgical principles, e.g., piecemealing the tumor by cutting through it in order to get it out through the endoscope. However, his long-term survival results were the same or better than results from traditional open surgical resections.[4] So for everyone who watched him operate and saw his patients start eating the first postoperative day, the future choice of surgical technique was obvious.

Significant progress has been made with regards to these surgical techniques over the last decades, and these treatment options are finally having some significant outcomes on the management of HNC. The endoscopic CO_2 laser was introduced for the larynx in the 1970s. As mentioned above, Steiner took the technique to the next level in the 1980s and 1990s with regard to oropharynx and pharynx. Since then, endoscopic removals of HNC have slowly taken head and neck surgery in a new direction. In many institutions that have adapted these techniques, we now see less need for large resections using an external approach and fewer free flaps. Shorter hospital stays, less need for feeding tubes, fewer tracheostomies, and better functional outcomes have made the switch easier, even though most institutions still rely heavily on major surgeries and reconstructive alternatives. Recently, Weinstein and O'Malley introduced robotic-assisted transoral resections that have given medical professionals who never originally jumped on the endoscopic train an option to secure a shortcut to minimally invasive surgery for mainly oropharynx cancers.

The discussion has intensified now that we see more and more HPV-related squamous cell HNC and subsequently younger patients without a history of smoking and drinking. These patients have a much-improved prognosis (85–90% 5-year survival vs. 65% as was the case in RTOG 91-11) and do better during treatment, since their performance status is much higher than traditional HNC patients. With better prognoses comes the dilemma of whether it is possible to scale down the aggressiveness of treatment. For instance, it may be that if primary surgery is chosen and favorable pathologic findings from the resection are present, chemotherapy and adjuvant radiation may not be necessary. Obviously, this would be dependent upon clear margins in the primary site and no extra capsular spread in the lymph nodes.

In this chapter, we will build on the technical introduction to transoral robotic surgery (TORS) that previous chapters have given. We will also expand the discussion into the pros and cons with the three dominating organ preservation options for oropharynx, pharynx, and larynx: chemoradiation, transoral laser microsurgery (TLM), and TORS.

Paradigm Shift

Prior to the current era of chemoradiation as the main treatment for oropharynx and larynx HNC, radical, but also disruptive, surgery and adjuvant radiation dominated. These major procedures could involve removal of the tongue base, mandible, and the neck lymphatics in one piece or leave large defects in the pharynx that needed to be reconstructed. After years where regional flaps, predominantly pectoralis major and, to some extent, latissimus dorsi and trapezuis flaps, were the work horses, more sophisticated and versatile free flaps became popularized. The radial forearm flap dominated for many years, and recently antero-lateral thigh flaps have gained popularity since the size can easily be personalized and donor site morbidity is less of an issue.

However, even with the introduction of these improved reconstructive alternatives, patients still had, and still have, suboptimal functional outcomes in many surgical scenarios. Reconstructing the pharynx with free flaps improved cosmetic and also functional outcomes, but the basic dilemma remained—any external approach to the pharynx involves disruption of normal structures, including but not limited to constrictor and other deep musculatures of the neck. In addition, external surgical approaches to the neck disrupt the normal sensory nerve functions of the pharynx. Subsequently, the procedure carries a 35% risk for chronic aspiration.

Chemoradiation changed that to some extent and gave patients hope for preserving the larynx and swallowing function. However, as time has passed and with improved survival rates thanks to the current increased incidence of HPV rather than smoking- and drinking-related tumors, the significant side effects, e.g., dysphagia and xerostomia, and the extended treatment time with often lengthy leave of absence for patients have prompted a discussion about whether the degree of aggressiveness in treatment can be scaled down. The introduction of intense modulated radiation therapy (IMRT), often in conjunction with concomitant chemotherapy, has certainly reduced side effects and improved prognostic outcomes, but we are still looking for ways to speed up treatment times and shorten rehabilitation.

Subsequently, when the minimally invasive techniques, described briefly above, were introduced and accepted, they certainly made an impact on HNC treatment. At first, small tumors of the larynx and oropharynx were operated upon, but as time passed larger and larger cancers have been successfully removed with improved functional outcomes. TLM for the larynx seemed to be easier to accept, but Steiner's transoral approach to larger oropharyngeal, supraglottic, and hypopharyngeal cancers was a much harder concept to accept for many institutions during the 1990s. There are many reasons for this; we have already mentioned the difficulties surgeons had in accepting the concept of piecemealing the tumor during resection. Another issue has been how to control the margins with somewhat limited visibility through an endoscope. Many surgeons seem to be resistant to trying alternative methods of head and neck surgery other than those for which they were trained.

With the introduction of TORS for HNC and its FDA approval in 2010, a minimally invasive alternative became available for all the head and neck surgeons who had never added TLM to their therapeutic arsenal. TLM is harder to learn and quite time consuming to incorporate into a practice, but TORS offers a leap in technology that had and still has an instant and profound impact on the acceptance for transoral resections in institutions all over the world. TORS, using the da Vinci/Intuitive equipment and techniques, is so intuitive that a well-trained head and neck surgeon can pick up and implement the technique after only a few training sessions.

We will discuss in more depth the differences and similarities between these two new minimally invasive surgical techniques for HNC in this chapter. As mentioned above, the prognosis is improving dramatically for the head and neck cancer population, thanks to HPV, which carries a much better response rate to radiation-based treatment. Subsequently, more focus needs to be on the issue of lowering morbidity. It is harder to accept significant lifelong side effects from therapies when you know the disease is not that difficult to cure anymore. Maybe chemotherapy should be skipped in certain cases, since HPV tumors are more radio sensitive than the alcohol- and tobacco-induced cancers on which the chemoradiation studies, e.g., RTOG 91-11, were based. Functionally superior curative minimally invasive surgical options should be considered more frequently, and postoperatively adjuvant therapy may be minimized. We might see reduced radiation fields and even reduced doses in the future, or these adjuvant therapies may be skipped altogether. A full treatment course of chemoradiation takes at least 7 weeks, with an additional 2–6 months of healing. Minimally invasive transoral head and neck surgery takes a few hours, and patients eat and drink the next day and heal from postoperative soreness within 1–2 weeks.

Transoral Laser Microsurgery

Since the early 1970s when CO_2 laser resections for the larynx gained popularity, regular direct laryngoscopy instruments have been used. Visualization through these rather narrow scopes is normally not a problem, unless the tumors are large, e.g., large T2 and higher T-stages. In the 1980s and 1990s, Steiner developed the technique further, and larger tumors of larynx, pharynx, and oropharynx became the target for transoral laser microsurgery (TLM).[5] From supraglottis and up to the oropharynx, the Steiner TLM set by Storz is the preferred method (Figure 1).

The short and long distention scopes work well for large tumors in the supraglottis/hypopharynx and oropharynx, respectively. Tumors up to 5 cm can be resected in one piece, and larger tumors can be piecemealed before being brought out through the endoscope. With the surgical microscope and the suction cautery instruments, visualization is adequate and hemostasis well controlled. The set also has left and right clip appliers required for bigger bleeders, especially those in the deep tongue base and lateral pharyngeal wall (branches off of the lingual and carotid arteries). Separate dissectors can be used to free up these vessels before clipping them. Retractors with suction channels for smoke evacuation from the CO_2 laser are useful for retraction that is essential for laser resections, just as they are essential for open surgeries.

A big advantage of TLM is that it can be performed without an assistant, but with an experienced OR technician. Any surgical problems are handled as you go, just like open surgeries. For example, the surgeon does not need to rely on an assistant to control sudden and large intra-operative bleedings from the pharynx, as is the case for TORS. This creates independence for the surgeon, making preoperative scheduling and intra-operative logistics easier. Another advantage of TLM is the tactile feedback the surgeons enjoy. An Aquaplast mouth guard should be used

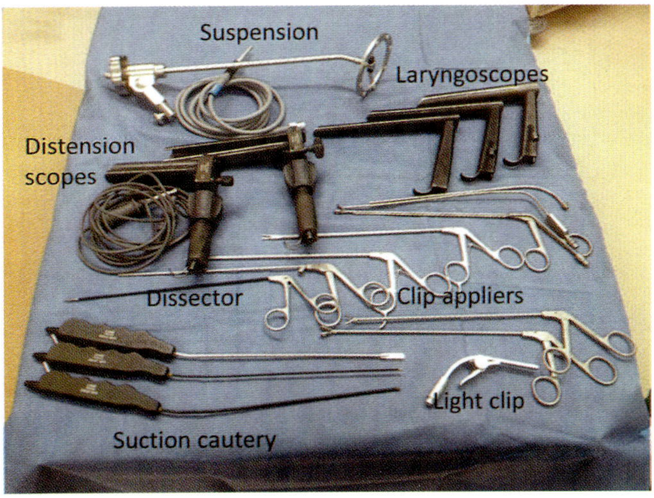

Figure 1. The Steiner set by Storz offers a wide variety of endoscopes, including several laryngeal scopes and two distension scopes for supraglottis and oropharynx. Left and right vessel clip appliers and suction cautery instruments are critical to TLM. In addition, graspers with smoke evacuation channels and left and right dissectors are also available.

to protect the teeth during the procedure, and standard laser precautions observed (ventilation for room air, wet eye patches, and facial towels).

Energy levels of 5–7 W are standard for surgery on the tongue but can and should be decreased when approaching the lateral pharyngeal wall and the large vessels of the neck. A 0.8 mm spot size of the CO_2 laser is recommended for optimal cutting capacity, but the spot size can certainly be increased in order to cause more carbonization and thus cauterization of the small to midsized blood vessels. The suction cautery should be used as both retractor and for hemostasis. The right foot of the surgeon can thus move seamlessly between the foot paddle of the laser and suction cautery.

For optimal visualization through the rather narrow space of the endoscope, the tumor should be flipped back and forth to provide the best possible sense of depth and anatomic relations. The CO_2 laser causes minimal thermal damage, which is an advantage over conventional Bovie. The consequence is significant; when working close to the epiglottis or larynx, mucosal edema can slow down the postoperative extubation process, which in turn can slow down recovery time. After TLM, the patient is normally intubated overnight, but not tracheotomized, and then is extubated the next morning if no bleeding or mucosal edema has been observed. A simple leak test, i.e., deflating the cuff and listening for air leak, is sufficient to make the extubation decision. If no mucosal swelling was observed intraoperatively, and the leak test on postoperative day 1 is positive, extubation can be performed without any risks.

A major disadvantage of TLM is the poor ergonomic position of the surgeon. The arms are raised, often for many hours, and sometimes the body position is compromised due to difficult anatomic circumstances (stiff neck, anterior larynx, etc.).

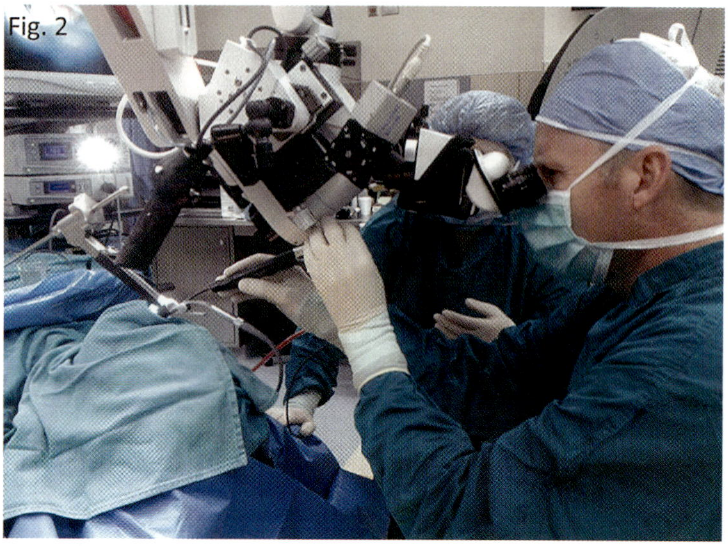

Figure 2. An example of transoral laser microsurgery, which is done by a single surgeon with a surgical technician, who can follow the surgery on a screen or with binocular vision through the microscope. The surgeon can work with the laser (left hand) and the suction cautery (right hand) simultaneously. The suction cautery can be utilized for retraction as well as hemostasis. Vessels larger than 3 mm have to be controlled by surgical clips.

Surgical Technique

TLM is performed after adequate visualization has been achieved. For larger tumors, the entire tumor cannot be visualized without moving the scope and the microscope, even though the distension scopes are used. Therefore, the resection has to start from the superior margin and move down. For tongue base, a horizontal cut above the tumor is recommended, into the tongue, to give the surgeon the option of advancing the anterior blade of the endoscope into that cut and, by doing so, dislodging the superior portion of the tumor and starting the process of dissecting around the tumor.

Lateral and medial cuts are made so that the tumor can be manipulated with graspers from side to side, thus exposing the deeper aspects of the tumor and its inferior margin. Margins are taken as the resection moves in an inferior direction, and positive margins should be addressed immediately. Vessels can be dealt with in two major ways—by suction cautery or by clipping them. Suction cautery is used for smaller vessels (3 mm and smaller) and the suction cautery should also be used to palpate the tissue and to retract. Clipping is for larger vessels, and normally the dissectors in the Steiner set are used to isolate vessels before clips are applied and transected.

In the original procedures, as described by Steiner, the tumors are transected or piecemealed. This does not need to be done unless the tumors are extremely bulky (above 5 cm). Steiner described cutting through the tumor and down into the deep margin to better assess the depth of invasion. Alternatively, the surface of the tumor can be resected first since most HNC are exophytic, which will give much better access to the base of the tumor without interfering with the margins. This will be especially useful since it keeps the deep margin intact, which is helpful for the pathologist when he or she receives the main specimen. Piecemealing is fine, but it demands a dedicated pathologist who fully understands where each piece of the tumor is located.

TORS

Despite its relatively short history,[6,7,8] TORS has already had a fundamental impact on HNC surgery. For setup of the OR and the equipment and for basic descriptions of the surgical techniques, see the previous chapter.

For head and neck surgeons who never adopted the more technically challenging TLM, TORS has become the method of choice. According to Weinstein et al., about 93% of patients who are screened for TORS can actually have the surgery. The remaining 7% have to have open procedures due to poor access.[10] Limitations to use of this technique are mainly related to poor access due to the patients' anatomic characteristics, e.g., small oropharynx or mouth, large teeth, and/or stiff neck. Cancers of the oropharynx are the low hanging fruit. The FK (Feyh-Kastenbauer) retractor, by Gyrus, gives good exposure down to the vallecula, but due to restrictions in angling the retractor and the resulting inability to follow the natural tract into the larynx, false cords and endolarynx are better handled with TLM.

For oropharynx, the 30 degree forward, wide-angle 3-D high-definition camera (Ikegami/Panasonic) offers great visualization of the anatomic subunits, including inferior tongue base, vallecula, and lateral pharyngeal walls. For a first-time user,

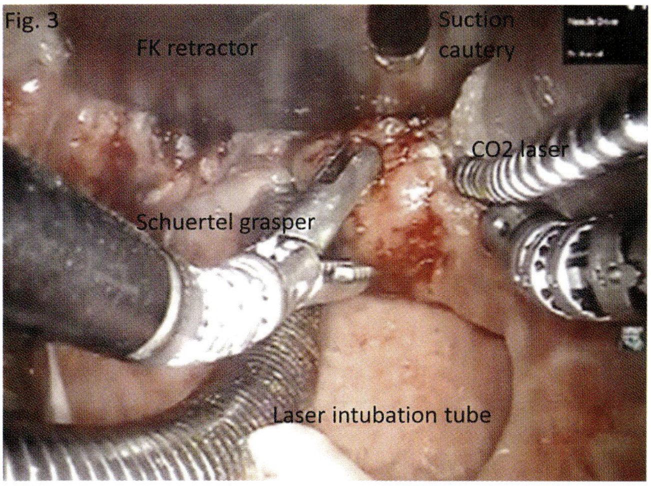

Figure 3. Transoral robotic surgery has become the surgical treatment of choice for oropharynx cancer. The surgeon sets up two robotic arms that have surgical instruments and a third arm that carries a 3-D high-definition wide-angle camera. Preferably the 30-degree upward camera should be considered for resections of the tongue base. The FK retractor is in place to provide wide exposure to the oral cavity and oropharynx.

the magnificent visualization is the first step toward "salvation." The second step is when the surgeon experiences the 540 degree movement of the instruments. By using the clutch, the surgeon can easily and completely intuitively reposition the instruments in order to get to basically any part of the oropharynx safely. The video at http://www.veengle.com/v/vSxfb shows a typical tongue base resection.

The only spot that offers serious challenges is the glosso-tonsillar sulcus. This area, if deep and if the oropharynx is small, can be hard to expose due to the above-mentioned limitations of the FK retractor. In such cases as this, the surgeon should have the Steiner TLM set handy and switch over, since the narrow endoscopes used by that technique can penetrate that particular space more efficiently.

The da Vinci system offers a standard Bovie device for cutting, with different blades available. In order to reduce the thermal trauma and to be able to cut more precisely, there are a few options for lasers that can be added to the system (OmniGuide [CO_2] and LISA [thallium] lasers). The OmniGuide CO_2 laser can be clipped onto the needle driver and works relatively well. The cutting is very precise, though, and with energy levels at 10–15 W, the tongue base can be easily resected. The downside is that the surgeon has to hold it as it extends from the driver and the combined driver-laser unit is somewhat clumsy.

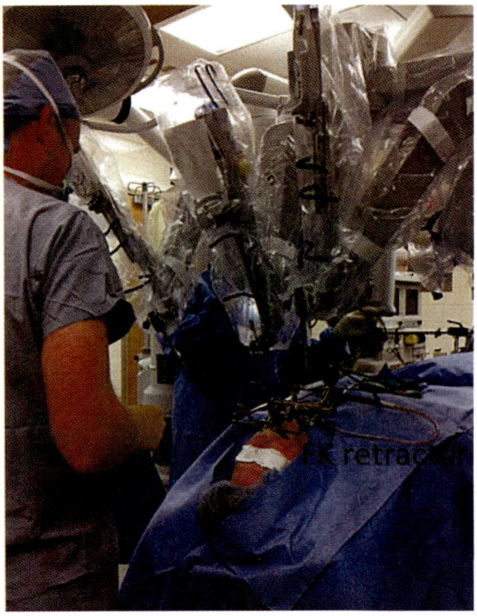

Figure 4. The OmniGuide CO_2 laser can be clipped onto the needle driver. Due to the size of the combined driver-laser device, it takes some experience to learn to maneuver the robotic arm so the tip of the device does not interfere with visualization.

Setup time for TORS procedures is mostly an issue for the first 10–20 cases and becomes shorter and more streamlined as standard procedures are established. Genden et al. reported a drop of setup time from 150 to 20 minutes over the first 20 cases.[9] This is also the case for surgical time. Even though the hand movements are intuitive and quickly become fluent, there is a learning curve to coordinate the work between surgeon, assistant, and the staff in the room.

Margins

During TLM or TORS, margins are best handled by taking them as the surgery moves along instead of waiting until the end of the case. There are two reasons for this. First, there will be 10–30 separate margins to analyze as frozen samples, which is a challenge for the pathologist to handle in a timely fashion. Second, if only a few samples are sent at a time, it is far easier for the surgeon to address the correct anatomic subunit when a frozen sample comes back positive. This saves time and helps the surgeon to plan the resection when he or she verifies that superior margins are negative, then lateral margins are negative, etc., as the procedure moves along.

There is a difference between taking margins with a CO_2 laser and a Bovie. The surgeon needs to excise more tissue with the latter since carbonization is much greater secondary to the thermal trauma. Another advantage with TLM is that the graspers are much finer and more precise margins can be taken. The TORS graspers are still much larger, e.g., Schertel, and, in addition, the lack of haptic/tactile feedback makes it harder to take very precise margins.

Comparison TLM vs TORS

Table 1 offers an overview when TLM and TORS are compared. Either technique is far superior to open procedures, especially with regard to functional outcome. With both techniques, PEG tube and tracheostomy frequencies are significantly lower. In addition, the patients are discharged much faster from the hospital straight to their home.[10]

That being said, there are technical differences between TLM and TORS. Each technique has advantages and disadvantages as discussed previously in this chapter. The main differences are single surgeon (TLM) vs. surgeon + skilled assistant (TORS); wide-angle visualization (TORS) vs. microscopic limited vision (TLM); and tactile feedback (TLM) vs. vision-based feedback (TORS). Switching intra-operatively from one modality to the other can be done in complex cases, e.g., during salvage surgery where tightness of the oropharynx is common after chemoradiation.

Table 1. Comparison of TLM and TORS for Minimally Invasive Surgery

	TLM	TORS
Tactile feedback	Yes	No
Access	Good	Great
Visualization		
Overview	Poor	Superior
Detailed	Superior	Good
Control of bleedings		
Cautery, clips	Yes	Yes
Need for assistant	No	Yes
Instruments (Bovie vs. laser)		
Bovie	No	Yes
Suction cautery	Yes (surgeon)	Yes (assistant)
Laser	Yes (CO_2)	Yes (CO_2, thallium)
Retractors	Yes (wide variety)	Yes (limited options)
Mouth gag	No	Yes (couple of options)
Skilled assistant needed	No	Yes (suction, retraction)
Ergonometric qualities	Poor	Superior
Teaching	Difficult	Easy

Discussion

Minimally invasive head and neck surgery for HNC is here to stay. The two current techniques, TLM and TORS, offer better functional outcome, faster recovery, decreased need for postoperative PEG and tracheostomy tubes, and are less expensive than traditional open surgery with reconstructions.

In this chapter we have discussed why minimally invasive head and neck surgery always should be discussed during the multidisciplinary treatment planning we offer complex, advanced HNC patients. The golden standard of chemoradiation has to be assessed in relation to a surgical option that offers faster recovery and fewer side effects.

Whether to choose TLM or TORS needs to be discussed in detail with our patients when minimally invasive resections are considered. Multidisciplinary conferences and clinics should be the forum for that discussion.

References

1. The Department of Veterans Affairs Laryngeal Cancer Study Group, Wolf G., et al. Induction chemotherapy plus radiation compared with surgery plus radiation in patients with advanced laryngeal cancer. *N Eng J Med.* 1991;324:1685–90.

2. Lefebvre JL, Chevalier D, Luboinski B, Kirkpatrick A, Collette L, Sahmoud T. Larynx preservation in pyriform sinus cancer: preliminary results of a European Organization for Research and Treatment of Cancer phase III trial. EORTC Head and Neck Cancer Cooperative Group. *J Natl Cancer Inst.* 1996;88:890–9.

3. Forastiere AA, Goepfert H, Maor M, et al. Concurrent chemotherapy and radiotherapy for organ preservation in advanced laryngeal cancer. *N Engl J Med.* 2003;27:2091–8.

4. Steiner W, Fierek O, Ambrosch P, Hommerich CP, Kron M. Transoral laser microsurgery for squamous cell carcinoma of the base of the tongue. *Arch Otolaryngol Head Neck Surg.* 2003;129:36–43.

5. Steiner W, Ambrosch P. *Endoscopic Laser Surgery of the Upper Aerodigestive Tract, with Special Emphasis on Cancer Surgery.* New York: Thieme; 2000.

6. Dean NR, Rosenthal EL, Carroll WR, et al. Robotic-assisted surgery for primary or recurrent oropharyngeal carcinoma. *Arch Otolaryngol Head Neck Surg.* 2010 Apr; 136(4):380–4.

7. White HN, Moore EJ, Rosenthal EL, et al. Transoral robotic-assisted surgery for head and neck squamous cell carcinoma: one- and 2-year survival analysis. *Arch Otolaryngol Head Neck Surg.* 2010 Dec;136(12):1248–52. View abstract.

8. Weinstein GS, Quon H, O'Malley BW Jr, Kim GG, Cohen MA. Selective neck dissection and deintensified postoperative radiation and chemotherapy for oropharyngeal cancer: a subset analysis of the University of Pennsylvania transoral robotic surgery trial. *Laryngoscope.* 2010 Sep;120(9):1749–55.

9. Genden EM, Desai S, Sung CK. Transoral robotic surgery for the management of head and neck cancer: a preliminary experience. *Head Neck.* 2009;39:293–99.

10. Weinstein GS, O'Malley BW Jr, Magnuson JS, et al. Transoral robotic surgery: a multicenter study to assess feasibility, safety, and surgical margins. *Laryngoscope.* 2012 Aug; 122(8):1701–7.

Chapter Sixteen

Anesthetic Considerations

James S. DeMeester, MD

Introduction

Minimally invasive surgery has grown enormously over the past twenty years and has brought improved patient outcomes in ways such as decreased morbidity and hospital length of stay. These laparoscopic techniques have become commonplace as has our understanding of their associated anesthetic concerns. The latest iteration of minimally invasive surgery can be seen now in the form of robotic-assisted surgery. This technology enables far more precision and degrees-of-freedom than that provided by conventional laparoscopic approaches.

The da Vinci Surgical System from Intuitive Surgical, Inc., is the most commonly used master-slave robotic system in the United States. The system, FDA approved for use in general surgery in 1997, has now been used for virtually all surgical specialties, including gynecologic, general, cardiac, thoracic, otolaryngology, colorectal, and urologic surgeries. The system is comprised of a robotic cart, a console, and a vision cart. The robotic cart is positioned at the bedside and has up to three articulating instruments and a fourth arm supporting an endoscope. The articulating instruments offer 7 degrees of freedom, as well as fine tremor filtering and motion scaling for precision greater than that of the human hand.

The vision system offers a stereoscopic three-dimensional magnified view. Control for these instruments comes from the surgeon at a console that is typically in the same room as the patient, though this is not required. These improvements exceed the standard capabilities of laparoscopic or thoracoscopic instruments and have allowed for the development of novel surgical approaches to disease that benefit patients in ways such as decreased morbidity and length of hospital stay. With these latest surgical developments, the anesthesiologist is also faced with new perioperative challenges.

Overview of Anesthetic Concerns: General Surgery

Anesthesia for robotic-assisted surgery typically includes longer operating room times, especially during the initial adoption phase of the technology. Anesthesia time is almost always longer given the additional time spent setting up the robotic equipment, patient positioning, and surgical inexperience. The learning curve, however, can be relatively short when compared to learning laparoscopic techniques coming from traditional open approaches.[1] With longer anesthesia times, the need for greater vigilance becomes ever important.

The start of any anesthetic procedure for robotic-assisted surgery includes placement of standard monitors for oxygenation, ventilation, circulation, and temperature. Specifically, these usually include pulse-oximetry, invasive or noninvasive blood pressure monitoring, capnography, and any modality of temperature monitoring. After routine safety checks and operating room (OR) briefings are conducted, a general anesthetic is induced and the airway is secured. The patient is then positioned specific to the particular surgical procedure, as each has its own positioning needs. This almost always includes tucking of both arms at the patient's side. Because of limited access to the patient, at least two intravenous lines are placed for most procedures and extensions are used for lines and monitors, if necessary. Not only does bilateral arm tucking limit patient access, but space limitations of the operating room and the need for proximity of the robotic cart and vision cart at the patient's side mean the anesthesia machine and anesthesiologist are displaced some degree from their usual position immediately at the patient's head. A flexible ventilator circuit is used to allow for increased distance to the patient. When the anesthesia machine is checked out prior to surgery, compliance checks with the circuit extended should be performed. All pressure points are checked and padded and any final positioning is completed. Warming measures are confirmed, including the use of an underbody fluid mattress or forced-air blankets, depending on the surgical exposure and duration.

After a sterile field is created, the robotic cart is brought to the bedside. The arms are brought through their expected range of motion, and the patient is inspected for any signs of potential injury from collision.[2] Muscle relaxation is essential at this time because once an incision is made and the robotic arms are "docked," any patient movement can cause significant injury. The operating room team needs to be adept at rapidly disengaging the robotic arms from the patient in the case of emergencies such as cardiac arrest and in instances of OR fires. For most surgeries, either a pneumoperitoneum or a capnothorax is created after incision to facilitate expansion of the surgical field.

Complications from robotic surgical techniques include many of those associated with laparoscopic techniques. Injury from initial trocar placement and effects of creating a pneumoperitoneum are just some examples. Arrhythmias are possible from increased vagal tone from peritoneal stretching or from severe hypercapnea. Such complications can include several seconds of asystole that only resolves with treatment and alleviation of abdominal insufflation.[3] Gas embolisms, usually venous, can occur from misplacement of an insufflation needle into a vessel or the needle may be inadequately advanced. Effects range from asymptomatic to catastrophic cardiovascular collapse and may be signaled by hypotension and a decrease in end-tidal carbon dioxide levels. Transesophageal echocardiography has been used to study venous gas embolisms and has found them in up to 69% of patients undergoing laparoscopic cholecystectomy, though these events are without significant cardiopulmonary effects.[4] Complications of pneumoperitoneum can be seen in Table 1.[5] Pneumothorax, though deliberately created in cardiothoracic procedures,

Table 1. Intraoperative Complications of Pneumoperitoneum

Vascular Injuries
- Veress needle/trocar insertion: aorta, IVC, iliac vessels, retroperitoneal hematoma

Gastrointestinal
- Veress needle/trocar insertion: small and large bowel, liver and spleen, mesenteric injury

Cardiac arrhythmias
- Hypercarbia
- Reflex increased vagal tone

Subcutaneous emphysema
- Intentional extraperitoneal insufflation: inguinal hernia repair/pelvic lymphadenectomy
- Unintentional: accidental extraperitoneal CO_2 insufflation

Pneumothorax/pneumomediastinum/pneumopericardium
- Embryonic defects
- Diaphragm defects
- Pleural tears
- Emphysematous bullae rupture
- CO_2 embolism

can be an inadvertent complication with abdominal insufflation that may result in severe injury if left unrecognized. Tension pneumothorax has been described with abdominal insufflation, which may result in unexplained increase in peak airway pressures on the ventilator, hypotension, or hypoxemia.[6] This effect may be more likely if higher pressures are used.

Peritoneal insufflation is created for abdominal and pelvic procedures, but for cardiac and thoracic procedures, a capnothorax is oftentimes necessary for retraction of the heart or lungs. Thoracic insufflation pressures range from 8–10 mmHg, in contrast to abdominal pressures that oftentimes approach 20 mmHg. Higher pressures in the hemithorax are unnecessary and poorly tolerated by the patient. Vassiliades showed a significant correlation between central venous pressure (CVP) and wedge pressure, both surrogates for volume status, and cardiovascular performance after CO_2 chest insufflation.[7] Patients with CVP <5 mmHg or wedge pressure <6 mmHg exhibited a dramatic fall in blood pressure and cardiac index. These effects were completely overcome by discontinuing insufflation and volume loading the patient such that CVP exceeded 10 mmHg. Subsequent gradual increases in insufflation up to 12 mmHg were well tolerated.[7] These changes were more pronounced when applied to the right chest as opposed to the left.[8] The effect of insufflation on cardiac output (CO) was determined by preoperative volume status and ejection fraction (EF). Patients with a normal volume status and EF of at least 30% had no significant decrease in cardiac output. In contrast, patients with hypovolemia and/or an EF <30% did not tolerate insufflation >6 mmHg. Such potential for hemodynamic insults justifies the universal use of invasive monitoring for our cardiothoracic procedures. Additional monitors such as a Swan-Ganz catheter or transesophageal echo probe are placed on an individualized basis.

Cardiac

Robotic-assisted minimally invasive cardiac surgery at our institution is mainly comprised of minimally invasive direct coronary artery bypass (MIDCAB) and da Vinci–assisted minimally invasive mitral valve repair. Other procedures, such as left atrial myxoma resection, are also performed with a similar anesthetic technique as that for mitral valve repair. The need to manage long periods of single-lung ventilation with associated hemodynamic compromise from cardiac manipulation makes these procedures the most challenging of all robotic-assisted procedures performed at our institution. An experienced cardiothoracic anesthesiologist with advanced TEE (transesophageal echocardiography) training is a prerequisite.

MIDCAB

Patient selection for MIDCAB has been previously discussed in the chapter describing the surgical technique, but generally consists of the following:

- BMI less than 40 kg/m^2
- Isolated left anterior descending (LAD) lesion with a target amenable to bypassing, or other targets amenable to hybrid procedure with percutaneous coronary intervention (PCI)
- Absence of left-main disease
- Pulmonary reserve sufficient to tolerate one-lung ventilation

In addition to the usual preoperative tests consisting of a coronary angiogram, CXR or CT chest, and carotid ultrasound, all patients also undergo pulmonary function testing. This is performed irrespective of past history, as the ability to tolerate single-lung ventilation is critical to the procedure. An FEV1 of 700 cc and a diffusion capacity (DLCO) greater than 50% is usually adequate to proceed.

Prior to proceeding to the OR, a preoperative evaluation is performed. Available preoperative studies and labs are reviewed and availability of blood is confirmed. The patient is then sedated and invasive monitors are placed. All patients receive a radial arterial line in either the right or left wrist. In addition to a large peripheral IV, a cordis introducer is placed, preferably in the right internal jugular vein under direct ultrasound guidance. Depending on patient comorbidities, a pulmonary artery catheter is placed for determination of cardiac output as well as monitoring pulmonary artery pressures.

After a preoperative check of allergies and patient identity, the patient is brought to the operating room. The patient is moved to the OR table with an underbody mattress warmer in place. Because no cardiopulmonary bypass is planned, maintaining normothermia with a body warmer is essential. This facilitates early extubation and prevents cold-induced coagulopathy. Standard monitors are then placed, and a general anesthetic is induced with a combination of narcotic, midazolam, and propofol or etomidate. Lung isolation is established, usually with a double lumen endotracheal tube or a bronchial blocker placed in the left main stem bronchus. The advantage of a double lumen tube over a bronchial blocker is the ability to

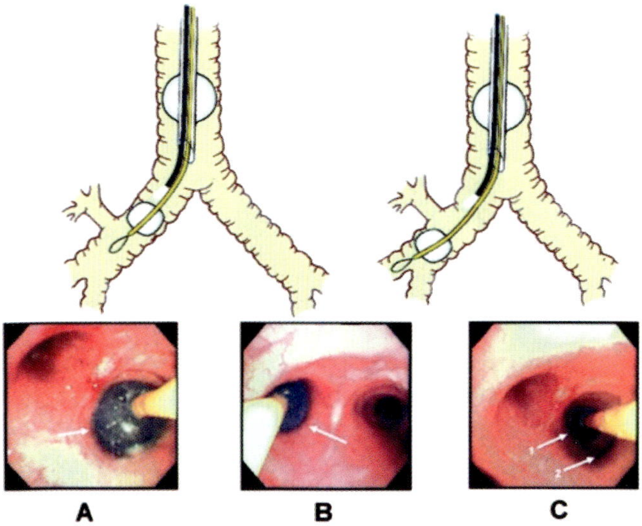

Figure 1. (A) Wire-guided endobronchial blocker (Arndt blocker), the optimal position of the Arndt blocker in the right, (B) the left main stem bronchus; and (C) as a selective lobar blocker when positioned into the bronchus intermedius. Arrow 1 indicates the outer surface of the inflated Arndt blocker cuff. Arrow 2 indicates a free entrance of the right upper lobe bronchus.

independently suction each lung. However, in patients with difficult airways, placement of the stiffer double lumen tube may be challenging, and using a single lumen tube with a bronchial blocker may be safer. Furthermore, a bronchial blocker precludes the need for replacement of the double lumen tube with a single lumen tube prior to transport to the ICU. Positioning is confirmed with broncoscopy. Figure 1 shows the technique of using a bronchial blocker.[9]

After induction and intubation, early lung isolation gives time for atelectasis to form and provides a more favorable operating environment for initial trocar placement. It also presents an opportunity to gauge tolerance to OLV and ensures proper placement before commencement of the procedure. If done prior to patient positioning, adequate lung isolation should be reconfirmed with broncoscopy. A one-lung ventilation strategy can been seen in Table 2.[10]

Patient positioning is accomplished with the left arm draped below the plane of the table in a fashioned "sling," so that the right robotic arm has unimpeded range of motion. Padding between the table and the arm is important to prevent ulnar neuropathy, and the shoulder and arm are inspected for excessive brachial plexus stretch. Occasionally, a roll is placed under the left scapula to rotate the chest to the right. External defibrillation pads are placed and neuromuscular blockade is confirmed prior to positioning the robot at the patient's side. A TEE probe is placed to provide additional cardiovascular monitoring. Preoperative evaluation of ventricular function can be compared to that at the time of LAD occlusion and at the conclusion of the procedure. This is also a direct monitor of preload and contractility.

Table 2. One-Lung Ventilation Strategy

1. Use FiO_2 of 100%
2. Use pressure control ventilation trying to keep plateau pressure <30 cm H_2O
3. Adjust minute ventilation such that $PaCO_2$ approximates 40 mmHg
4. Check arterial blood gas
5. Apply continuous positive airway pressure to nonventilated lung
6. Apply positive end-expiratory pressure to ventilated lung

Prior to incision, volume status is augmented and the left lung is isolated in anticipation of CO_2 insufflation. Constant communication between the surgeon and anesthesiologist is important throughout the procedure. Patients who have poor ventricular function or are hypovolemic may not tolerate initial insufflation and this needs to be conveyed to the surgical team while corrective measures are taken.

During the period of internal mammary artery (IMA) takedown, an infusion of nitroglycerin at 10 mcg/min is started to prevent spasm of both the native coronary arteries and the IMA. Norepinephrine is titrated to maintain blood pressure to within 20% of baseline, or as dictated per the surgical conditions. Prior to IMA ligation, heparin is administered and titrated every 15 minutes to an activated clotting time between 225 and 250 seconds. As a final act prior to the robotic approach, a pericardiotomy is performed prior to ligation of the IMA. Next, a mini-thoracotomy is made at the left fifth intercostal space after undocking of the robot and trocar removal. The IMA to the left anterior descending coronary artery (LAD) anastomosis is facilitated by placement of a stabilization device and arterial ligation. During this time, TEE and EKG are used to identify myocardial ischemia. It should be noted, however, that ST analysis might not be accurate in the setting of a capnothorax, as the electrical axis of the heart may have shifted.[11] Hemodynamic instability is uncommon, as a shunt is placed routinely in the LAD during creation of the anastomosis. Should hypotension occur, it is usually treated effectively with crystalloid volume administration and titration of norepinephrine.

One-lung ventilation is continued throughout this entire period until chest closure and final inspection of trocar sites for bleeding. A final TEE interrogation for wall motion and function is performed. Any new wall motion abnormality is communicated to the surgeon, which might prompt reexamination of the anastomosis. Prior to leaving the operating room, the double lumen tube is exchanged to a single lumen tube for safety. ICU personnel are not accustomed to the management of double lumen tubes and leaving them in place can lead to additional morbidity. The patient is then brought to the ICU sedated, but prepared for early extubation.

Minimally Invasive Mitral Valve Repair

The first robotic-assisted mitral valve repair performed in the United States was in 2000 by Chitwood et al., at East Carolina University.[12] Prior to this, "minimally invasive" meant smaller thoracotomy incisions with thoracoscopic instruments. The change to robotics and an almost completely "closed" chest required further modification of conventional cross-clamp and cardioplegia delivery strategies to the periphery and a reliance on the anesthesiologist to a greater extent for placement of these peripherally placed devices.

Candidates for minimally invasive mitral valve repair (MIMVR) must be able to tolerate prolonged periods of one-lung ventilation (OLV) and meet the criteria discussed previously. Because the combination of a capnothorax, elevated ventilation pressures, and hypercarbia during OLV is likely to precipitate hemodynamic instability, patients with severe pulmonary hypertension or right ventricular dysfunction are not candidates. Likewise, severe left ventricular dysfunction is also a contraindication. Preoperative testing for MIMVR includes those used for MIDCAB, in addition to routine preoperative echocardiography and CT angiogram. A preoperative echo describes mitral valve pathology for the surgeon for preoperative planning. It also, in addition to the CT angiogram, evaluates for severe aortic atheromatous disease, which increases risk for plaque embolism with femoral cannulation or deployment of an endovascular balloon cross-clamp.

The anesthetic approach to mitral valve repair is more complex than for MIDCAB procedures. Cardiopulmonary bypass (CPB) is used and additional monitors and vascular access lines are required. Our surgeons prefer a balloon endovascular aortic clamp (EndoClamp by Edwards Lifesciences) to conventional aortic clamping, and also retrograde cardioplegia delivered via an EndoPlege (Edwards Lifesciences) coronary sinus catheter placed via an introducer in the right internal jugular vein. The patient is first seen in the preoperative holding area and sedated for bilateral arterial line placement. A large peripheral IV is placed in the left arm. In the operating room, a general anesthetic is induced after preoxygenation with fentanyl, midazolam, and isoflurane. A muscle relaxant is given and one-lung ventilation is established. A TEE exam is then performed in order to confirm mitral valve pathology and to evaluate ascending aortic dimensions and pathology. Ascending aorta dimensions >40 mm and mobile or protruding atheroma >5 mm are contraindications for EndoClamp use. The atrial septum is interrogated for a patent foramen ovale, which the femoral venous cannula and coronary sinus catheters can both easily traverse.

It is important at this time to also rule out a persistent left superior vena cava. Retrograde cardioplegia in this setting will be ineffective. Finally, the coronary sinus is found in multiple views. The right neck is prepped and two guide wires are placed under ultrasound guidance. A cordis introducer is inserted over the more distal guide wire in Seldinger fashion, so that an EndoPlege catheter can be placed. This is guided into the coronary sinus using both live fluoroscopy and echocardiography. Care is taken to place the catheter in the distal coronary sinus so that the cardioplegia solution spreads uniformly through the myocardium. Figure 2 shows correct placement of the EndoPlege catheter.[13] A 3-D echo view of the EndoPlege catheter coming from the SVC (top left corner), passing a patent foramen ovale, and entering the coronary sinus away from the viewer is shown in Figure 3.

Next, a 16–20F superior vena cava bypass cannula is placed over the second guide wire next to the existing EndoPlege catheter. This is sized according to patient

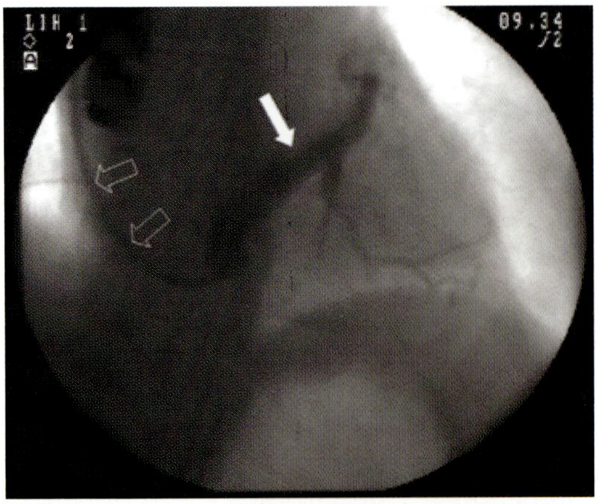

Figure 2. Correct placement of the EndoPlege catheter. The solid arrow points to contrast filling the coronary sinus, and the hollow arrows show the course of the EndoPlege catheter.

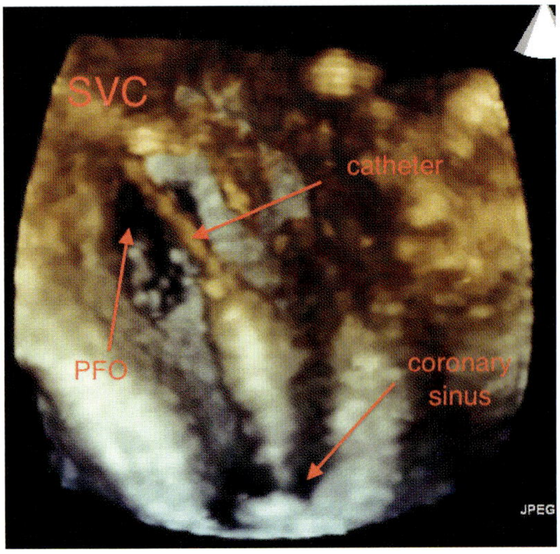

Figure 3. A 3-D echo view of the EndoPlege catheter coming from the SVC (top left corner), passing a patent foramen ovale, and entering the coronary sinus away from the viewer.

anatomy and body mass index. Although drainage on cardiopulmonary bypass can be successful with only femoral cannulation, inadequate decompression hinders adequate surgical exposure and leaves the potential for SVC compression from the left atrial retractor. Central venous pressure (CVP) is generally transduced off the introducer side-port and monitors for cerebral venous congestion, in addition to volume status. External defibrillator pads are placed, followed by positioning of the patient to the right of the operating room table with the right arm hanging in a "sling" below the plane of lie. The pelvis may be "bumped" so that it angles to the left, exposing the right groin for venous and arterial cardiopulmonary bypass cannulation. The surgeon determines the location of the port access sites, the heart is exposed, and the pericardium incised. Heparin is administered according to our protocol, followed by advancement of the venous cannula guided by TEE. Figure 4 shows a bicaval view with the IVC on the left and the cannula (arrows) being advanced into the SVC/RA junction.[13]

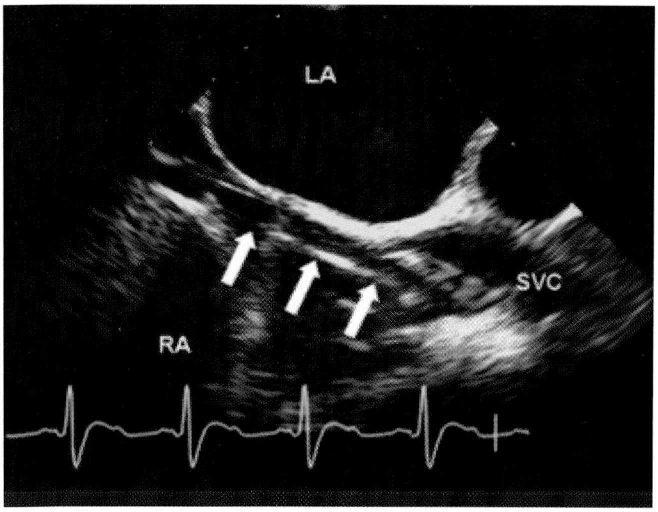

Figure 4. Bicaval view with the IVC on the left and the cannula (arrows) being advanced into the SVC/RA junction.

The arterial cannula is then placed, followed by initial placement of the Endo-Clamp. This serves as a mechanism both to enable "cross-clamping" of the aorta by balloon occlusion and delivery of antegrade cardioplegia. Once cardiopulmonary bypass is initiated, the EndoClamp is fully inflated. This critical process takes several minutes to accomplish successfully. Live TEE ensures that the balloon is seated properly in the proximal ascending aorta. During full cardiopulmonary bypass, the anesthesiologist must continually monitor for balloon excursion into the coronary sinus, as this could prevent cardioplegia delivery down the coronary arteries and prevent adequate myocardial protection. Likewise, balloon excursion into the arch can occlude the innominate artery and result in cerebral hypoperfusion and neurologic injury. TEE is unable to image the arch at this level, so the right radial arterial pressure is evaluated for a fall in pressure. Any deviation in pressure between both right and left radial arteries is cause for reexamination of the balloon location.

Prior to termination of the CPB, TEE is used to evaluate the mitral valve for function and any residual regurgitation. The left ventricular outflow tract is inspected for systolic excursion of the mitral valve, causing a dynamic flow obstruction, otherwise known as systolic anterior motion (SAM). The ventricles are also inspected for intracardiac air. Although with robotic cardiac surgery there is no direct way to remove intracardiac air, the use of CO_2 insufflation in the hemithorax tends to displace the air that does enter the cardiac chambers. Large breaths are given on the ventilator to flush out any residual air in the pulmonary veins. This is typically all that is required in the de-airing process.

One of the benefits of minimally invasive mitral valve repair is improved overall patient satisfaction. However, patients still experience significant postoperative pain[14] that is not significantly different from cardiac surgery with sternotomy.[15] At our institution, because of pain and respiratory insufficiency, patients are brought to the ICU sedated on a propofol infusion and given an IV PCA for postoperative pain control. We typically are able to extubate the majority of our patients within six hours of arrival. Some institutions, however, have become more aggressive in their handling of postoperative pain and perform multiple paravertebral nerve blocks before surgery in conjunction with ketorolac to achieve intraoperative extubation.

Urologic Surgery: Radical Prostatectomy

Robotic-assisted laparoscopic radical prostatectomy (RALP) has become the second most performed robotic-assisted surgery worldwide.[16] Outcome data, such as erectile dysfunction, incontinence, positive margin rate, and transfusion rate, compare favorably with that of laparoscopic or open radical retropubic approaches.[17] Though operative time is usually longer, it can approach that of traditional open surgery once the operator gains experience.

The significant anesthetic concerns surrounding RALP are related to the steep 30–45 degree Trendelenburg (T-burg) position with the use of pneumoperitoneum for surgical exposure. This exaggerated position, in conjunction with increased intra-abdominal pressure, has several physiologic sequelae. The first of these is airway edema. The anesthesia team needs to be judicious about crystalloid volume administration. Though estimating blood loss can be challenging in this position, as shed blood is out of the field of view, RALP has been associated with significantly less blood loss than open procedures. Overzealous volume administration only serves to worsen facial, pharyngeal, and laryngeal edema and may also obscure the operative field during vesico-urethral anastomosis.[18] We typically limit IVF administration to <2000 cc, which has been found to be associated with fewer postoperative complications.

Cerebrovascular effects from T-burg positioning result from an increase in intracranial pressure as a result of transmitted CVP. The head-down position increases CVP, which is compounded by creation of a pneumoperitoneum. In patients with cerebrovascular disease or uncontrolled hypertension, maintenance of cerebral perfusion pressure (mean arterial pressure – [CVP or ICP]) is critical to preventing neurologic compromise.

Another potential neurologic complication is blindness from ischemic optic neuropathy. One such case associated with RALP has been reported in the literature.[19] Injury was attributed to long procedure times in conjunction with excessive fluid administration, resulting in increased CVP and destruction of the perfusion gradient, leading to ischemia.

Respiratory obstacles related to RALP are due largely to the resultant increase in airway pressures from positioning. Not only does atelectasis increase and functional residual capacity decrease, but chest binding, in order to prevent the patient from sliding off the operating table, also reduces chest compliance by as much as 68%.[18] Such physiologic perturbations are particularly relevant to those with lung disease and can be the difference between extubation in the operating room versus delayed extubation in the recovery area. Optimization of lung function, and even consultation with a pulmonologist, should be a priority. Those with severe disease, such as bullous emphysema and severe COPD, are relatively contraindicated. High airway pressures place bullae at risk of rupture, and longer expiratory times necessary for those with severe COPD may not be attainable in a CO_2 insufflation setting, thus also risking pneumothorax.

The hemodynamic effects of RALP not only include elevated CVP, but also increased mean arterial and wedge pressures. These increases are due more from positioning than from peritoneal insufflation and can be two times greater in magnitude from the supine position. Right and left heart stroke work index is also increased, suggesting greater cardiovascular strain that may not be tolerated by patients with compromised cardiac function. As discussed previously, reflex bradycardia and venous gas embolism are also potential complications.

Practical considerations for the positioning of patients for RALP, apart from physiologic concerns, are also of utmost importance. At our institution, tape is used to create an X-like pattern across the shoulders to prevent the patient from sliding off the table. Pressure point and brachial plexus injuries can occur if tape is used in places other than bony prominences, such as the acromio-clavicular joint. This avoids compression of the upper trunk of the brachial plexus and the associated stretch that can occur.[20] Because of the limited access and duration of the procedure, greater vigilance should be given to other pressure points that may result in ulnar or lateral femoral cutaneous nerve injury.

Otolaryngology (ENT)

The adoption of da Vinci robotic assistance in otolaryngology has lagged behind that of other fields. A possible explanation for this is that the da Vinci system was developed primarily with other surgical subspecialties in mind. Adapting this technology to surgeries of the head and neck, with equipment optimized for a larger operating field, has taken time to develop.[21] Despite this, however, there are some procedures where the robotic system has been shown to improve access and visualization, namely for tongue base tumors and supraglottic carcinoma.[22] These are two of the more common procedures performed at our institution, including uvulopalatopharyngoplasty.

The anesthetic implications of robotic head and neck surgery include all of those associated with conventional approaches, with the addition of the more general considerations surrounding robotic surgery as discussed previously. With any ENT procedure, the primary concern of the anesthesiologist is airway control and prevention of airway surgical fire. Prior to delivery of any anesthetic, there is a pre-procedure checklist that includes a discussion of fire risk and preventative measures to be taken. Airway control is discussed, with the surgeon regarding ventilation strategies, type of endotracheal tube required, use of laser instrumentation, need for apneic oxygenation, and any other relevant airway considerations. Other concerns include airway edema, laryngospasm, and airway soiling from bleeding or secretions. Similar to other robotic surgeries, the anesthesiologist is removed from the usual place at the head of the patient. Airway circuit and IV tubing extensions are necessary to provide room for the robotic manipulator at the head of the bed. It is also essential that the patient remain still for the duration of robotic manipulation, as any "bucking" or movement on the part of the patient while the instruments are "docked" can lead to severe injury. This can be accomplished with either a deep level of anesthesia or, more commonly, use of a muscle relaxant. Apart from these concerns, the anesthetic management of otolaryngologic procedures deviates little from traditional procedures.

Conclusion

In this chapter, I have attempted to address the anesthetic concerns most unique to robotic-assisted procedures. Though there are many more surgical uses for the da Vinci Robotic System than what is covered here, most of the salient concerns from an anesthetic planning perspective have been addressed. For example, though gynecologic procedures were not specifically discussed, the anesthetic concerns are very similar to those of urologic surgery. Both use similar steep Trendelenburg positioning, both require creation of a pneumoperitoneum, and resultant cardiopulmonary embarrassment between the two is similar. Furthermore, patient access issues such as vascular access and proximity to airway are nearly universal across all robotic-assisted procedures. Nearly all procedures require displacement of the anesthesia workstation from the patient, and virtually all require bilateral arm-tucking. With the exception of, perhaps, robotic-assisted cardiac surgery, most of the concerns are not novel or foreign, but simply require a higher index of awareness. Robotic surgery in many disciplines has already shown improved metrics with regard to various patient outcomes. Considering that robotic use is still in its infancy, many new and exciting surgical developments surely lie ahead.

References

1. Yohannes P, Rotariu P, Pinto P, et al. Comparison of robotic vs. laparoscopic skills: is there a difference in the learning curve? *Urology.* 2002;60(1):39–45.

2. Parr KG, Talamini MA. Anesthetic implications of the addition of an operative robot for endoscopic surgery: a case report. *J Clin Anesth.* 2002;14:228–233.

3. Reed DN Jr, Nourse P. Untoward cardiac changes during CO_2 insufflation in laparoscopic cholecystectomies in low-risk patients. *J Laparoendosc Adv Surg Tech A.* 1998; 8(2):109–114.

4. Derouin M, Couture P, Boudreault D, et al. Detection of gas embolism by transoesophageal echocardiography during laparoscopic cholecystectomy. *Anes Analg.* 1996; 82:119.

5. Barash PG. *Clinical Anesthesia.* 5th ed. Philadelphia: Lippincott Williams & Wilkins; 2005, 1066.

6. Dawson R, Ferguson CJ. Life-threatening tension pneumothorax during laparoscopic cholecystectomy. *Surg Laparosc Endosc.* 1997;7:271.

7. Vassiliades TA Jr. The cardiopulmonary effects of single-lung ventilation and carbon dioxide insufflation during thoracoscopic internal mammary artery harvesting. *Heart Surg Forum.* 2002;5(1):22–24.

8. Ohtsuka T, Nakajima J, Kotsuka Y, et al. Hemodynamic responses to intrapleural insufflation with hemipulmonary collapse. *Surg Endosc.* 2001;15(11):1327–1330.

9. Campos JH. An update on bronchial blockers during lung separation techniques in adults. *Anes Analg*. 2003;97(5):1266–74.

10. Miller RD, *Miller's Anesthesia*. 7th ed. Philadelphia: Churchill Livingstone; 2010, 2395.

11. Sugantha G. Anaesthesia for minimally invasive cardiac surgery. *Best Pract Clin Anaesthesiol*. 2002;16:63–80.

12. Chitwood WR Jr, Nifong LW, Elbeery JE, et al. Robotic mitral valve repair: trapezoidal resection and prosthetic annuloplasty with the da Vinci surgical system. *J Thor Cardiovasc Surg*. 2000;1171–1172.

13. Rehfeldt, KH, Mauermann WJ, Burkhart HM, et al. Robot-assisted mitral valve repair. *J Cardiothorac Vasc Anesth*. 2011;25(4):721–730.

14. Woo YJ. Robotic cardiac surgery. *Int J Med Robot*. 2006;2:225–232.

15. Cogan J, Lebon J, Rochon A, et al. Pain levels after minimally invasive cardiac surgery: results for the first 7 days. *Anesth Analg*. 2010;110:1–101.

16. *Intuitive Surgica, Inc.*, Sunnyvale, CA, USA. Annual Report 2010.

17. Tewari A, Srivasatava A, Menon M. A prospective comparison of radical retropubic and robot-assisted prostatectomy: experience in one institution. *BJU*. 2003;92:205–210.

18. Danic MJ, Chow M, Gayload A, et al. Anesthesia consideration for robotic-assisted laparoscopic prostatectomy: a review of 1500 cases. *J Robotic Surg*. 2007;1:119–123.

19. Weber ED, Colyer MH, Lesser RL, et al. Posterior ischemic optic neuropathy after minimally invasive prostatectomy. *J Neuro-Opthalmol*. 2007;27:285–287.

20. Phong SVN, Koh LKD. Aneaesthesia for robotic-assisted radical prostatectomy: considerations for laparoscopy in the Trendelenburg position. *Anaesth Intensive Care*. 2007;35:281–285.

21. Maan Z, Gibbins N, Al-Jabri T, D'Souza AR. The use of robotics in otolaryngology–head and neck surgery: a systematic review. *Am J Otolaryngol*. 2012;33:137–146.

22. Tanna N, Joshi AS, Glade RS, et al. Da Vinci robot-assisted endocrine surgery: novel applications in otolaryngology. *Otolaryngol Head Neck Surg*. 2006;135:633–635.

Acknowledgments

Essentials of Robotic Surgery would not have been written without a robust program to discuss; and we wouldn't have a robust program to discuss without the leadership who supported this vision and work from the beginning. Many thanks to our executives and physician leadership, including Garry C. Faja; Robert Casalou; Walter M. Whitehouse Jr., MD; and Suzette Bouchard-Isackson, RN, for your support to build this incredible program.

All of the surgeons would like to thank the Surgical Operating Room Teams whose dedication on a daily basis makes the Center for Robotic Surgery at St. Joseph Mercy Ann Arbor a Center of Excellence. We are thankful for you and the work you do every day.

Many thanks to Michele Szczypka for making *Essentials of Robotic Surgery* come to fruition. Her many hours, from the initial concept to project oversight and keeping forward momentum, are why this book is available today. Also to Lauren Smoker and the Marketing & Communications Team who shared ideas and managed projects to help move the process along.

Special thanks to Don Montgomery of Montgomery & Associates for the front and back cover artwork and design; Chris Stranad of Chris Stranad Photography for the front and back cover photos; and M. LaWaun Hance for illustrations found throughout the book.

Many thanks to Steven Thiry, MD, Chair, Family Medicine, for his time to review and endorse the book and to Sandy Hess, Physician Relations, who helped review and distribute *Essentials of Robotic Surgery* to physicians.

Special thanks to Stefan Leichtle, MD, for seeing this vision with me and staying on for the ride anyway.

To the many patients who were willing to take a leap with this great technology and have healed quicker and enjoyed the benefits of robotics, thank you for entrusting us with your care.

Finally, a special thanks to my wife and four lovely children who help keep things in perspective. You are a wonderful reminder that being a surgeon is only part of my life.

With gratitude,
Manak Sood, MD

Editor's Note

It has been remarkable to watch the evolution of robotically assisted surgery at our institution. Perhaps the most enjoyable aspect of being a surgeon is the continuous opportunities for learning available to us, and I have the utmost respect for surgeons and surgical teams who have dedicated the time and effort to become successful in the world of robotics. It has been extremely rewarding for us to be able to impact recovery and optimize results for our patients at St. Joseph Mercy Hospital in Ann Arbor, Michigan.

Robotic applications will continue to infiltrate the world of surgery, and there will be three tiers of hospitals in the future: those who refrain from the robotic approach, those who purchase a robot to remain competitive, and hospitals that truly embrace this technology and offer minimally invasive surgery to their patients in a safe and efficient manner. St. Joseph Mercy Hospital in Ann Arbor will remain in the latter category and continue to serve as leaders and educators in the field.

The robots will undergo many improvements. They will become smaller, more dexterous, and eventually provide sensory feedback. The ultimate beneficiary will be the patients.

On a personal level, I have witnessed an unprecedented level of cooperation and collegiality among the specialists who sit on the console, and many colleagues have become friends as we shared this common path.

It is an exciting time to be a surgeon. The future is very bright for our patients.

Manak Sood, MD, FACS
Medical Director,
Center for Robotic Surgery,
St. Joseph Mercy Hospital Ann Arbor

Index